# Cardiovascular Nursing
## DeMYSTiFieD

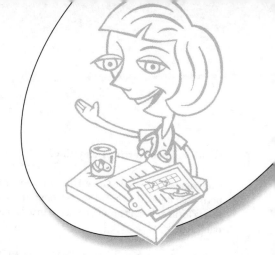

# Cardiovascular Nursing
## DeMYSTiFieD

Jim Keogh RN-BC, MSN

x

New York   Chicago   San Francisco   Athens   London   Madrid
Mexico City   Milan   New Delhi   Singapore   Sydney   Toronto

*9-15-15*
*LN*
*$30.00*

**Cardiovascular Nursing Demystified**

1 2 3 4 5 6 7 8 9 0   DOC/DOC   20 19 18 17 16 15

ISBN    978-0-07-1849180
MHID    0-07-1849181

This book was set in Minion Pro by Cenveo® Publisher Services.
The editors were Andrew Moyer and Cindy Yoo.
The technical editor was Anne Marie Flatekval RN, MSN, NE-BC.
The production supervisor was Richard Ruzycka.
Project management was provided by Tanya Punj, Cenveo Publisher Services.
RR Donnelley was printer and binder.

This book is printed on acid-free paper.

**Library of Congress Cataloging-in-Publication Data**

Keogh, James Edward, 1948- , author.
    Cardiovascular nursing demystified / Jim Keogh.
        p. ; cm.
    Includes index.
    ISBN 978-0-07-184918-0 (paperback : alk. paper)—ISBN 0-07-184918-1 (paperback : alk. paper)
    I. Title.
    [DNLM: 1. Cardiovascular Diseases—nursing—Examination Questions.   2. Cardiovascular Diseases—nursing—Outlines.   3. Diagnostic Techniques, Cardiovascular—nursing—Examination Questions.
    4. Diagnostic Techniques, Cardiovascular—nursing—Outlines.   WY 18.2]
    RC674
    616.1′0231076—dc23
                                                          2015010454

McGraw-Hill Education books are available at special quantity discounts to use as premiums and sales promotions or for use in corporate training programs. To contact a representative, please visit the Contact Us pages at www.mhprofessional.com.

*This book is dedicated to Anne, Sandy, Joanne, Amber-Leigh Christine, Shawn, Eric, and Amy. Without their help and support, this book couldn't have been written.*

—Jim Keogh, RN-BC, MSN

# About the Author

**Jim Keogh, RN-BC, MSN,** is Board Certified in Psychiatric-Mental Health and has written McGraw-Hill's *Nursing Demystified* series. These include *Behavioral Health and Psychiatric Nursing Demystified, Healthcare Informatics Demystified, Pharmacology Demystified, Microbiology Demystified, Medical-Surgical Nursing Demystified, Medical Billing and Coding Demystified, Nursing Laboratory and Diagnostic Tests Demystified, Dosage Calculations Demystified, Medical Charting Demystified, Pediatric Nursing Demystified, Nurse Management Demystified, Schaum's Outline of ECG Interpretations, Schaum's Outline of Medical Terminology,* and *Schaum's Outline of Emergency Nursing.* His books can be found in leading university libraries, including Yale School of Medicine, Yale University, University of Pennsylvania Biomedical Library, Columbia University, Brown University, University of Medicine and Dentistry of New Jersey, Cambridge University, and Oxford University. He is a former member of the faculty at Columbia University and is a member of the faculty of New York University School of Nursing and Saint Peter's University in New Jersey.

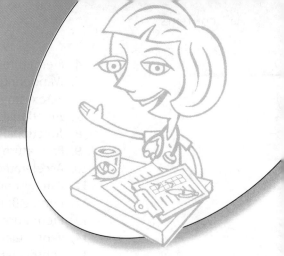

# Contents

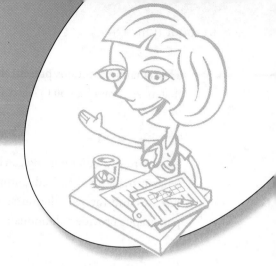

# Introduction

Every patient knows how to seek medical help when his or her chest discomfort becomes too much to bear. However, how does the health care provider determine what is wrong and what to do to restore the patient to good health? The answer depends on the patient's signs and symptoms and the results from medical tests. In this book you will learn to identify these signs and symptoms, interpret the medical test results, and perform the nursing interventions that will assist in solving or alleviating the patient's cardiovascular problem.

*Cardiovascular Nursing Demystified* contains 10 chapters, each providing a roadmap to the cardiovascular system and the diseases and disorders that can affect that system. The discussion of each disease or disorder is divided into the following sections:

- What Went Wrong?
- Prognosis
- Hallmark Signs and Symptoms
- Interpreting Test Results
- Treatment
- Nursing Diagnoses
- Nursing Intervention
- Crucial Diagnostic Tests

The "What Went Wrong?" section presents a brief description of how the body is affected when the particular disease or disorder occurs. The "Prognosis" section discusses the possibilities of curing this disease and permanent damage that can occur.

The remaining sections present the information as lists of symptoms, diagnoses, etc that make it easy for you to learn and that also serve as a useful tool for later reference.

## A Look Inside

Since cardiovascular nursing can be challenging for the beginner, this book was written to provide an organized, outline approach to learning about major cardiovascular diseases and the part the nurse can play in the treatment process. The following paragraphs provide a thumbnail description of each chapter.

## Chapter 1 Cardiovascular Anatomy and Physiology

Think of the **vascular system** as a distribution mechanism that consists of blood vessels (pipes) and the heart (pump). Visualizing the vascular system as "pipes" and a "pump" helps you understand signs and symptoms of cardiovascular disorders and diseases.

Blood vessels touch every organ and tissue in the body, providing oxygen and nutrients such as glucose needed for cells to work. Work is performed inside the cell by enzymes. An enzyme causes a chemical reaction to occur quickly. The chemical reaction causes the cell to do the cell's specific task in the body. The by-product of the chemical reaction—waste—is removed from the cell into the blood vessel where the waste is carried to organs (eg, kidneys) and excreted from the body.

Blood is composed of cells and fluid called plasma that provides oxygen and nutrients to cells throughout the body and removes waste from cells. An average adult has about 5 L of blood. The high concentration of blood moves across cell membranes through the process of diffusion. Diffusion is a process by which a high concentrated area (ie, blood) moves to a low concentrated area (ie, inside the cell). Cell waste moves outside of the cell and into blood where the waste is transported to the kidneys and lungs for excretion. Blood pressure called hydrostatic pressure pushes blood from the blood vessels, enabling diffusion into the cells. Oncotic pressure keeps blood inside blood vessels to maintain constant blood volume. Oncotic pressure is controlled by the amount of albumin dissolved in the blood.

The heart is a muscle that pumps blood throughout the vascular system. Health care providers need a thorough understanding of what can go wrong with the cardiovascular system; in this chapter you will learn to recognize the anatomy and physiology of the cardiovascular system.

## Chapter 2 Cardiovascular Assessment and Tests

The cardiovascular assessment is a focused assessment that typically follows a comprehensive assessment of the patient. The focused assessment follows up information that leads the nurse to suspect that the patient may have a cardiovascular disorder or is at risk for developing a cardiovascular disorder.

The cardiovascular focused assessment begins with a review of the patient's medical history. The patient's medical history can reveal symptoms of a cardiovascular disorder or risk factors that, if left unaddressed, can lead to cardiovascular disorders.

The patient's cardiovascular history will guide you through a focused cardiovascular physical examination. For example: A patient may report chest pain or other symptoms associated with cardiovascular disease, which is why the patient is being assessed. This is referred to as an episode, which causes the nurse and practitioner to focus on the reported problem rather than the overall health of the patient.

Cardiovascular tests and procedures are a key element in assessing the patient for cardiovascular disease. The cardiovascular history and physical assessment may or may not identify signs and symptoms of cardiovascular disease. The patient may report symptoms or you may identify signs that lead you to believe that cardiovascular disease may exist. However, the patient may be asymptomatic and your physical assessment may not reveal any signs of a cardiovascular problem. The practitioner may order cardiovascular tests to rule out a cardiovascular problem and may perform procedures if such a problem exists.

In this chapter you will learn how to perform a cardiac assessment and how to use cardiac tests to assess the cardiovascular system.

## Chapter 3 Electrophysiology and Electrocardiogram

Electrophysiology is the study of electrical properties of tissues and cells that cause the heart muscles to contract (depolarize) and relax (repolarize), forcing blood throughout the body. The electrophysiological activity of the heart is measured and recorded by an electrocardiograph (ECG). The heart is composed of striated involuntary muscles called cardiac muscles consisting of cells called cardiomyocytes commonly referred to as pacemaker cells.

The ECG tracing is an image of the electrophysiology of cardiac muscle in the form of a line that is automatically drawn on graph paper by the ECG. Initially, the line is aligned to a baseline on the graph paper. This is referred to as zeroing or calibrating the ECG and is performed before recording a patient's ECG.

The baseline is called the isoelectric line, which is a straight horizontal line on the graph paper commonly called a flat line. The graph paper consists of small and large boxes. Each small box is 1 mm$^2$. There are five small boxes in one large box. The patient's cardiac function is analyzed by measuring both the height (deflection) of the isoelectric line and the width of the wave (duration of the deflection). In this chapter you will learn how to apply concepts of electrophysiology and how to use an ECG.

## Chapter 4 Cardiac Arrhythmias

All cells in the heart are capable of stimulating the heart to contract. In a regular cardiac rhythm, the sinoatrial (SA) node of the heart stimulates cardiac contractions. An arrhythmia is an irregular cardiac rhythm caused when a cardiac cell other than the SA node stimulates cardiac contractions. The SA node is called the ectopic pacemaker. There are three common ectopic pacemakers. These are atrial ectopic: atrial ectopic pacemaker located in the atria; junctional ectopic: junctional ectopic pacemaker located in the atrioventricular (AV) junction; and ventricular ectopic: ventricular ectopic pacemaker located in the ventricles. In this chapter you will learn how to recognize different cardiac arrhythmias using the ECG.

## Chapter 5 Cardiac Inflammatory Disorder

The heart can become inflamed resulting in cardiac malfunction. Inflammation is the immune response to a localized infection caused by a microorganism; however, the immune response typically continues after the infection resolves. The extended immune response may impair cardiac contractions resulting in decreased flow of the blood throughout the body, and increase the risk of blood clots because of pooling blood.

Myocarditis is inflammation of the middle layer of the heart wall called the myocardium. Pericarditis is inflammation of the fluid sac that contains the heart called the pericardium. The increase in blood by the inflammation process causes the pericardium to swell, resulting in layers of the pericardium rubbing together causing irritation. Endocarditis is an infection of the inner lining of the heart called the endocardium. Endocarditis is less common in patients who do not have a history of cardiac defects.

In this chapter you will learn how to recognize and treat cardiac inflammatory disorders.

## Chapter 6 Cardiac Valve Disorder

There are four chambers of the heart: right atrium, right ventricle, left atrium, and left ventricle. The right atrium receives deoxygenated blood from the circulatory system and sends deoxygenated blood to the right ventricle. The right ventricle sends deoxygenated blood to the lungs. The left atrium receives oxygenated blood from the lungs and sends oxygenated blood to the left ventricle. The left ventricle sends oxygenated blood to the circulatory system.

Each chamber of the heart has a one-way valve that allows blood to flow in one direction. The valve also prevents blood from flowing backward. These valves are the tricuspid, pulmonary, mitral, and the aortic valves. The tricuspid valve allows blood to flow from the right atrium into the right ventricle. The pulmonary valve allows blood to flow from the right ventricle to the pulmonary artery. The mitral valve allows blood to flow from left atrium to the left ventricle. The aortic valve allows blood to flow from the left ventricle to the aorta.

A cardiac valve disorder is a condition when a valve malfunctions. In this chapter you will learn how to recognize and treat cardiac valve disorders.

## Chapter 7 Hematology and Hematologic Disorders

The hematologic system refers to the blood and blood-forming organs. The formation of red blood cells (RBCs), white blood cells (WBCs), and platelets begins in the bone marrow. Stem cells are produced in the bone marrow. Initially, these cells are not differentiated and may become RBCs, WBCs, or platelets. In the next stage of development, the stem cell becomes committed to a particular precursor cell, to become either a myeloid or lymphoid type of cell, and will differentiate into a particular cell type when in the presence of a specific growth factor.

In this chapter you will learn about the hematologic system, and how to recognize and treat hematologic disorders.

## Chapter 8 Vascular Disorders

Vascular disease is a disruption of blood flow through the blood vessels, which prevents adequate blood to reach tissues and organs. As a result, tissues and organs are deprived of nutrition and oxygen leading to tissue necrosis and organ failure. Vascular disease can involve the arteries and veins. Nearly half the population will experience vascular disease as result of age, obesity, and type 2 diabetes.

A buildup of fat and cholesterol on the walls of blood vessels, referred to as plaque, decreases blood flow through the vessel for patients who have atherosclerosis. Eventually plaque could block blood flow referred to as a blockage. A blocked blood vessel can be called an ischemic attack that results in the patient becoming symptomatic. Some ischemic attacks last for a fraction of a second. These are referred to as transient ischemic attack (TIA) that usually has no prolonged effect on the patient.

Other ischemic attacks can have long-term effects. Ischemic attack of coronary arteries causes chest pains (angina) that can lead to a heart attack. Ischemic attack of the carotid arteries that supply blood to the brain can lead to a stroke. Ischemic attack of arteries supplying the legs can result in cramps during activities (claudication), leg pain, and can lead to ulcers, gangrene, and amputation. Ischemic attack of renal arteries can lead to hypertension, congestive heart failure, and kidney failure.

In addition to disorders that decrease circulation, there are other vascular diseases that affect circulation, which you will learn about and how to treat vascular disorders in this chapter.

## Chapter 9 Cardiac Disorders

A *cardiac disorder* is a term used to describe many different conditions that cause the heart to function abnormally. A cardiac disorder disrupts the heart's ability to pump blood throughout the body. As a result, the patient may experience shortness of breath, light-headedness, and irregular heart beats and chest pains.

There are a number of underlying causes of a cardiac disorder. These include trauma, infection, postoperative effects, myocardial infarction, and heart disease. These underlying causes may lead to fluid retention in the lungs, around the heart, and in the legs. Some cardiac disorders are idiopathic and have no obvious underlying cause. In this chapter you will learn about how to recognize and treat cardiac disorders.

## Chapter 10 Cardiovascular Emergencies

A cardiovascular emergency is a condition that has the potential of disrupting circulation throughout the patient's body, resulting in decreased blood flow to organs causing malfunction of other systems in the body. This can be from hypertension, thrombosis, embolus—anything that disrupts the oxygen and nutrients from reaching tissues and organs.

A cardiac emergency is a condition that disrupts the function of the heart. The patient is asymptomatic or experiences discomfort, chest pain, back pain, jaw pain, increased urination at night, swelling of the ankles and feet, heart pounding, missing heart beats, and shortness of breath. However, there are times when a patient is in respiratory distress or respiratory arrest. This is not a cardiac emergency because the patient's heart is working although respiratory arrest can lead to a cardiac emergency if rescue breathing does not occur. In this chapter you will learn about how to recognize and treat cardiovascular emergencies.

# chapter 1

# Cardiovascular Anatomy and Physiology

## LEARNING OBJECTIVES

1. Vascular System
2. Blood
3. The Heart

## KEY TERMS

Blood Flow Through the Heart
Blood Group
Blood Pressure (BP)
Blood Supply to the Heart
Blood Transfusions
Blood Vessels
Blood Vessel Walls Arterioles
Cardiac Contractions
Electrolytes

Mean Arterial Pressure (MAP)
Narrow Pulse Pressure
Plasma
Platelets (Thrombocytes)
Pulse Pressure
Red Blood Cells (Erythrocytes)
White Blood Cells (Leukocytes)
Wide Pulse Pressure

# Vascular System

Think of the **vascular system** as a distribution mechanism that consists of blood vessels (pipes) and the heart (pump). Visualizing the vascular system as "pipes" and a "pump" helps you understand signs and symptoms of cardiovascular disorders and diseases.

**Blood vessels** touch every organ and tissue in the body, providing oxygen and nutrients such as glucose needed for cells to work. Work is performed inside the cell by enzymes. An **enzyme** causes a chemical reaction to occur quickly. The chemical reaction causes the cell to do the cell's specific task in the body. The byproduct of the chemical reaction—waste—is removed from the cell into the blood vessel where the waste is carried to organs (ie, kidneys) and excreted from the body.

## Blood Vessels

The vascular system consists of a network of high-pressure "pipes" (arteries) and low-pressure "pipes" (veins). **Arteries** carry oxygenated blood under high pressure away from the heart. Arteries close to the heart are large and gradually reduce in diameter as arteries branch out away from the heart and closer to organs and tissues. Small arteries are called *arterioles* that deliver blood to capillaries.

### NURSING ALERT

A superficial cut typically results in blood oozing from capillaries. A deeper cut may result in blood slightly pulsating from the wound. The pulsation implies that blood is flowing from an arteriole.

*Capillaries* are small and thin blood vessels that border organs and tissues and exchange with the cells oxygen and nutrients for waste products through capillary action, which is the ability of fluid (blood) to pass through a thin membrane.

Capillaries are connected to small veins called *venules*, which in turn are connected to progressively larger veins that return deoxygenated blood to the heart and waste to organs that process and excrete the waste.

Veins work differently than arteries. Arteries are relatively thick, strong enough to handle fluid (blood) that is under pressure from the heart. Pressure drops appreciably at the capillaries. There is little pressure from the heart to move blood through the veins. Think of looking at the end of a long garden hose where the water is slowly pouring out and this is similar to what happens at the capillaries.

Veins move blood back to the heart through gravity and contractions of skeletal muscles when a person moves around. Movement is not consistent. Sometimes we sit for a while and then move. Inconsistent flow within the veins can result in blood flowing backward. Many veins have **one-way valves** that prevent backflow of blood. These valves are similar to one-way valves used in sewage systems to prevent the backflow of waste.

---

### NURSING ALERT

Blood has difficulty returning to the heart when a patient is immobile such as when a patient lies in bed. Blood pools in the vein, becoming stagnated. Stagnated blood can clot along the walls of the veins, which is called a *thrombosis*. Veins further away from the heart such as in the feet are at high risk for thrombosis called *deep vein thrombosis* (DVT). The clot increases in size the longer the blood stagnates. The clot can dislodge—called an *emboli*—and travel through the bloodstream blocking small blood vessels in the brain, resulting in a stroke, or in the lungs.

---

## Blood Vessel Walls

Blood vessel walls have three layers:

- **Outer layer (tunica externa):** The outer layer is made of collagen. *Collagen* is a long fibrous protein that strengthens blood vessels and anchors nerve fibers, lymphatic vessels, and capillaries that support the blood vessel.

- **Inner layer (tunica media):** The middle layer contains smooth muscle and neurons that collectively constrict and dilate the blood vessels in response to physiological activities.

- **Inner layer (tunica interna):** The inner layer, called the *endothelium*, is smooth and delicate, enabling free flow of blood.

---

**NURSING ALERT**

*Cholesterol* is a waxy, fat-like substance regulated by the liver that is needed to form hormones and substances that help digest food. *Low-density lipoproteins* (LDLs) are proteins that carry cholesterol from the liver to organs and tissues via blood vessels. *High-density lipoproteins* (HDLs) are proteins that carry cholesterol from organs and tissues throughout the body to the liver for recycling via blood vessels. Cholesterol can break off and fatty streaks of cholesterol can attach to the inner layer of blood vessels—a precursor to cholesterol plaque. White blood cells (WBCs) digest the cholesterol. However, WBCs become intertwined with cholesterol, forming **cholesterol plaque**. Over years cholesterol plaque builds up, reducing blood flow in a process called *atherosclerosis*. Cholesterol plaque can break off, forming emboli that could block small blood vessels.

---

# Blood

**Blood** is composed of cells and fluid called *plasma*; it provides oxygen and nutrients to cells throughout the body and removes waste from cells. An average adult has about 5 L of blood. The high concentration of blood moves across cell membranes through the process of diffusion. *Diffusion* is a process by which a substance moves from an area of high concentration (ie, blood) to an of low concentration (ie, inside the cell). Cell wastes move outside of the cell and into the blood, where the waste is transported to the kidneys and lungs for excretion. Blood pressure called **hydrostatic pressure** pushes blood from the blood vessels, enabling diffusion into the cells. **Oncotic pressure** keeps blood inside blood vessels to maintain constant blood volume. Oncotic pressure is controlled by the amount of albumin dissolved in the blood. **Albumin** is a protein in plasma that keeps blood from leaking out of blood vessels. Albumin also binds to hormones and drugs, carrying them throughout the body.

## Plasma

**Plasma** is the yellowish fluid portion of blood, making up of half the volume of blood. Plasma is 90% water; the remaining 10% is dissolved substances that are needed for cells throughout the body to function.

> **NURSING ALERT**
>
> Depending on the nature of a blood test, the blood sample is allowed to clot, causing blood cells and the clotting factors to fall to the bottom of the test tube and serum to rise to the top of the test tube. **Serum** is then analyzed for amounts of various substances.

Plasma contains substances that float in it. These are red blood cells (RBCs) (see Red Blood Cells [Erythrocytes]), WBCs (see White Blood Cells [Leukocytes]), and platelets (see Platelets [Thrombocytes]).

Plasma contains substances that are dissolved in it. The **dissolving process** causes a substance to become part of the liquid. There are many substances dissolved in plasma, including glucose, hormones, cholesterol, and vitamins. The two primary substances dissolved in plasma are listed follows:

1. **Proteins (10%):** Proteins attract water and are larger than water molecules, giving proteins a unique ability to maintain plasma levels within the blood vessels. Proteins have a relatively difficult time leaking from blood vessels because of their size. Proteins are used for oncotic pressure, transport nutrients and other substances throughout the body, to maintain pH balance, and to foster chemical reactions. The primary proteins in plasma are the following:

   • Albumin that is produced in the liver and is used for oncotic pressure (60% of the proteins)

   • Globulins for the immune system (see White Blood Cells [Leukocytes])

   • Fibrinogen for clotting

2. **Electrolytes:** Electrolytes (see Electrolytes) are substances required for nerve conduction, blood clotting, fluid balance, muscle contraction, and pH balance. Electrolytes dissolved in plasma are the following:

   • Sodium

   • Potassium

   • Chloride

   • Bicarbonate

   • Calcium

   • Magnesium

> **NURSING ALERT**
>
> Three percent of oxygen from the lungs is dissolved in plasma.

## Red Blood Cells (Erythrocytes)

**Red blood cells** make up 40% of the volume of blood and contain hemoglobin. **Hemoglobin** is a protein that attaches to oxygen and carbon dioxide. The number of RBCs that are produced is determined by the hormone **erythropoietin**. When the oxygen level is low, there is an increased production of erythropoietin by the kidneys. Erythropoietin stimulates pluripotential hematopoietic stem cell production and the speed at which these cells mature.

Mature RBCs remain in plasma for 120 days. Afterward RBCs are removed from plasma in the spleen and liver.

Folate, iron, and vitamin $B_{12}$ are required for RBC production. Iron atoms in the hemoglobin bind with oxygen. Iron also gives RBCs their color.

Chemical reactions in cells produce **carbon dioxide** that leaves the cells, enters the plasma, and attaches to hemoglobin. The carbon dioxide is carried to capillaries in the lung where it is exchanged for oxygen. An insufficient amount of hemoglobin (**anemia**) results in fatigue due to low levels of oxygen available in the blood. An abnormally high amount of hemoglobin (**polycythemia**) results in a high risk of clots due to the thickness of blood. RBCs change shape without rupturing and can pass through capillaries.

> **NURSING ALERT**
>
> Kidney disease can lead to anemia due to the decline in erythropoietin production.

## White Blood Cells (Leukocytes)

White blood cells are a primary component of the immune system. Plasma transports WBCs to organs and tissues that are damaged or infected. WBCs make up 1% of blood and protect the body from infection. The number of WBCs increases as an inflammation response by the immune system to an infection or injury to the body. There are six main types of WBCs, listed as follows:

1. **Neutrophils (58%):** Neutrophils kill and ingest bacteria in a process called *phagocytosis*. Neutrophils can have a nucleus that is **segmented**, **multi-lobed**, or **polymorphonuclear** in form, leading to neutrophils described as **segs**, **PMNs**, or **polys**.

2. **Bands (3%):** Immature neutrophils form **bands**. There is an increase in bands and neutrophils when the patient has a bacterial infection.

3. **Lymphocytes (4%):** Lymphocytes move freely between blood, lymph fluid, and lymph tissues and can live for 1 year. Lymphocytes recognize bacteria and viruses that have previously invaded the body, enabling lymphocytes to target specific bacteria and viruses. There are three main types of lymphocytes, listed as follows:

    i. **T cells:** T cells develop from bone marrow or liver stem cells and mature in the thymus, which is located between the breastbone and heart. T cells are involved in cell-mediated immunity. There are four types of T cells, listed as follows:

    ii. **Helper T cells:** Helper T cells, referred to as *CD4*, identify viral infected cells. Helper T cells then secrete lymphokines that cause stimulation of killer T cells and B cells that attack the pathogen. The AIDS virus infects and kills helper T cells.

        a. **Cytotoxic T cells:** Cytotoxic T cells release chemicals and kill invading microorganisms.

        b. **Memory T cells:** Memory T cells can identify specific microorganisms that have previously invaded the body and remain in blood to swiftly attack should the microorganisms invade the body again.

        c. **Suppressor T cells:** Suppressor T cells reduce the immune response once the invading microorganism has been destroyed. This prevents the immune system from attacking normal cells.

    iii. **B Cells:** B cells develop from bone marrow stem cells and mature in the bone marrow. B cells transform into plasma cells when an invading microorganism is detected. B cells produce antibodies referred to as *immunoglobulins* or *gamma globulins* that are considered **humoral immunity**. There are five types of immunoglobulins, listed as follows:

        a. **Immunoglobulin A (IgG):** Found in mucous membranes, lining of the gastrointestinal tract, lining of the respiratory system, tears, and saliva.

        b. **Immunoglobulin M (IgM):** First to fight a new infection and found in the plasma and lymph fluid.

        c. **Immunoglobulin E (IgE):** Reacts to allergens and found in mucous membranes, lungs, and skin.

    d. **Immunoglobulin G (IgG):** Protects against bacterial and viral infections (most abundant).

    e. **Immunoglobulin D (IgD):** Found in the blood (least amount in blood).

Antibodies bind to the microorganism, causing them to clump together and break open. B cells also activate the complement system. The **complement system** consists of enzymes that attack and activate neutrophils and macrophages, which attack the invading microorganism. There are also memory B cells that remain active, looking for the reappearance of the microorganism.

4. **Monocytes (4%):** Monocytes defend against many infectious microorganisms, including bacteria, and ingest damaged cells. Monocytes remain in blood for up to 20 hours before entering tissues throughout the body, where they can remain active for years.

5. **Eosinophils (2%):** Eosinophils respond to allergies and kill parasites. Eosinophils are referred to as *granulocytes*. A granulocyte has digestive enzymes used to kill microorganisms.

6. **Basophils (1%):** Basophils are a type of WBC that contain histamine and serotonin. Basophils react to allergens by releasing histamine, which causes blood vessels to dilate, resulting in increased blood flow to tissues affected by the allergen.

## Platelets (Thrombocytes)

Platelets are particles that form a platelet plug to seal a ruptured blood vessel and promote the clotting process. A low number of platelets (**thrombocytopenia**) results in bruising and bleeding that takes a long time to stop. A high number of platelets (**thrombocythemia**) places the patient at risk for blood clots unless the patient is actively bleeding.

Blood cells are produced by red bone marrow through a process called *hematopoiesis*. Blood cells begin as a stem cell called a *pluripotential hematopoietic stem cell* that can form RBCs, WBCs, or platelets.

> **NURSING ALERT**
>
> Aging of bones diminishes the ability of bone marrow to produce blood cells to parts of the extremities, ribs, pelvis, sternum, and spine. **Yellow bone marrow** does not produce any stem cells.

## Blood Group

A blood group, also known as a *blood type*, is a classification of blood based on a substance on the surface of RBCs called an *inherited antigen* (also *agglutinogens*). This is referred to as the *ABO blood group system*. The blood type of a person is contributed from both parents. Table 1–1 contains the four major blood groups. Plasma contains the antibody opposite of the antigen that is on the surfaces of RBC, which is called *agglutinin*. These antibodies are formed during infancy but are not present at birth.

The **Rh blood group system** is another classification of blood based on the Rh antigen. The **Rh antigen** may be present on the surface of RBCs. There are many Rh antigens, but the most common is the **D antigen**. The Rh blood group system classifies blood as:

- **Rh+:** The Rh antigen is present (85% of the population in the United States).

- **Rh−:** The Rh antigen is not present (15% of the population in the United States).

> **NURSING ALERT**
>
> A person with Rh− blood can develop the Rh antibodies through a blood transfusion. A pregnant woman who is Rh− and has a fetus who is Rh+ can develop Rh+ antibodies through the placenta, which results in **hemolytic disease of the newborn (HDN)** or **erythroblastosis fetalis**.

**TABLE 1–1**  ABO Blood Groups and Anti-Blood Type Antigens

|  | Blood Group | Anti-Blood Type Antigen in Plasma |
|---|---|---|
| A | The A antigen is on the surface of RBCs | Anti-type-B |
| B | The B antigen is on the surface of RBCs | Anti-type-A |
| AB | Both the A and B antigens are on the surface of RBCs | No anti-type |
| O | Neither the A nor the B antigen is on the surface of RBCs | Anti-type-A and anti-type-B |

## Blood Transfusions

A blood transfusion is replacement of all or a portion of blood with either the patient's own blood prior to surgery or from donor blood. Before a patient undergoes the scheduled surgery, one or more pints of a patient's blood are taken in a process called *apheresis*. Specific components are removed from the blood and used as needed during and after the surgery.

A patient can experience a transfusion reaction if it contains RBCs. Antibodies in the patient's plasma can react to antigens on the donor's RBCs if donor blood is a different blood type from the patient's blood type. Antibodies attach to the antigen causing RBCs to clump together. RBCs are then destroyed in a process called *hemolysis,* causing hemoglobin to enter the bloodstream, and eventually metabolized into bilirubin.

Blood type O negative is called the *universal donor* because anyone can receive it because the blood has no antigen. Blood type AB is called the *universal recipient* because the recipient has no antibodies.

Blood components that can be used in a blood transfusion are the following:

- **Packed red blood cells:** RBCs are thawed and transfused when the patient has severe anemia or has lost a massive amount of blood.
- **Fresh frozen plasma:** Fresh frozen plasma is transfused when the patient has a bleeding disorder, liver failure, or is overly medicated with anticoagulant medication (ie, Coumadin) that results in severe bleeding.
- **Platelets:** Platelets are transfused when the patient experiences a low platelet count (thrombocytopenia).
- **White blood cells:** WBCs are rarely transfused except when a patient has extremely low WBCs placing the patient at risk for infection.
- **Albumin:** Albumin is infused when the patient experiences severe bleeding, severe burns, or has liver failure resulting in decrease blood volume and other fluids have not worked.
- **Immunoglobulins:** Immunoglobulins are transfused when the patient has hepatitis.
- **Cryoprecipitate:** Cryoprecipitate is the part of plasma that contains fibrinogen and other substances that create blood clots and is transfused when the patient has low blood clotting factors.
- **Whole blood:** Whole blood consists of all components of blood and is transfused when there is massive bleeding when more than 10 units of RBCs are required in a 24-hour period.

> **NURSING ALERT**
>
> A hemorrhage is the loss of blood categorized by four classes based on the total blood volume lost.
>
> - **Class I:** 15% blood volume loss with no change in vital signs. The patient does not require replacement fluids.
> - **Class II:** 16% to 30% blood volume loss with patient experiencing pale cool skin, tachycardia, and narrowing of the difference between systolic and diastolic blood pressure. The patient requires normal saline or lactated Ringer solution.
> - **Class III:** 31% to 40% blood volume loss with the patient experiencing tachycardia, decrease in blood pressure, decrease in capillary refill, and unstable mental status. The patient requires normal saline or lactated Ringer solution and a blood transfusion.
> - **Class IV:** Greater than 40% blood volume loss requires aggressive resuscitation.

## Electrolytes

*Electrolytes* are salts found in food and fluids that are ingested and dissolved in plasma. Electrolytes are required to conduct electrical impulses for nerve and muscle functions. In addition to being in plasma, electrolytes are also found inside cells and in fluid that surrounds cells. A balance of electrolytes maintains the voltage across the cell membrane.

The body maintains the balance in the levels of water and electrolytes. Levels of electrolytes are maintained by the kidneys. The kidneys filter electrolytes from plasma, excreting excess electrolytes in the urine.

Electrolyte balance is also controlled by antidiuretic hormone, parathyroid hormone, and aldosterone. **Antidiuretic hormone** (ADH, vasopressin) stimulates reabsorption of water in the kidneys and increases the uptake of electrolytes when the electrolyte level is low in the body. The **parathyroid hormone** (PTH) controls the level of calcium in the blood. A low level of calcium in the blood causes an increase in PTH moving calcium from other parts of the body such as bone into the blood. A high level of calcium in blood causes it to leave the blood and move into other parts of the body. The **aldosterone hormone** produced at the adrenal cortex of the adrenal glands causes the kidneys to retain sodium and secrete potassium, resulting in increased reabsorption of water, leading to an increase in blood pressure.

> ## NURSING ALERT
>
> An *electrolyte panel* is a blood test that determines the level of electrolytes in plasma. An imbalance of electrolytes can explain a patient's signs and symptoms and indicate an underlying cause that can lead to appropriate treatment of the patient.

### Electrolyte Imbalance

The most common electrolyte imbalances are the following:

**Sodium**

- **Low sodium (hyponatremia)**
  - *Cause:*
    - Kidney disease
    - Drinking too much water
  - *Symptoms:*
    - Headache
    - Fatigue
    - Weakness
    - Nausea
      - Severe symptoms:
        - Confusion
        - Seizure
        - Coma
        - Death
  - *Treatment:*
    - Normal saline (sodium and water) IV
- **High sodium (hypernatremia)**
  - *Cause:*
    - Diarrhea
    - Excessive vomiting
    - Excessive fluid loss
    - Diabetes
    - Adverse side effect of medication

- *Symptoms:*
  - Thirst
  - Headache
  - Fatigue
  - Weakness
  - Nausea
    - Severe symptoms:
      - Confusion
      - Seizure
      - Coma
      - Death
- *Treatment:*
  - Oral intake of water
  - $D_5W$ IV or 0.45 saline IV

**Potassium**

- **Low potassium (hypokalemia)**
  - *Cause:*
    - Diarrhea
    - Excessive sweating
    - Dietary deficiency
    - Adverse side effect of diuretic medication
  - *Symptoms:*
    - Muscle pain
    - Irritability
    - Paralysis
    - Weakness
    - Irregular heartbeat
  - *Treatment:*
    - Ingest food high in potassium
    - Potassium supplements
    - Potassium chloride IV
- **High potassium (hyperkalemia)**

- *Cause:*
  - Kidney failure
  - Adverse side effect of medication
- *Symptoms:*
  - Tingling in the extremities
  - Numbness
  - Weakness
  - Irregular heartbeat
- *Treatment:*
  - 50% dextrose with insulin IV
  - Bicarbonate IV
  - Magnesium sulfate IV

## Blood Pressure

The heart pushes blood through arteries, creating a force that is measured as **systolic blood pressure**. Normal systolic blood pressure is below 120 mm Hg. A systolic blood pressure between 120 and 139 mm Hg is considered **borderline hypertension**. A systolic blood pressure 140 mm Hg or above is considered **hypertension**.

Pressure in arteries between contractions—when the heart is at rest—is measured as **diastolic blood pressure**. Normal diastolic blood pressure is less than 80 mm Hg. Diastolic blood pressure between 80 and 89 mm Hg is considered borderline hypertension. A diastolic blood pressure above 90 is considered hypertension.

Blood pressure changes during the day depending on a number of factors that cause blood vessels to contract or dilate. It rises when smooth muscles in the inner layer of the blood vessel contract, and decreases when these muscles relax. There are a number of factors that cause muscles in the inner layer of the blood vessel to contract and relax; for example, caffeine and nicotine cause blood vessels to contract, thereby increasing blood pressure. Aerobic exercise causes blood vessels to dilate lowering blood pressure.

Anything that disrupts the flow of blood through blood vessels may cause an increase in blood pressure; for example, obesity may increase pressure from the outside of blood vessels, resulting in high blood pressure in the blood vessels. The buildup of cholesterol plaque on the inner walls of blood vessels may interrupt blood flow.

**Mean arterial pressure (MAP)** is a good indicator of perfusion to vital organs. MAP is the average pressure in the patient's arteries during one cardiac cycle. The true MAP can only be determined by invasive monitoring, although some blood pressure machines estimate the MAP based on the patient's blood pressure. An MAP of 60 mm Hg is sufficient to perfuse vital organs.

**Pulse pressure** is the difference between the systolic and diastolic pressure and represents the force generated each time the heart contracts. A normal blood pressure of 120/80 mm Hg has a pulse pressure of 40 mm Hg. An adult who is healthy and sitting has a pulse pressure range between 30 and 40 mm Hg.

A low pulse pressure, referred to as a **narrow pulse pressure** between 25 and 29 mm Hg, may indicate a drop in the left ventricular stroke volume. A pulse pressure of 25 mm Hg or less may indicate shock or congestive heart failure.

A high pulse pressure, referred to as a **wide pulse pressure**—greater than 40 mm Hg—is common during and following aerobic exercise. However, a resting pulse pressure consistently higher than 100 mm Hg may indicate stiffness in the major arteries.

---

### NURSING ALERT

Emotions also affect blood pressure. Blood pressure rises when a patient is anxious as the fight or flight mechanism activates. Some patients are anxious during a physical assessment or at the thought of seeing a practitioner. This is referred to as **white coat syndrome**, which can produce false high blood pressure readings. Practitioners typically ask the patient to take their own blood pressure at home twice a day for a couple of weeks to obtain an accurate blood pressure measurement.

---

Blood pressure is measured in the arm with the arm level with the heart; however, it can be measured at any limb. Blood pressure is measured when the patient is lying, sitting, and standing. There should be only minor variations in blood pressure in each position.

Arterial blood pressure is also measured by inserting an arterial catheter that is connected to a pressure transducer. The *arterial catheter* is a tube that is inserted into an artery in an extremity. Pressure of blood flowing from the heart is detected by the arterial catheter and is translated into an electrical signal by the **pressure transducer.** The electrical signal corresponds to the blood pressure, which is displayed on an electronic device and/or printed paper.

## The Heart

The *heart* is a muscle that pumps blood throughout the vascular system. The heart is located in a fluid-filled sac called the *pericardium* that protects the heart by acting like a shock absorber. The outer layer of the heart is the *myocardium*. The inner layer of the heart is the *endocardium*.

- **Right atrium (RA):** The right atrium receives deoxygenated blood from the circulatory system and sends deoxygenated blood to the right ventricle (Figure 1–1).
- **Right ventricle (RV):** The right ventricle sends deoxygenated blood to the lungs.
- **Left atrium (LA):** The left atrium receives oxygenated blood from the lungs and sends oxygenated blood to the left ventricle.

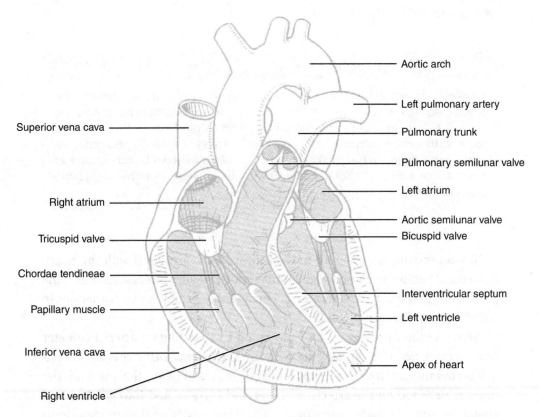

**FIGURE 1–1** · The heart has four chambers: the right atrium, right ventricle, left atrium, and left atrium. (Reproduced, with permission, from Keogh J, Reed D. *Schaum's Outline of ECG Interpretation*. New York: McGraw-Hill Education, 2011:4. Figure 1.3.)

- **Left ventricle (LV):** The left ventricle sends oxygenated blood to the circulatory system.

The heart contracts (**systole**), forcing blood from the heart, and then relaxes (**diastole**), during which blood enters the heart. The heart contracts in two stages. First the right and left atria contract causing blood to move into the right and left ventricles. Next, the ventricles contract forcing blood from the heart. The right ventricle forces deoxygenated blood through the pulmonary artery to the lungs, and the atrium sends oxygenated blood through the aorta to the circulatory system.

Each chamber has a **one-way valve** that allows blood to flow in one direction and prevents the blood from flowing backward. These valves are the following:

- **Tricuspid valve:** The tricuspid valve allows blood to flow from the right atrium into the right ventricle.
- **Pulmonary valve:** The pulmonary valve allows blood to flow from the right ventricle to the pulmonary artery.
- **Mitral valve:** The mitral valve allows blood to flow from the left atrium to the left ventricle.
- **Aortic valve:** The aortic valve allows blood to flow from the left ventricle to the aorta.

## Blood Flow Through the Heart

Deoxygenated blood flows into the heart from the superior vena cava (SVC) and the inferior vena cava (IVC). The **IVC** returns blood from the legs and lower body. The SVC returns blood from the head, arms, and upper body. Blood from the vena cava flows into the right atrium (Figure 1–2).

When the right atrium contracts, blood flows through the tricuspid valve into the right ventricle. Contraction of the right ventricle causes blood to pass through the pulmonary valve to the **pulmonary artery** leading to the lungs. The pulmonary artery is the only artery that contains deoxygenated blood.

Oxygenated blood flows from the lungs through the **pulmonary vein** into the left atrium. The pulmonary vein is the only vein that contains oxygenated blood. Contraction of the left atrium causes blood to flow through the mitral valve into the left ventricle.

When the left ventricle contracts, oxygenated blood flows through the aortic valve into the aorta and out into a network of arteries that supply oxygenated blood to organs and tissues.

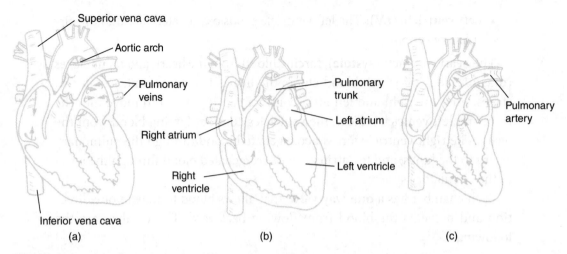

**FIGURE 1–2** · Deoxygenated blood flows into the heart, and then out to the lungs. It returns to the heart and is forced out to the body. (Reproduced, with permission, from Keogh J, Reed D. *Schaum's Outline of ECG Interpretation*. New York: McGraw-Hill Education, 2011:7. Figure 1.5.)

## Cardiac Contractions

A group of cardiac cells called the *sinoatrial node* (SAN) (Figure 1–3), located in the right atrium, is the **natural pacemaker** of the heart. The SAN separates charged particles and spontaneously leaks charged particles into cells,

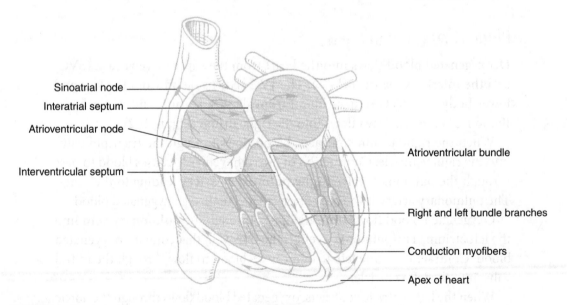

**FIGURE 1–3** · The cardiac conduction system controls contraction of cardiac muscles. (Reproduced, with permission, from Keogh J, Reed D. *Schaum's Outline of ECG Interpretation*. New York: McGraw-Hill Education, 2011:6. Figure 1.4.)

creating the electrical activity that causes other cardiac muscle cells to contract. The impulse travels from the SAN to the right and left atria in 0.04 second, causing the atria to contract. This gives the ventricles time to fill with blood.

The impulse travels along specialized fibers to the **atrioventricular node** (AVN) and then to the **bundle of His**. The bundle of His branches to the **left bundle branch** to the left ventricle and the **right bundle branch** to the right ventricle. Impulses along this path cause the ventricles to contract.

---

### NURSING ALERT

Any cardiac tissue can become a pacemaker and can replace the SAN should the SAN fail. The SAN creates a faster impulse than other cardiac tissues and therefore is the primary pacemaker.

---

The normal heart contracts 72 times per minute. However, the rate of contractions and the force of the contraction can be influenced by the autonomic nervous system. The autonomic nervous system is involuntary and part of the peripheral nervous system that controls involuntary actions.

The **autonomic nervous system** is divided into the sympathetic nervous system and the parasympathetic nervous system. The **sympathetic nervous system** increases the rate and force of contractions. The **parasympathetic nervous system** decreases the rate and force of contractions.

## Blood Supply to the Heart

Cardiac tissue requires a supply of oxygenated blood and nutrients as does all tissue in the body. Oxygenated blood is supplied to cardiac tissue by the **coronary arteries** (Figure 1–4). There are two primary coronary arteries: the **left main stem coronary artery** and the **right stem coronary artery.** Both receive blood from the aorta. The left main stem coronary artery branches into the **left anterior descending branch** and the **left circumflex arteries**.

Deoxygenated blood returns from the heart through cardiac veins. The primary cardiac veins are the **great cardiac vein**, the **small cardiac vein**, the **middle cardiac vein**, and the **posterior vein** attached to the left ventricle. There is also the **oblique vein** attached to the left atrium. Cardiac veins flow into the **coronary sinus** leading to the right atrium.

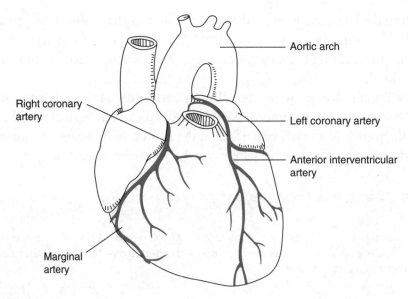

**FIGURE 1-4** · The coronary circulation system supplies blood to the heart. (Reproduced, with permission, from Keogh J, Reed D. *Schaum's Outline of ECG Interpretation*. New York: McGraw-Hill Education, 2011:8. Figure 1.6.)

---

### NURSING ALERT

Lack of oxygenated blood to the heart caused by a blockage in one or more coronary arteries results in chest pain called *angina*. A complete blockage of a coronary artery can cause death of the corresponding cardiac tissue serviced by the coronary artery. This is commonly referred to as a *heart attack*.

---

## Collateral Coronary Circulation

Collateral coronary circulation provides blood to the heart if the coronary arteries are blocked providing a pathway for blood to bypass the primary coronary circulation system. The collateral coronary circulation system may or may not provide sufficient oxygenated blood to the cardiac tissue. Insufficient oxygenation results in death (necrosis) of cardiac tissue.

# CASE STUDY

## CASE 1

The practitioner asks you to meet with the family of a 68-year-old woman who has had repeated cardiac episodes. After confirming with the patient, the practitioner has a preliminary diagnosis of coronary artery disease and atrial fibrillation. Here are the questions asked by the family. What is the best response?

QUESTION 1. Why does the patient get chest pain?
ANSWER: Chest pain is called *angina* and is caused by the lack of oxygenated blood to the heart through coronary arteries. The lack of oxygenated blood is caused by a blockage in one or more coronary arteries.

QUESTION 2. Why does the patient's heart beat irregularly at times?
ANSWER: The portion of the heart called the *SA node* is commonly referred to as the *pacemaker* and sets the heart rhythm for all cardiac tissues. However, any cardiac tissue is capable of becoming the pacemaker. This keeps the heart working if the SA pacemaker fails. Sometimes an area of cardiac tissue creates its own pulse different from that of the SA pacemaker, resulting in an irregular heartbeat.

QUESTION 3. What is the atrium of the heart?
ANSWER: The heart is divided into four chambers. The two top chambers are the atria and the two bottom chambers are the ventricles. The right atrium receives deoxygenated blood from the rest of the body and sends the deoxygenated blood to the right ventricle where the deoxygenated blood goes to the lungs. The lungs replace carbon dioxide in the blood with oxygen and send the oxygenated blood to the left atrium. The oxygenated blood then flows into the left ventricle and then out to other parts of the body.

QUESTION 4. The practitioner told us that atrial fibrillation means that the atria quiver. Why would the atrium quiver?
ANSWER: *Quivering* is the irregular beating of the atria caused by disruption in the pace-making system in the heart, resulting in chaotic electrical signals between the atria and the ventricles. The atria beat faster than the ventricles.

## FINAL CHECKUP

1. **A 32-year-old man who was diagnosed with deep vein thrombosis following major foot surgery asks you how he might have developed this condition. What is your best response?**

   A. The clot occurred because you played football in college and were repeatedly tackled.

   B. You smoked two packs of cigarettes a day for the last year.

   C. Your leg was immobilized after surgery.

   D. Circulation in your legs decreased because you were immobilized following surgery, causing a blood clot to form.

2. **A 36-year-old woman reported increased fatigue. She tells you that her practitioner said her RBCs were low and that she had anemia. The patient asks you why she is fatigued. What is your best response?**

   A. You are fatigued because you have anemia.

   B. RBCs carry oxygen throughout your body. You are fatigued because your body is not receiving sufficient oxygen because there aren't enough RBCs.

   C. You must take an iron supplement so your body can create more RBCs.

   D. You need a $B_{12}$ injection.

3. **A 28-year-old man was told that his blood pressure was high during a routine physical examination. The practitioner suggested that he purchase a blood pressure machine and take his blood pressure twice a day for a week and then bring the results to his next appointment. The patient was confused and asked why the practitioner made the request. What is the best response?**

   A. You should ask the practitioner.

   B. Blood pressure taken at home is a better measurement than if taken in the practitioner's office.

   C. The practitioner wanted to rule out "white coat syndrome."

   D. Three blood pressure readings taken at different times are necessary to determine a diagnosis of hypertension.

4. **A 63-year-old man was admitted to the unit for symptoms that indicated that he was experiencing an electrolyte imbalance. The practitioner ordered an electrolyte panel, which confirmed that an electrolyte imbalance exists. The practitioner ordered a renal panel. The patient asks you why the renal panel was ordered. What is your best response?**

   A. The levels of electrolytes are maintained by the kidneys.

   B. The practitioner must know if your kidneys are functioning well before ordering medication to treat your condition.

   C. These tests are to determine how well your kidneys are working.

   D. The practitioner wants to know the amount of kidney function that you lost.

5. **A 45-year-old patient was admitted to your unit with a 103°C temperature. The practitioner ordered a CBC blood test. She calls you asking for the WBC count. You report 15,000 WBCs. She then asks you about the number of bands. What is the rationale for asking that question?**

   A. Increased band formation indicates a viral infection.

   B. Bands are immature lymphocytes and are present when there is a bacterial or virus infection.

   C. Bands are immature neutrophils that increase when there is a bacterial infection.

   D. The practitioner needs to identify the proper medication to prescribe.

6. **A 42-year-old female patient tells you that her good cholesterol is normal and that her bad cholesterol is a little high. What is mistaken about the patient's statement?**

   A. HDL is commonly referred to as *good cholesterol* and LDL as *bad cholesterol*. These are not cholesterols. HDL and LDL are proteins that carry cholesterol to and from organs and tissues.

   B. There is no such thing as good or bad cholesterol.

   C. LDL is commonly referred to as *good cholesterol* and HDL as *bad cholesterol*. These are not cholesterols. HDL and LDL are proteins that carry cholesterol to and from organs and tissues.

   D. The patient is on statin therapy that alters the real state of her cholesterol levels.

7. **A 52-year-old man diagnosed with alcohol abuse has a low albumin level. Why should this be of concern for the practitioner?**

   A. Albumin controls hydrostatic pressure in blood vessels that keeps blood from leaking out of blood vessels. A low level can lead to ascites.

   B. Albumin controls oncotic pressure in blood vessels that keeps blood from leaking out of blood vessels. A low level can lead to atherosclerosis.

   C. Albumin controls the protein level in blood. A low level can lead to poor distribution of hormones and medications.

   D. Albumin controls oncotic pressure in blood vessels that keeps blood from leaking out of blood vessels. A low level can lead to ascites.

8. **A 34-year-man diagnosed with thrombocythemia tells you that he is relieved because he thought he had too low a platelet level and was at risk for bleeding. Should the patient feel relieved?**

   A. No, because thrombocythemia is the medical term for low platelet level.

   B. No, because the patient is at risk for blood clots.

   C. Yes, because having a low platelet count places the patient at risk for bruising and bleeding.

   D. Yes, because the practitioner has placed the patient on medication therapy for thrombocythemia.

9. **A 35-year-old man was on Coumadin and for some unknown reason took an unusually large amount of Coumadin that resulted in severe bleeding. The practitioner ordered an infusion of fresh frozen plasma. What is the rationale for this order?**

   A. Plasma contains clotting factors.

   B. Fresh frozen plasma causes vasoconstriction that narrows blood vessels resulting in decreased bleeding.

   C. Fresh frozen plasma is composed mostly of clotting factors that will stop bleeding.

   D. The practitioner is replacing all the blood that the patient lost.

10. **A 41-year-old man was brought to the emergency department bleeding from an open wound on his arm. The front of his clothes was covered in blood. You report to the practitioner that vital signs are stable. What do you think the practitioner will order next?**

    A. Normal saline IV because the patient has a class III hemorrhage.

    B. Blood transfusion because the patient has a class II hemorrhage.

    C. No fluid replacement. Treat the wound and monitor the patient. The patient has a class I hemorrhage.

    D. Blood transfusion and lactated Ringer solution because the patient has a class III hemorrhage.

## CORRECT ANSWERS AND RATIONALES

1. D. Circulation in your legs decreased because you were immobilized following surgery causing a blood clot to form.

2. B. RBCs carry oxygen throughout your body. You are fatigued because your body is not receiving sufficient oxygen because there aren't enough RBCs.

3. C. The practitioner wanted to rule out "white coat syndrome."

4. A. The levels of electrolytes are maintained by the kidneys.

5. C. Bands are immature neutrophils that increase when there is a bacterial infection.

6. A. HDL is commonly referred to as *good cholesterol* and LDL as *bad cholesterol*. These are not cholesterols. HDL and LDL are proteins that carry cholesterol to and from organs and tissues.

7. D. Albumin controls oncotic pressure in blood vessels that keeps blood from leaking out of blood vessels. A low level can lead to ascites.

8. B. No, because the patient is at risk for blood clots.

9. A. Plasma contains clotting factors.

10. C. No fluid replacement. Treat the wound and monitor the patient. The patient has a class I hemorrhage.

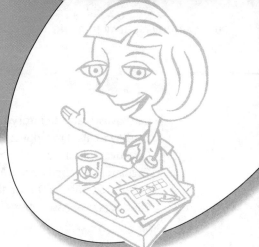

chapter 2

# Cardiovascular Assessment and Tests

## LEARNING OBJECTIVES

1. Cardiovascular Patient History
2. Cardiovascular Episode Assessment
3. Cardiovascular Physical Assessment
4. Cardiovascular Documentation
5. Cardiovascular Tests and Procedures

# Cardiovascular Patient History

The cardiovascular assessment is a focused assessment that typically follows a comprehensive assessment of the patient. The focused assessment follows up information that leads the nurse to suspect that the patient may have a cardiovascular disorder or is at risk for developing a cardiovascular disorder.

The cardiovascular assessment begins with a review of the patient's medical history. This history can reveal symptoms of a cardiovascular disorder or risk factors that, if left unaddressed, can lead to cardiovascular disorders.

The patient's cardiovascular history will guide you through a focused cardiovascular physical examination. Ask the patient about a history of:

- Hypertension
- Elevated blood cholesterol
- Elevated triglycerides
- Recurring anemia
- Rheumatic fever
- Congenital heart disease
- Heart murmurs
- Unexplained joint pain during childhood
- Diagnosed cardiovascular disorders and related treatments

Also inquire about any cardiovascular tests that might have been performed in the past or recently by another practitioner. These include blood tests, a stress test, and an electrocardiogram (ECG). The nurse may be able to obtain the results from other health care practitioners with permission of the patient. These results can serve as a baseline that can be compared with current test results.

Next, focus on the patient's current and past lifestyle, which helps you identify factors that expose the patient to the risk of cardiovascular disorders. Inquire about the following:

- **Smoking:** Does the patient currently smoke cigarettes or other tobacco products? Has the patient smoked in the past, if not currently smoking? How many years has the patient smoked?

- **Alcohol:** How much alcohol does the patient consume per day or per week?

- **Drugs:** Identify all prescribed and over-the-counter medications, herbal supplements, and street drugs that the patient is taking and has taken in the past.

- **Exercise:** Inquire about the patient's exercise program and frequency, if any.

- **Nutrition:** Ask about the patient's diet and recent changes in his/her weight.

---

### NURSING ALERT

The Cancer Treatment Centers of America developed a measurement of smoking called "pack-year" history that is used to assess the amount of cigarettes a patient smokes. Here is the formula used to calculate pack-year.

Packs per day × years smoked = pack-year history

For example,

2 packs per day × 20 years = 40 pack-year history

---

## Cardiovascular Episode Assessment

A patient may report chest pain or other symptoms associated with cardiovascular disease, which is why the patient is being assessed. This is referred to as an *episode*, which causes the nurse and practitioner to focus on the reported problem rather than the overall health of the patient.

Practitioners use the **PQRST** mnemonic when examining the cardiovascular system when the patient reports chest pain or discomfort.

- **Provocative:** What makes the pain, discomfort, or symptom better or worse?

  - Meals, emotional stress, cold, and smoking may increase symptoms of angina.

- Chest pain that decreases when sitting or leaning forward is suggestive of pericarditis.
- Chest pain that subsides with rest suggests coronary artery ischemia.
- Discomfort during or after eating is likely to be caused by an upper gastrointestinal disorder.
- Discomfort from swallowing might infer an esophageal disorder.
- **Quality:** Describe the quality of the symptom.

  - *Constriction:* The patient clenches his fist against the chest. This is referred to as the Levine sign.
  - *Burning:* Feeling of indigestion or heartburn is a sign of myocardial infarction especially in women.
  - *Pressure:* An elephant sitting on the chest.
  - *Frequency:* Recurring episodes with a higher level like quality of chest pain indicate coronary heart disease.
  - *Squeezing:* A band is squeezing the chest.
  - *Tightness:* A knot present in the center of the chest.

> **NURSING ALERT**
>
> Emotional stress, meals, smoking, exertion, and cold can cause ischemic pain.

- **Region:** Where does the pain or discomfort begin and does it travel to another area of the body?
  - *Localized pain:* Pain within a small area of the chest is less likely related to underlying cardiac conditions and is more likely related to a condition of the chest wall or possibly the pleural area.
  - *Shoulder, upper extremity, throat, neck, and lower jaw pain:* Pain in these areas is associated with myocardial ischemia.
  - *Diffused pain:* Pain that is difficult to localize to one area and reports generally in the chest area is likely to be ischemic cardiac pain.
  - *Radiating pain:* Pain that radiates to several areas is likely to be a symptom of myocardial infarction (MI).
- **Severity:** On a scale from 0 to 10 with 10 being the worst, how would you rank the pain or discomfort?
  - *10-Point Numeric Pain Scale:* 0 is no pain; 10 is excruciating pain. The rating does not indicate the degree of ischemia. Nearly a third of

patients who have ischemia may not report pain. Also, some patients have difficulty assigning a number to the severity of pain.

- *Adjective Pain Rating Scale:* Permit the patient to describe the pain in words.

- *Wong-Baker FACES Pain Rating Scale:* A patient, usually a child, is shown a series of faces progressively depicting severity of pain and is asked to pick the face that corresponds to the pain that the patient is experiencing.

- *FLACC Scale:* The Face, Legs, Activity, Cry, Consolability Scale is used for children from age 2 months to 7 years and for patients who are unable to communicate the severity of pain, such as patients in the intensive care unit (ICU). A pain scale score from 0 to 2 is assigned based on the patient's presentation (Table 2–1).

- **Time:** Is the pain or discomfort associated with an activity such as eating, movement, or exercise?

  - *Gradual pain:* Myocardial ischemic pain typically starts gradually and increases in intensity over time.

  - *Abrupt pain:* Pain that starts suddenly with the most intensity and then gradually decreases is typically associated with aortic dissection, pneumothorax, or an acute pulmonary embolism.

**TABLE 2–1**  The FLACC Pain Scale Is Used to Assign a Pain Rating Between 0 and 2 for Patients Who Are Unable to Communicate Pain

| Criteria | 0 | 1 | 2 |
| --- | --- | --- | --- |
| Face | No particular expression or smile | Withdrawn, uninterested, occasionally grimacing | Clenched jaw, frequent or constant quivering |
| Legs | Normal relaxed position | Tense, uneasy, restless | Legs drawn up, kicking |
| Activity | Normal position, moves easily, lies quietly | Squirming, tense | Arched, rigid, or jerking motion |
| Cry | No crying | Moans, whimpers, occasional complaints | Screams, sobbing, constantly crying, complains frequently |
| Consolability | Content | Distractible and can be reassured by touching or talking | Difficult to console |

- *Crescendo pain:* Pain that increases in intensity over a short time may be related to esophageal disease.
- *Short duration pain:* Myocardial ischemia pain typically lasts for a few minutes.
- *Prolonged duration pain:* Myocardial infarction pain is prolonged.
- *Morning pain:* Myocardial ischemia is likely to occur in the morning. However, patients taking beta-blockers or patients diagnosed with diabetes may experience myocardial ischemia pain at various times.

---

### NURSING ALERT

Myocardial ischemia may also produce the following symptoms: nausea, vomiting, sweating (diaphoresis), fainting (syncope), palpitations, difficulty breathing on exertion (exertional dyspnea), and fatigue.

Elderly patients may also report myocardial ischemia as confusion, difficulty breathing at rest, or loss of appetite (anorexia).

---

## Factors to Consider During the Cardiovascular Assessment

There are symptoms related to an underlying cardiac condition that may not be reported or are underreported by the patient. These are as follows:

- **Decreased ability to breathe when lying down (orthopnea):** The patient typically uses several pillows to keep his head raised during sleep. Ask the patient the number of pillows used when sleeping.
- **The need for fresh air after a few hours of sleeping (paroxysmal nocturnal dyspnea [PND]):** The patient may feel that waking up suddenly with the need for fresh air is caused by anxiety. When a patient lies down, blood volume increases in the thoracic cavity. Normally, the heart compensates by reducing the volume that has accumulated in the thoracic cavity. However, the heart is not strong enough to pump sufficient blood for a patient with congestive heart failure. Therefore, blood accumulates in the thoracic cavity, signaling the brain to awaken the patient with the need to breathe fresh air.
- **Fatigue:** The patient frequently feels tired and considers the problem as being "out of shape," an expected result of aging, or the result of mild depression. Depression causes fatigue all day whereas cardiovascular disorders typically cause fatigue in the evening.
- **Swelling in the legs (edema):** Some patients may consider swelling of the legs related to aging. Bilateral leg swelling is likely caused by an underlying

cardiovascular condition such as congestive heart failure. Swelling is usually less noticeable in the morning because the patient's legs were raised while sleeping and more noticeable in the evening after a day of standing, walking, and normal activities.

- **Getting up at night to urinate (nocturia):** There are many reasons why a patient awakens to urinate, one of which is an underlying cardiovascular disorder such as heart failure. Failure of the heart to pump blood effectively can result in excess fluid building up in the cardiovascular system. Lying in bed sleeping (**recumbency**) encourages reabsorption of fluid. When the bladder is nearly full, the patient's brain awakens the patient, signaling a need to urinate.

## Pediatric History

Infants and children can display symptoms of cardiovascular disease but are usually unable to recognize symptoms because they believe that the symptoms are normal. Here are the factors to investigate when asking parents about their child.

- **The number and lengths of naps:** Frequent or long naps may indicate fatigue, possibly caused by an underlying cardiovascular disorder.
- **Family history:** Does anyone in the family have congenital heart disease?
- **Milestones:** Is the child reaching expected developmental milestones?
- **Activity:** Is the child able to perform activities with playmates of the same age?
- **Blue spells (cyanotic):** Does the child appear bluish at any time, especially on exertion?

# Cardiovascular Physical Assessment

The process of the cardiovascular physical assessment follows a pattern that ensures that all areas of the patient's cardiovascular system are examined. The cardiovascular physical examination is conducted in the following sequence.

## Neck Physical Assessment

- **Inspect:** Inspect the patient's jugular veins by having the patient lie face up (supine) on the examination table and elevate the head of table 45°. Observe the patient's neck. You should not see any pulsations from the jugular veins. Pulsating jugular veins may indicate a cardiovascular disorder.

- **Listen (auscultate):** Place the bell or diaphragm of the stethoscope over blood vessels in the patient's neck. Listen for a swishing sound (**bruit**) that occurs when there is disruption in blood flow (**turbulence**), which might indicate a vascular disorder.

- **Palpate:** Lightly press the side of the patient's neck 0.75 inches deep (**light palpation**); press deeper 2 inches (**deep palpation**). You should feel a smooth contour with a normal pulse, normal moisture, and normal temperature. Any tenderness or abnormal contour might be a sign of an underlying cardiovascular disorder.

### NURSING ALERT

Ask the patient to momentarily hold his/her breath to prevent you from confusing breath sounds with vascular sounds. The bell of the stethoscope is used to hear low-pitched sounds and the diaphragm is used to hear high-pitched sounds. Palpate the carotid arteries gently and separately.

## Circulatory System Physical Assessment

- **Inspect:** Observe the patient's skin. Constriction of blood vessels (**vasoconstriction**) is suspected if the patient has cool, clammy skin. A pale color might indicate peripheral vascular resistance as seen in **atherosclerosis**. Dilation of blood vessels (**vasodilation**) is suspected if the skin is warm and moist. Redness (**dependent rubor**) in the legs may indicate arterial insufficiency common in peripheral arterial disease (PAD). View the patient's oral mucous membranes for bluish color (**cyanosis**). Lips, extremities, and nail beds may also reveal a bluish color, but the blue color may not be apparent depending on the patient's skin tone. Look for swelling (**edema**) in the extremities. Swelling in both legs (**bilateral edema**) may indicate thrombophlebitis, heart failure, or liver failure. Note lack of hair on the patient's legs, which may indicate arterial insufficiency.

### NURSING ALERT

Test for dependent rubor by laying the patient supine and elevating the legs to 45° for 1 minute. If the soles become pale, suspect that the patient has ischemia. Ask the patient to sit upright. If the patient's feet gradually turn pink or look like red cooked lobster, suspect that the patient has ischemia.

- **Auscultation:** Circulatory auscultation is performed by taking the blood pressure. Blood pressure increases with age, stress, weight gain, and anxiety. Systolic blood pressure represents pressure created when the left ventricle contracts. Diastolic blood pressure represents pressure in the patient's arteries between left ventricle contractions. Blood pressure readings should be taken at three different occasions before reaching a diagnosis of hypotension or hypertension. The objective is to determine a trend of at least three data points rather than from a single data point. However, critical blood pressure values should be treated immediately. Table 2–2 contains values used to diagnose hypertension.

- **Palpation:** Palpation is feeling the contour and amplitude of peripheral arteries. The **pulse contour** indicates the shape and boundary of the artery. The **pulse amplitude** indicates the pulse strength and the elasticity

| TABLE 2–2 Classification of Hypertension Based on the Systolic and Diastolic Readings | | |
|---|---|---|
| Category | Systolic | Diastolic |
| Normal | <120 | <80 |
| Pre-hypertension | 120-139 | 80-89 |
| Stage I | 140-159 | 90-99 |
| Stage II | >160 | >100 |

of the arterial wall. Compare the corresponding left and right peripheral arteries. They should feel similar. Any difference should be noted and investigated. Begin with the **radial** (wrist) then progress to the **brachial** (upper arm), **femoral** (upper thigh), **popliteal** (back of the knee), **dorsalis pedis** (top of the foot), and **posterior tibial** (inside ankle).

## Precordium Physical Assessment

- **Inspect:** Inspect the area of the chest above the heart (**precordium**) for pulsations from the **apical pulse** (the central pulse from the apex of the heart), which is in the fourth or fifth intercostal space. The apical pulse may or may not be visible.

- **Auscultation:** Use the diaphragm of the stethoscope to listen to the patient's heart (Figure 2–1). The heart produces two normal sounds commonly referred to as sounding like "lub dub." The "lub" is the first heart sound, called $S_1$, and the "dub" is the second heart sound, called $S_2$. $S_1$ is turbulence caused by closure of the mitral and tricuspid values at the start of **systole**. $S_2$ is caused by the closure of the aortic and pulmonic values at the end of systole. Ventricles fill between the $S_2$ ("dub") and $S_1$ ("lub"), which is called *diastole*. Visualize the position of the heart when placing the stethoscope on the patient's chest (see Figure 2–1). Abnormal heart sounds may be heard. The most common are called a *murmur* and are referred to as $S_3$ and $S_4$. $S_3$ sound occurs shortly after $S_2$ and gives the rhythm of three heart sounds "lub-DUB-ta" rather than "lub dub." $S_3$ is also called the *ventricular gallop* caused by the ventricles rapidly filling. The ventricle is not completely empty during diastole. $S_4$ is heard right before $S_1$ and gives the rhythm of a gallop (**atrial gallop**) sounding like "ta-lub-DUB." $S_4$ is caused by the decreased ability of the ventricle to function, causing a resistance in flow of blood. Document the quality of abnormal heart sounds based on the following:

  - **Timing:** The sound is closer to $S_1$ (systole) or closer to $S_2$ (diastole).
  - **Location of maximum intensity:** Location of the abnormal sound.
  - **Radiation:** The abnormal heart sound can be heard in other locations such as the neck.
  - **Frequency:** High/low pitch.
  - **Quality:** Described as blowing, harsh, or soft.
  - **Intensity:** Based on the intensity scale (Table 2–3).

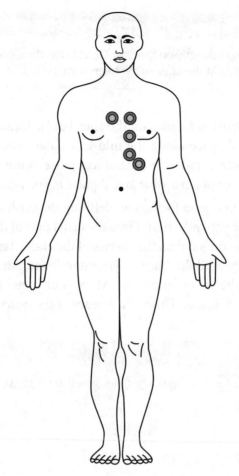

**FIGURE 2–1 ·** Move the stethoscope in a Z position when listening to heart sounds.

| TABLE 2–3 Murmur Intensity Scale | |
|---|---|
| Grade | Intensity |
| 1 | Faint |
| 2 | Barely heard |
| 3 | Same as $S_1$ or $S_2$ |
| 4 | Loud with no thrill |
| 5 | Loud with thrill |
| 6 | Extremely loud—detectable without the stethoscope touching the chest. |

> **NURSING ALERT**
>
> Place the stethoscope directly on the skin. Don't listen through clothing. S$_3$ heart sounds are heard best at the apex of the heart with the bell of the stethoscope.

- **Palpation:** Palpation focuses on the apical pulse located in the fourth or fifth intercostal space along the mid-clavicular line. You should feel a short tap; however, palpating the apical pulse is not possible for many patients. Absence of a palpable apical pulse is not significant.
- **Percussion:** Percussion focuses on defining the cardiac border. Visualize the heart in the patient's chest. Place the distal part of the middle finger of your nondominant hand on the surface of the chest. Tap the middle finger quickly with the middle finger of your dominant hand. You should hear dullness over the area of the heart. Move your finger to the point where you don't hear dullness. This is the border of the heart.

> **NURSING ALERT**
>
> The outline of the heart is typically determined by a chest X-ray rather than percussion.

## Cardiovascular Documentation

The physical assessment must be documented in the patient's record. Some health care facilities use paper charts where some or all of a patient's information is written on paper. Many health care facilities have converted to electronic medical records using an electronic medical records system provided by a third party vendor. Each electronic medical records system provides a mechanism for collecting similar patient information; however, the interface (ie, screens) for these systems is unique to each vendor.

The trend is for documentation to be less narrative and to use more uniform terminology. Instead of writing a narrative about the assessment, the nurse is presented with assessment categories and a list of findings in the form of a checkbox or drop-down list as shown in Figure 2–2, which depicts cardiovascular assessment documentation. Some assessment categories are required, depending on the health care facility's policies. The nurse is not permitted to exit the assessment documentation screen until the required categories are documented.

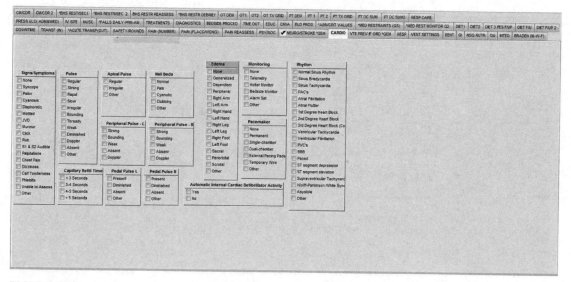

**FIGURE 2–2** · The cardiovascular assessment is documented by selecting the appropriate findings under each assessment category.

Not all cardiovascular documentation appears on the same screen. Some vendors divide the cardiovascular document into other screens where either assessment categories and/or assessment findings are long. For example, it is common for a neuro/stroke assessment to be on a same screen as shown in Figure 2–3.

The neuro/stroke assessment is performed and documented daily or each shift for every cardiovascular patient, depending on the health care facility's policy. The screen is also used to document that a patient shows sign of a stroke.

## Cardiovascular Tests and Procedures

Cardiovascular tests and procedures are key elements in assessing the patient for cardiovascular disease. The cardiovascular history and physical assessment may or may not identify signs and symptoms of cardiovascular disease. The patient may report symptoms or you may identify signs that lead you to believe that cardiovascular disease may exist. However, the patient may be asymptomatic and your physical assessment may not reveal any signs of a cardiovascular problem.

The practitioner may order cardiovascular tests to rule out a cardiovascular problem and may perform procedures if such a problem exists. The following

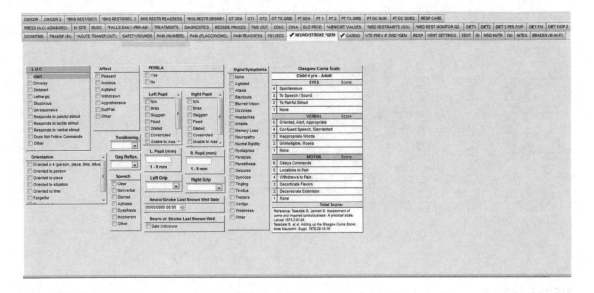

**FIGURE 2–3** • The neuro/stroke assessment is documented by selecting the appropriate findings under each assessment category.

are cardiovascular tests and procedures that a practitioner may order for a patient.

## Pulse Oximetry

Pulse oximetry assesses the arterial oxygen saturation of the patient's blood by passing an infrared beam of light through the patient's nail bed or skin. The amount of infrared light absorbed by the patient's blood provides an estimate of arterial oxygen saturation. This is referred to as an *abbreviated arterial oxygen saturation value.*

The pulse oximetry value should be between 95% and 100% if the patient is breathing room air and does not have chronic pulmonary disease such as chronic obstructive pulmonary disease (COPD). A patient who has COPD may have a lower pulse oximetry value, which might be normal for the patient. A patient who is sedated or sleeping may also have a low pulse oximetry, which is not alarming because the cause of the low value is known.

A patient who has supplemental oxygen should have a pulse oximetry value between 95% and 100%. A lower value may indicate a cardiac or respiratory problem. It may also indicate that a mechanical problem prevents the patient from receiving the supplementary oxygen such as an obstructed nasal cannula tube.

A value less than 95% on room air or on supplemental oxygen indicates there is instability in the cardiorespiratory system. If the underlying cause is not obvious, such as the patient hyperventilating, then the health care provider is likely to order an arterial blood gas.

## Cardiovascular Laboratory Tests

There are several laboratory tests that are ordered to assess the patient's risk for cardiovascular disease and whether or not the patient experienced a cardiovascular event. These laboratory tests are as follows:

- **Platelet function test:** Platelets (see Chapter 1) are fragments of cells that clump together to prevent bleeding. Platelets can also accumulate on deposits of plaque in arteries, which can lead to strokes or a heart attack. The platelet function test measures the rate at which the patient's blood clots. A practitioner may prescribe antiplatelet medications if the rate of clotting is relatively high.

- **Cholesterol test:** The cholesterol test provides a lipoprotein profile that measures the cholesterol levels (see Chapter 1) in the patient's blood. The lipoprotein profile measures three elements. These are as follows:

  i. **High-density lipoprotein (HDL):** HDL prevents the buildup of cholesterol in blood vessels. A value of 40 mg/dL or higher is a preferred value. A value that is lower than 40 mg/dL increases the patient's risk for cardiovascular disease.

  ii. **Low-density lipoprotein (LDL):** LDL causes plaque buildup in arteries. A patient without cardiovascular disease should have an LDL level lower than 130 mg/dL. However, a patient who has cardiovascular disease might require an LDL level lower than 70 mg/dL.

  iii. **Triglycerides:** Triglycerides (see Chapter 1) are fat (lipid) that is converted when the patient eats food. Sometimes this is referred to as *unused calories*. Triglycerides are stored in fat cells (**adipose cells**). A hormone causes triglycerides to be released from fat cells between meals to provide energy for the body. Triglyceride levels may be high (hypertriglyceridemia) if the patient eats more carbohydrates and fats than are being used by the body. A normal level is less than 150 mg/dL.

- **Cardiac markers test:** A cardiac marker is a blood test that measures specific enzyme, protein, or myoglobin levels in the blood to determine if the patient has experienced a cardiac disorder such as a myocardial infarction (heart attack). Enzymes, proteins, and myoglobin are inside cells. When cells rupture, enzymes, proteins, and myoglobin enter the bloodstream. The cardiac marker test includes the following:

  - *Creatine phosphokinase (CPK):* CPK enzymes are found in cardiac muscles and skeletal muscles. Elevated levels of CPK indicate muscle injury, but not necessarily injury of the cardiac muscle.

  - *Creatine kinase (CK-MB):* CK-MB enzyme is found in cardiac muscle. Normally there are undetectable levels in blood. Elevated levels of CK-MB are detected between 3 and 6 hours after the patient reports chest pain and peak between 12 and 24 hours. CK-MB returns to normal levels between 48 and 72 hours.

  - *Troponin:* There are two troponin tests. These are troponin I (TnI) and troponin T (TnT). One of the troponin tests can be ordered along with other cardiac tests. Troponin is a specific protein found in cardiac muscle; therefore, a the slight elevation in the patient's blood may indicate heart damage. The practitioner may order a series of troponin tests over several hours. Troponin levels can remain elevated for up to 2 weeks following a heart attack.

  - *Myoglobin:* Myoglobin elevates in blood 2 to 3 hours after muscle injury, including a heart attack, and peaks at 8 to 12 hours after the injury. Myoglobin returns to normal levels 24 hours after the muscle injury. Practitioners order a myoglobin test because myoglobin is detected sooner than troponin.

---

### NURSING ALERT

Practitioners use the troponin test when available rather than the CK-MB test, although the CK-MB test is still in use. Kidney failure can also cause elevated CK-MB levels in blood. Strenuous exercise may increase troponin values.

---

- **C-reactive protein (CRP) test:** CRP is used to measure vascular inflammation and the risk for peripheral arterial disease, heart attack, and stroke. A value of less than 1 mg/L indicates a low risk, and a value greater than 3 mg/L indicates a high risk.

- **Renin assay test:** The renin assay test is used to identify the underlying cause of hypertension. Blood pressure is regulated by the renin-angiotensin system (RAS). Low blood pressure causes the secretion of the renin enzyme by the kidneys, which increases angiotensin I that constricts blood vessels, resulting in increased blood pressure. The renin assay test measures the level of renin in blood. High renin assay test results may indicate malignant high blood pressure, kidney disease, blocked artery, cirrhosis of the liver, Addison disease, or hemorrhage. The renin stimulation test may be ordered if the renin level is low. The renin stimulation test stimulates secretion of the renin enzyme to determine if the kidney is functioning properly.

- **Electrolyte panel:** An electrolyte panel is ordered as part of basic blood chemistry. An electrolyte is a mineral present in blood and other bodily fluids as well as inside cells. **Electrolytes** are used by heart cells to maintain electrical balance across the cell walls and to carry electrical impulses necessary for contraction of the heart. Electrolyte balance must be maintained to ensure proper cardiac function. The electrolyte panel measures the levels of each electrolyte to determine if electrolytes are balanced.

- **Brain natriuretic peptide (BNP):** BNP is an amino acid that is secreted by the ventricles when the ventricles are excessively stretched (**cardiomyocytes**). The practitioner orders the test when the patient presents with swelling of both legs (peripheral edema), is fatigued, and has shortness of breath. Increased BNP along with corresponding symptoms may indicate heart failure. The level of BNP indicates the severity of heart failure. Normal levels in conjunction with symptoms indicate a condition other than heart failure is causing the symptoms.

## Cardiovascular Tests

There are several nonlaboratory tests that are ordered to diagnose cardiovascular disease. These tests are as follows:

- **Heart monitors:** A heart monitor records activities of the heart. There are several types of heart monitors, including:
  - *Electrocardiogram (ECG):* An electrocardiogram depicts the electrical activity of the heart in the form of a graph. Chapter 3 explores recording the electrical activity of the heart in detail.

- *Holter monitor:* A Holter monitor is a device that records the electrical activity of the heart constantly from 24 to 48 hours. The Holter monitor is worn by the patient during activities of daily living.

- *Event monitor:* An event monitor is a wearable device that records data only when a cardiac event occurs. The patient can wear the event monitor for up to a month.

- *Implantable loop recorder:* An implantable loop recorder is a device placed beneath the skin of the chest that monitors the electrical activity of the heart for up to 2 years. This is used when the patient reports infrequent cardiac symptoms.

- **Venous ultrasound:** A venous ultrasound uses a transducer to send sound waves along the blood vessels in the body. Based on the returning sound detected by the transducer, a computer generates an image of blood vessels showing a narrowing or blockage.

- **Transcranial Doppler (TCD):** Transcranial Doppler is an ultrasound test performed at the base of the brain to assess the risk for a stroke and is used to measure the rate of blood flow through blood vessels.

- **Chest X-ray:** Chest X-rays are done to detect size and position of the heart and structural abnormalities of the lungs. An X-ray machine directs X-rays through the chest and onto film positioned behind the patient's back. As X-rays are directed to the patient, some X-rays are absorbed by the body and others pass through to the X-ray film. Areas of the body that absorb X-rays appear light on the X-ray film. Dark areas on the X-ray film represent X-rays that pass through the body.

- **Echocardiogram:** An echocardiogram uses sound waves to produce images that show how well the heart is beating. There are four types of echocardiograms as follows:

    i. **Transthoracic:** This is the standard echocardiogram where a transducer is placed on the patient's chest and sends sound waves through the chest. The transducer detects sound waves that bounce back; these waves are converted into moving images by a computer.

    ii. **Transesophageal:** This is used when the transthoracic echocardiogram doesn't produce a clear image of the heart. The transesophageal echocardiogram requires that the transducer be inserted into the esophagus. Sound waves are transmitted through the esophagus, and returning sound waves are used to generate a moving image of the heart.

   iii. **Doppler:** A Doppler echocardiogram is used to measure the speed and direction of blood flow in the heart. Results are colorized on the monitor and are used to detect problems with blood flow.

   iv. **Stress:** Stress echocardiogram is taken before and after the patient walks on a treadmill. Sometimes the practitioner will use medication that stresses the heart instead of using a treadmill. This is useful for patients who are unable to walk on a treadmill.

- **Cardiac catheterization (angiography):** This is an invasive procedure used to examine coronary arteries and intracardiac structures and measure cardiac output, intracardiac pressures, and oxygenation. A radiopaque dye is injected through a catheter into the femoral artery in the patient's left leg or in the antecubital fossa of the arm and flows to the coronary arteries. The flow of the radiopaque dye is viewed and recorded using a fluoroscope, enabling the physician to determine obstructions to the flow and the structures of the heart. Before the test, ensure the following:

  - Inquire if the patient is allergic to seafood or iodine. If so, notify the physician immediately because the patient might also be allergic to the radiopaque dye.

  - Obtain written consent from the patient. Risks and benefits of the test need to be explained to the patient before commencing the angiography.

  - NPO for 4 to 6 hours before the test to reduce the risk of aspiration.

  - Explain the procedure to the patient and its possible side effects such as flushing of the face, nausea, urge to urinate, and chest pain, which are usually reactions to the dye.

  - Record baseline vital signs, so you can later assess for changes.

  - Record the pedal pulse baseline, so you can later assess for changes.

- After the test, ensure the following:

  - Assess for bleeding at the injection site since a major artery has been accessed. If bleeding, apply pressure until bleeding stops.

  - Keep patient on bed rest for 8 hours, so as not to dislodge a clot from the artery used for the catheter.

  - Keep pressure on injection site for 8 hours to ensure clotting at the site.

  - If femoral artery is used, keep left leg straight for 8 hours to minimize the risk of dislodging clot.

  - If antecubital fossa is used, keep arm strain for 3 hours to minimize the risk of dislodging clot.

- Monitor vital signs to assess for changes.
- Increase fluid intake to assist the kidneys in excreting the dye.

- **Echocardiograph:** Echocardiograph is an ultrasound of the heart that provides a noninvasive examination of intracardiac structures and blood flow. Sound waves are directed to and deflected by the heart, causing an echo that is detected by the echocardiograph, which is interpreted by a physician. The patient must lie still for 30 minutes during the test to ensure an accurate picture of the structures.

- **Nuclear cardiology:** Nuclear cardiology is a group of tests that determines myocardial perfusion and contractility of the heart, ischemia, infarction, wall motion, and ejection fraction. Radioisotopes are injected through the intravenous (IV) line. The radiation detector monitors the flow of the radioisotope as it flows through the heart. Assess for bleeding at the injection site after the test is performed.

## Cardiovascular Procedures

There are several cardiac procedures used to restore blood flow to the heart and reestablish cardiac rhythm. These are as follows:

- **Percutaneous transluminal coronary angioplasty (PTCA):** This is a nonsurgical procedure used to open a blocked coronary artery by inserting a balloon-tipped catheter into the femoral artery and moving the catheter into the blocked coronary artery using a fluoroscope to help guide the catheter into position. Once in position, the balloon is inflated, pushing the plaque that is causing the blockage against the coronary artery wall and allowing blood to flow again.

- **Coronary artery bypass graft (CABG):** This is a surgery procedure performed when a patient experiences myocardial ischemia. Before this procedure is performed, the patient typically undergoes catheterization to determine the severity of the myocardial ischemia. In severe ischemia, the blockage is bypassed by grafting a segment of the saphenous vein from the leg.

- **Cardioversion:** This is a nonsurgical procedure used to treat atrial fibrillation, atrial flutter, supraventricular tachycardia, and ventricular tachycardia. A low energy level shock is administered that is synchronized with the patient's heart cycle, causing interruption of the reentry circuit and enabling control to resume by the sinoatrial node.

- **Transcutaneous pacemaker:** This is a nonsurgical procedure that uses an external electrical generator to send impulses through electrodes placed on the patient's chest to the patient's heart to provide external impulses to the heart in an emergency. The transcutaneous pacemaker remains active until a transvenous pacemaker is implemented.

## CASE STUDY

### CASE 1

You are a nurse in an acute psychiatric unit where many of the patients are being stabilized on psychiatric medication. Patients remain inpatients for relatively longer periods than on a medical unit since it takes several weeks before the patient receives the therapeutic effects of many psychiatric medications. During their stay, patients freely walk the unit engaging in social activities (ie, television, recreation) with other patients. Each morning when the patients first awaken, you assess each patient by recording vital signs and therapeutic questioning. Your 56-year-old patient's blood pressure was 190/100 mm Hg. Other vital signs were not remarkable. He reports no symptoms and walked to you with a quick steady gait. He reports that yesterday in gym he felt slight pressure over this chest area while playing volleyball. He said he sat for a while and the chest discomfort resolved itself. What would your best response be to the following questions?

QUESTION 1. What would you ask the patient about his blood pressure?
ANSWER: Ask the patient if he has high blood pressure. If so, then ask him if he has taken his blood pressure medication this morning. You may not be the nurse who administered medication to the patient. It is likely that the patient has chronic hypertension and has not yet taken his blood pressure medication. You should record the blood pressure reading and retake the patient's blood pressure an hour after he has taken his blood pressure medication. You should also review the patient's previous blood pressure readings in the patient's chart to identify the trend of the patient's blood pressure.

QUESTION 2. What would you do about the patient's report of chest discomfort?
ANSWER: Notify the practitioner, conveying that the discomfort took place while the patient was playing volleyball and also noting that the discomfort resolved when the patient sat down. It is also critical to inform the practitioner about your current assessment of the patient. You should ask the patient to refrain from activities that will cause exertion until the practitioner follows up with the patient.

QUESTION 3. How do you expect the practitioner to respond?

ANSWER: The practitioner is likely to order an ECG and cardiac markers, both of which may show signs of an underlying cardiac disorder and myocardial infarction. The practitioner is also likely to order the patient to refrain from any activity that will cause exertion and to report any discomfort immediately. It is also highly likely that the practitioner will order the patient to undergo a stress test.

QUESTION 4. What would you do if you reported your findings to the resident-on-call and the resident-on-call ordered stat sublingual nitroglycerin, 100% $O_2$ nasal cannula, stat ECG and cardiac markers, and to prepare the patient to be immediately moved to the cardiac care unit?

ANSWER: Restate your assessment and ask the resident-on-call to confirm that he understood your assessment. Emphasize that the patient is being treated for hypertension and was just administered blood pressure medication, and that the patient was asymptomatic for any cardiac discomfort during your assessment. In fact, the patient walked briskly with a steady gait. If the resident-on-call does not modify his original orders, process the order for the ECG and cardiac markers and report the situation to your supervisor immediately and ask for direction. The patient likely experienced an angina attack caused by narrowing of one or more coronary arteries that blocked blood flow during exertion. Angina resolved when the patient relaxed and continued with normal activities. The patient is currently asymptomatic. His oxygen saturation is 100%; therefore, supplementary oxygen is contraindicated. Administering nitroglycerin may harm the patient who is asymptotic and has just taken blood pressure medication. Your supervisor is likely to consult with the attending-on-call or the hospitalist who will likely place all but the ECG and cardiac markers on hold and then consult with the resident-on-call.

# FINAL CHECKUP

1. **A 32-year-old man who is unable to speak is seen with his legs drawn up near his chest and sobs constantly. Which is your best assessment of the patient?**

    A. The patient is looking for attention.

    B. The patient is experiencing discomfort associated with a gastrointestinal disorder.

    C. The patient is experiencing a pain rating of 2 on the Wong-Baker Pain Scale.

    D. The patient is experiencing a pain rating of 2 on the FLACC Pain Scale.

2. **A 53-year-old woman reports swelling of her legs. You notice both legs are swollen. What is next question you should ask the patient?**

   A. Do you abuse alcohol?

   B. Are you experiencing shortness of breath?

   C. Do you have dependent rubor?

   D. Do you spend hours on your feet at work?

3. **A 48-year-old woman was brought to the emergency department complaining of lower jaw pain. The practitioner ordered a myoglobin test and a troponin test. What is the best rationale for ordering the myoglobin test?**

   A. Myoglobin elevates in blood after muscle injury including a heart attack sooner than troponin levels.

   B. Troponin elevates in blood after muscle injury including a heart attack sooner than myoglobin levels.

   C. Myoglobin returns to normal levels 24 hours after the muscle injury.

   D. Troponin levels can remain elevated for up to 2 weeks following a heart attack.

4. **A 20-year-old man reported "a funny feeling in his chest occasionally." The patient's ECG is within normal range. The practitioner ordered that the patient wear an event monitor. The patient asks you why the event monitor was ordered. What is your best response?**

   A. An event monitor is a wearable device that records your heart activity for up to 48 hours.

   B. An event monitor is a wearable device that records data only when a cardiac event occurs and you can wear the event monitor for up to a month.

   C. An event monitor is a wearable device that records your heart activity.

   D. An event monitor is a wearable device that records data only when a cardiac event occurs and will record your heart activity the next time you have a "funny feeling" in your chest.

5. **A 45-year-old male patient reports pain in a small area of his chest. He has unremarkable vital signs. What is your best response?**

   A. Ask the patient if he has a history of cardiovascular disease.

   B. Ask the patient if he feels tightness around his chest.

   C. Ask the patient what he was doing in the past 24 hours.

   D. Ask the practitioner if he/she wants to order a stat ECG and markers and place the patient on 100% oxygen immediately.

6. **A 42-year-old woman tells you during a cardiac assessment that she sleeps with four pillows under her head and without a blanket at night. What is your best response?**

    A. Do you get cold when sleeping?

    B. Do you have difficulty breathing?

    C. Have you tried sleeping with three pillows?

    D. Are your legs swollen?

7. **A 52-year-old woman tells you that her BNP was elevated, according to her practitioner. She asks why BNP elevation is concerning. What is your best response?**

    A. BNP is secreted by ventricles of your heart when the ventricles are excessively stretched. Elevated BNP may indicate heart failure with symptoms indicate a condition other than heart failure.

    B. It is best to ask your practitioner that question.

    C. BNP is secreted by the ventricles of your heart when the ventricles are excessively stretched. Elevated BNP may indicate heart failure.

    D. BNP is an electrolyte found inside the cells. Elevation of BNP may indicate increased cell necrosis.

8. **A 54-year-old man who has smoked two packs of cigarettes per day for 20 years reports mild chest discomfort and is short of breath at times during the day. His practitioner ordered a chest X-ray to rule out a potential heart condition. The patient asks how a chest X-ray could determine the condition of his heart. What is your best response?**

    A. A chest X-ray is used to detect the size of the heart.

    B. A chest X-ray is used to rule out lung disease.

    C. You should ask your practitioner to answer this question.

    D. A chest X-ray shows contractions of your heart.

9. **What is the rationale for comparing left and right corresponding peripheral arteries?**

    A. You are able to detect any fistula.

    B. Comparing left and right corresponding peripheral arteries is an efficient way of assessing peripheral arteries.

    C. Corresponding peripheral arteries should have relatively the same contour and amplitude when palpated.

    D. You are able to detect a shunt.

10. **What is the rationale for palpating the dorsalis pedis?**

    A. The dorsalis pedis is located in the upper thigh and is the farthest peripheral artery from the heart. You are assured that the patient's legs are receiving sufficient arterial blood flow if the dorsalis pedis can be palpated.

    B. The dorsalis pedis is located at the back of the knee and is the farthest peripheral artery from the heart. You are assured that the patient's legs are receiving sufficient arterial blood flow if the dorsalis pedis can be palpated.

    C. The dorsalis pedis is located at the top of the foot and is the farthest peripheral artery from the heart. You are assured that the patient's legs are receiving sufficient arterial blood flow if the dorsalis pedis can be palpated.

    D. The dorsalis pedis is located at the top of the foot and is the farthest peripheral artery from the heart.

# CORRECT ANSWERS AND RATIONALES

1. D. The patient is experiencing a pain rating of 2 on the FLACC Pain Scale.
2. B. Are you experiencing shortness of breath? Bilateral edema may be an indication of heart failure, which would be accompanied by shortness of breath.
3. A. Myoglobin elevates in blood after muscle injury including a heart attack sooner than troponin levels.
4. D. An event monitor is a wearable device that records data only when a cardiac event occurs and will record your heart activity the next time you have a "funny feeling" in your chest.
5. C. Ask the patient what he was doing in the past 24 hours. Pain in a small area of the chest is a localized pain that is more likely related to a condition other than an underlying cardiac condition such as a bruise or pulled muscles.
6. B. Do you have difficulty breathing? A patient who sleeps with her head raised may experience orthopnea, which is the decreased ability to breathe when lying down.
7. C. BNP is secreted by ventricles of your heart when the ventricles are excessively stretched. Elevated BNP may indicate heart failure.
8. A. A chest X-ray is used to detect the size of the heart.
9. C. Corresponding peripheral arteries should have relatively the same contour and amplitude when palpated.
10. C. The dorsalis pedis is located at the top of the foot and is the farthest peripheral artery from the heart. You are assured that the patient's legs are receiving sufficient arterial blood flow if the dorsalis pedis can be palpated.

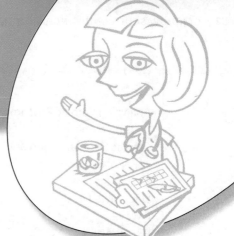

chapter **3**

# *Electrophysiology and Electrocardiogram*

## LEARNING OBJECTIVES

1. Electrophysiology
2. Electrocardiograph
3. Cardiac Monitoring Equipment and Lead Placement
4. Reading an Electrocardiograph
5. The Conduction System

# Electrophysiology

**Electrophysiology** is the study of electrical properties of tissues and cells that cause heart muscles to contract (**depolarize**) and relax (**repolarize**) forcing blood throughout the body. The electrophysiological activity of the heart is measured and recorded by an **electrocardiograph** (ECG).

The heart is composed of striated involuntary muscles called *cardiac muscles* consisting of cells called *cardiomyocytes* commonly referred to as *pacemaker cells*. Cardiomyocytes have the following three properties:

1. **Automaticity:** Cardiomyocytes are able to initiate an electrical impulse without receiving an impulse from the nervous system; they can contract without impulses from the nervous system.

2. **Excitability:** The nervous system sends impulses to increase or decrease contractions based on the body's needs.

3. **Conductivity:** Impulses generated by cardiomyocytes are transmitted to other cardiomyocytes resulting in coordinated depolarization and repolarization of cardiac muscles.

## Cardiac Depolarization and Repolarization

*Depolarization* is the action that causes cardiac muscles to contract. *Repolarization* is the action that causes cardiac muscles to return to a relaxed state. Depolarization and repolarization are caused by movement of electrolytes into and out of cardiac cells (cardiomyocytes).

- **Electrolytes:** An *electrolyte* is a substance that contains free ions making the substance conductive. An ion is a molecule where the total number of electrons is not equal to the total number of protons. Sodium and potassium are electrolytes used for electrical activity in cells.

- **Sodium-potassium pump:** The sodium-potassium pump controls the electrical activity of cardiac cells by moving free ions of electrolytes into and from cardiac cells. The sodium-potassium pump uses the enzyme **adenosine triphosphatase** (ATP) as a catalyst to transport the free ions across the cell membrane.

- **Depolarization:** Cardiac muscle contracts (depolarizes) when there is a higher concentration of potassium (K) inside the cardiac cell than in blood. As a result, the sodium-potassium pump exchanges potassium with sodium (Na), which has a higher concentration in blood than inside the cardiac cell. This exchange causes cardiac muscle to contract.

- **Repolarization:** When a higher concentration of potassium in blood than inside the cardiac cell exists, the sodium-potassium pump exchanges sodium with potassium, causing a higher concentration inside the cardiac cell than in blood. This exchange causes cardiac muscle to relax.

## Electrolyte Levels

Depolarization and repolarization may be altered by abnormal levels of electrolytes in the body and can affect the conduction of impulses throughout the heart. Electrolytes that are critical to proper cardiac function are as follows.

**Sodium:** This is the primary cation located in the extracellular space. A *cation* is a positively charged ion. Sodium is responsible for regulating blood and body fluids, transmission of nerve impulses, and cardiac activity. Abnormal levels can have a profound effect on the neurological status of the patient. Normal levels of sodium particles in 1 L of blood are 135 to 145 mEq/L.

- **Hyponatremia:** This occurs when there is less than a normal level of sodium in blood serum, and is defined as a serum sodium level of less than 135 mEq/L. Several underlying conditions can cause hyponatremia. These are as follows:

  - *Medications:* Some medications can cause the patient to urinate or perspire more than normal such as diuretics and antidepressants.

  - *Congestive heart failure:* Congestive heart failure causes fluids to accumulate in the body, resulting in dilution of sodium in body fluids.

  - *Kidney disease:* Kidney disease may prevent the kidneys from excreting urine, resulting in accumulation of fluid in the body.

- *Liver disease:* The liver produces albumin. Albumin is a protein found in blood that prevents it from leaking from blood vessels into other parts of the body such as the peritoneal cavity. Liver diseases prevent normal production of albumin, resulting in fluid accumulation.

- *Increased water consumption:* Drinking too much water disrupts the balance between bodily fluids and sodium.

- *Syndrome of inappropriate antidiuretic hormone (SIADH):* SIADH results in an increased production of antidiuretic hormone that causes the body to retain fluids.

- *Chronic vomiting or diarrhea:* Severe ongoing vomiting and diarrhea result in increased loss of sodium and other electrolytes.

- **Assessment of underlying cause of hyponatremia:** The underlying cause of hyponatremia is assessed by measuring the serum and urine osmolality. Osmolality is the concentration of particles of a substance in a fluid.

- *Serum osmolality:* This is used to differentiate between hyponatremia (low sodium), pseudohyponatremia (low serum sodium in the present of normal plasma tonicity), and hypertonicity (high concentration of solutes in plasma).

  - Pseudohyponatremia or hypertonicity: This can be caused by elevated glucose, glycine, or mannitol.

- *Urine osmolality:* This is used to differentiate between primary dehydration and impaired free water excretion.

  - Urine osmolality >20 mmol/L and patient is dehydrated.

    - Addison disease

    - Excess diuresis

    - Renal failure

  - Urine osmolality >500 mmol/L and the patient is not edematous or dehydrated.

    - SIADH

    - The patient is not edematous or dehydrated

      - Water intoxication

      - Severe hypothyroidism

      - Glucocorticoid insufficiency

- *Urine sodium concentration:* This is used to differentiate between hypo-volemia, hyponatremia, and SIADH.
  - Urine sodium <20 mmol/L and patient is dehydrated.
    - ⊚ Loss through diarrhea and/or vomiting, burns, trauma, and small bowel obstruction
    - ⊚ Patient is edematous and not dehydrated.
      - Nephrotic syndrome
      - Cirrhosis
      - Renal failure

**Potassium:** Very low or very high levels of potassium can result in a life-threatening situation.

- **Hypokalemia:** Serum potassium level <3.5 mEq/L
  - *Amplifies other medical conditions:* Hypokalemia amplifies other medical conditions on the ECG such as digitalis-induced arrhythmias, myocardial infarction (MI), or hypomagnesemia.
  - *Not cause for arrhythmias:* Hypokalemia does not cause arrhythmias.
  - *ECG:*
    - T wave: Flattened and/or inverse
    - QT wave: Prolonged
    - U wave: Prominent
- **Hyperkalemia:** Serum potassium level >5.5 mEq/L
  - *Hyperkalemia:* Hyperkalemia is a life-threatening condition because it decreases cardiac conduction.
  - *ECG* (Figure 3–1):
    - May see changes when serum potassium level reaches 6.6 mEq/L.
    - Always see changes when serum potassium level is >8.0 mEq/L.
    - T wave: begins with a peak in $V_2$ and $V_3$ leads.
    - P wave: Amplitude lost.
    - PR interval: Prolonged. Increased interval indicates cardiac conduction is decelerating leading to a complete heart block (CHB); >0.20 second in first-degree heart block.

Magnesium: This is an electrolyte required for the operation of the sodium-potassium pump. Magnesium is also an intrinsic calcium blocker.

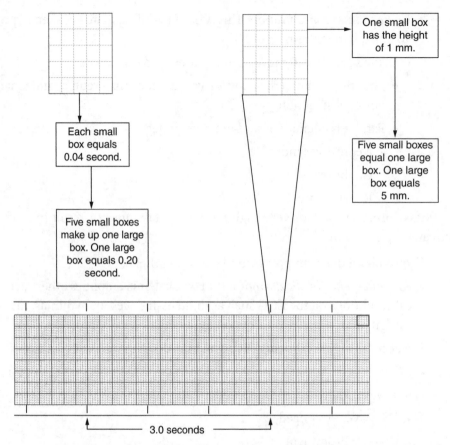

**FIGURE 3–1** • An ECG graph is divided into a grid, making the measurement of wave tracing simple. (Reproduced, with permission, from Keogh J, Reed D. *Schaum's Outline of ECG Interpretation*. New York: McGraw-Hill Education, 2011:58. Figure 5.1.)

- **Hypomagnesemia:** Serum magnesium level <1.4 mEq/L may cause the following:
  - *Resulting in tachyarrhythmias:* Early depolarization resulting in tachyarrhythmias especially torsades de pointes (polymorphous ventricular tachycardia), which is life-threatening, and prolonged QT interval (QTI).
  - Underdiagnosed: Most commonly underdiagnosed electrolyte abnormality.
  - *Can be a side effect of the following:*
    - Diuretic therapy
    - Antibiotic therapy (decreased reabsorption of magnesium when aminoglycosides are administered to the patient)
    - Diarrhea

- **Hypermagnesemia:** Serum magnesium level >2.0 mEq/L may cause the following:

  - *Decreased serum calcium:* High levels of magnesium decrease serum calcium.

  - *Hypermagnesemia is caused by the following:*
    - Renal impairment
    - Adrenal insufficiency
    - Hyperparathyroid
    - Lithium intoxication
    - Diabetic ketoacidosis (DKA)

  - *Hypermagnesemia can cause the following:*
    - Hyporeflexia (low reflexes) at serum levels >4 mEq/L
    - First-degree atrioventricular (AV) block at serum levels >5 mEq/L.
    - CHB at serum levels >10 mEq/L
    - Cardiac arrest at serum levels >13 mEq/L

**Calcium:** This is an abundant electrolyte in the body and is involved in coagulation, neuromuscular transmission, and smooth muscle contraction. Ionized calcium is the biologically active form of calcium. Total serum calcium corrected to albumin levels is as useful as ionized calcium.

- **Ionized hypocalcemia:** Serum level of ionized calcium is <1.3 mmol/L.

  - *Caused by the following:*
    - Depletion of magnesium
    - Sepsis
    - Alkalosis
    - Transfusions
    - Medication
      - Mithramycin (plicamycin), bisphosphonates, calcitonin, and oral or parental phosphate preparations and prolonged therapy with anticonvulsants such as diphenylhydantoin (phenytoin) or phenobarbital
    - Renal failure
    - Pancreatitis

  - *Causes:*
    - Hypotension

- Decreased cardiac output
- Ventricular ectopy (extra heartbeat originating in the lower chamber of the heart)
- Heart blocks
  - *Cardiovascular effects:*
    - Rarely seen in serum levels of 0.8 to 1.0 mmol/L
    - Typically seen in serum levels of <0.65 mmol/L
- **Ionized hypercalcemia:** Serum level of ionized calcium is >2.5 mmol/L
  - *Less common than hypocalcemia*
  - *Severe hypercalcemia:*
    - Total serum calcium: >14 mmol/L
    - Ionized serum calcium: >3.5 mmol/L
    - Caused by the following:
      ◉ Thyrotoxicosis (related to hyperthyroidism)
      ◉ Malignancy
      ◉ Medication
      - Excessive intake of vitamin D, alkaline antacids, diethylstilbestrol (DES), long-term use of diuretics, estrogens, and progesterone
  - Cardiovascular effects:
    ◉ Hypovolemia
    ◉ Hypotension
  - ECG (see Figure 3–1):
    ◉ **QTI:** Shortened

## Electrocardiograph

Electrical conduction of the heart is recorded by the ECG as a **waveform** (Figure 3–1). Normal electrical conduction produces a **normal waveform**. Abnormal electrical conduction produces changes in the normal waveform that infer an underlying cause of the abnormal cardiac electrical conduction.

The ECG tracing is an image of the electrophysiology of cardiac muscle in the form of a line that is automatically drawn on graph paper by the ECG. Initially, the line is aligned to a baseline on the graph paper. This is referred to as *zeroing* or *calibrating* the ECG and is performed before recording a patient's ECG.

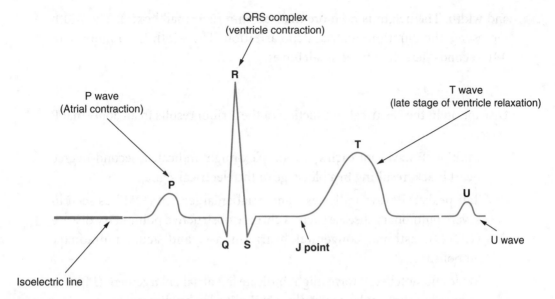

**FIGURE 3–2** · PQRST sequences form the normal cardiac waveform.

The baseline is called the *isoelectric line* (Figure 3–2), which is a straight horizontal line on the graph paper commonly called a *flat line*. The graph paper consists of small and large boxes. Each **small box** is 1 mm². There are five small boxes in one large box (see Figure 3–1).

The ECG moves the graph paper at a rate of 12 mm/s when recording electrical conduction of the heart. Each small box passes the stylus every 40 milliseconds, and one large box, every 200 milliseconds.

Electrodes placed on the patient's body detect changes in the electrical conduction of the heart, which are transmitted through wires to the ECG. Electrical changes cause the ECG stylus to move vertically on the graph paper drawing a line image that reflects the corresponding electrical changes in the heart over time. This is called the *PQRST sequence* (see Figure 3–2).

# P Wave

The **P wave** is the first deflection of the isoelectric line and begins with electrical activity at the sinoatrial (SA) node. This is atrial depolarization. There is one P wave for every QRS complex.

## Normal P Wave

The normal P wave starts when the stylus leaves the isoelectric line and ends when the stylus returns to the isoelectric line. The P wave is measured in height and width. The height is no more than 2.5 mm (2.5 small boxes). The width represents the duration of atrial depolarization. The width is no more than 0.10 second—less than three small boxes.

### Abnormal P Wave

Disruption in the electrical conduction of the atrium results in an abnormal P wave.

- Multiple P waves for each QRS complex might indicate a second-degree heart block, resulting in a blockage of the electrical signal.
- Tall-peaked P wave indicates right atrial enlargement (RAE) as seen in severe pulmonary disease such as chronic obstructive pulmonary disease (COPD), asthma, congenital heart disease, and acute pulmonary embolism.
- Wide and notched P wave might indicate left atrial enlargement (LEA) as seen in left ventricular myopathies and mitral valve disease.
- Inverted or absent P wave might indicate that the initial electrical impulse is originating other than from the SA node (ectopic in nature) and is seen in junctional rhythms.

## PR Interval

The **PRI** (Figure 3–3) is the period between the end of the P wave and the beginning of the QRS complex. This is the time the electrical impulse takes to travel to the ventricles after atrial repolarization. The PRI is measured from the time the P wave returns to the isoelectric line to the start of the Q wave in the QRS complex.

### Normal PRI

The normal PRI is between 0.12 and 0.20 second (three to five small boxes).

### Abnormal PRI

Shortened PRI (<0.12 second) indicates the following:

- A shorter path was taken to send the impulse to the ventricles.
- An accessory pathway was used to send the impulse other than through the AV node such as in Wolff-Parkinson-White disease.
- The impulse begins from a site other than the SA node (ectopic site), which is closer than the SA node is to the AV node.

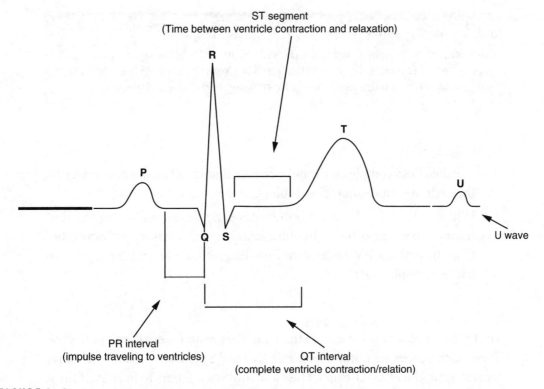

**FIGURE 3–3** · Intervals in a normal cardiac waveform.

Prolonged PRI (>0.20 second) indicates the following:

- Slower conduction of the impulse through the AV node is seen in the following:
  - Toxicity of medication that slows conduction (ie, digitalis toxicity)
  - Aging
  - Hypothyroidism
  - First-degree heart block rhythm

## QRS Complex

The **QRS complex** traces the electrical impulse leaving the AV node, through the bundle of His and then reaching the ventricles, causing them to depolarize. The QRS complex is measured from the beginning of the Q wave to the return of the S wave to the isoelectric line. This is commonly referred to as the *J point.*

> **NURSING ALERT**
>
> The end of the S wave might be difficult to identify because of elevated or depressed ST segment. The isoelectric line is thicker than the QRS line. The difference in thickness can be used to help identify the end of the S wave.

## Abnormal QRS Complex

- Notched QRS complex indicates a bundle branch block where conduction through the bundle branches is blocked.
- Widened QRS (>0.12 second) indicates early depolarization of the ventricles caused either by the impulse following an accessory pathway other than through the AV node or the initiating impulse beginning in the ventricles (ectopic beat).

## QRS Complex Notation

The QRS complex may have more than one R wave and more than one S wave. These occurrences are noted as R prime (R′) and S prime (S′). Label each wave separately on the ECG. Use uppercase and lowercase letters to indicate if the R prime and S prime waves are above or below the isoelectric line. A height (amplitude) below the isoelectric line (<5 mm) is represented in lowercase (r′ or s′). A height above the isoelectric line >5 mm is represented using uppercase (R′ or S′).

> **NURSING ALERT**
>
> The QRS complex is larger than the P wave because a voltage higher than that for the arteries is required to depolarize the ventricles.

## ST Segment

The **ST segment** is the time between the end of ventricular depolarization and ventricular repolarization. The ST segment begins when the S wave returns to the isoelectric line (end of ventricular depolarization) and ends with the beginning of the T wave (ventricular repolarization). The ST segment is measured from the end of the QRS complex and the beginning of the T wave, which should be one small box (0.04 second) past the end of the QRS complex.

## Abnormal ST Segment

- *Elevated ST segment:*
  - Elevation >1 mm (one large square) in two or more leads has clinical significance.
    - Convex elevation indicates a MI.
    - Concave elevation (>2 mm) indicates a non-acute myocardial infarction (AMI) relating to benign early ventricular repolarization or might indicate pericarditis.
    - Horizontal elevation indicates a MI.
    - Distribution of ST elevations is related to ECG leads that detect the non-AMI.
    - Elevated ST segments in all leads indicate a cause other than MI such as pericarditis.
    - Hyperkalemia and vasospasms (ie, Prinzmetal angina) also cause ST elevations.
- *Depressed ST segment:*
  - Can have a scooped out appearance, a horizontal depression, or a downsloping depression.
  - Can be the result of reciprocal changes where corresponding leads have mirrored changes (one lead shows a depressed ST segment and another lead shows an elevated ST segment).
  - Indicates a possible
    - Non-Q wave MI
    - Subendocardial MI
    - Ischemia (transient) resolved with rest, nitrates, and morphine encourages reperfusion
    - Hypokalemia (depression is less than 1 mm and has a normal T wave that is called nonspecific ST abnormality)
    - Hypothermia (also lengthens the PRI and the QTI)

# T Wave

The **T wave** begins at the end of the ST interval and gradually flows upward from the isoelectric line followed by a quick drop to the isoelectric line. The T wave represents the late phase of ventricular repolarization.

A normal T wave has a height (amplitude) of less than 5 mm.

### Abnormal T Wave

- Generalized tall-peaked T wave indicates hyperkalemia.
- Localized tall-peaked T wave indicates MI.
- Inverted T wave indicates the following:
  - Evolving infarction
  - Chronic pericarditis
  - Conduction block
  - Ventricular hypertrophy
  - Acute cerebral disease
  - Flattened T wave is nonspecific.

## QT Interval

The **QTI** is from the beginning of the QRS complex to the end of the T wave and represents the complete cycle of ventricular depolarization/repolarization. The QTI has an inverse relationship with the heart rate. As the heart rate increases, the QTI decreases. As the heart rate decreases, the QTI increases.

The QTI must be corrected according to the patient's heart rate. The corrected QTI is noted as **QTc**. Most 12-lead ECG machines automatically correct the QTI. The practitioner can also manually make this correction by doing the following:

- Count the number of small boxes that make up the QTI.
- Multiple this number by 0.04 second.
- Count the number of small boxes that make up the R-R interval (the distance between the R waves).
- Multiple this number by 0.04 second.
- Calculate the square root of the R-R interval in seconds.
- Divide the QTI in seconds by the square root of the R-R interval in seconds.
- The result is the QTc interval value.
- The QTc interval value should be ½ of the R-R interval.

### Abnormal QTI

Prolonged QTI indicates there is a delay in ventricular repolarization. The heart is spending more than the normal time depolarized (relative refractory period), making the heart vulnerable to torsades de pointes (R on T phenomenon) resulting in ventricular tachycardia. This can be caused by the following:

- Medication such as amiodarone, sotalol, Haldol, or quinidines
- Long QT syndrome
- Hypothyroidism
- Hypocalcemia
- Hypomagnesemia
  - Hypothermia
  - Bradyrhythmia

## U Wave

The **U wave** (Figure 3–4) is a small wave that may not be present at times especially in patients with slow heart rates. Absence of the U wave is not clinically significant. The U wave, when present, should measure less than 2 mm.

### Abnormal U Wave

If a U wave measures more than or equal to 2 mm, it is called an *abnormal U wave*. This may be caused by the following:

- Hypokalemia
- Hypercalcemia
- Thyrotoxicosis
- Intracranial hemorrhage

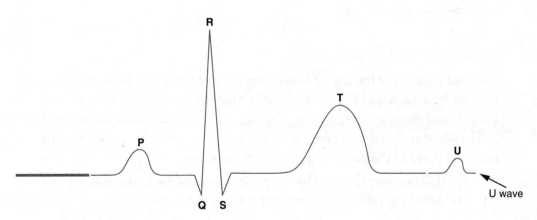

**FIGURE 3–4** · The U wave may or may not be present.

# Cardiac Monitoring Equipment and Lead Placement

A *cardiac monitor* is a device that traces the electrophysiology of the heart deflecting the isoelectric line in response to cardiac electrical impulses.

Wires called *leads* connect the cardiac monitor to transducers called *electrodes* that are strategically placed on the patient's body. A **transducer** (electrode) is an electrical/mechanical device that detects electrical activity of the heart and translates the activity into electrical waves used by the cardiac monitor to form the tracing.

Three commonly used cardiac monitors are as follows:

1. **12-Lead ECG:** A *12-lead ECG* is a device that produces 12 different tracings on graph paper enabling the practitioner to have a 12-view snapshot of the heart, which is used to accurately diagnose degrees and locations of acute coronary syndrome (ACS), such as ischemia versus infarct.

2. **Three-lead or five-lead cardiac monitor:** These monitors (**three-lead or five-lead cardiac monitor**) display the tracing on a screen usually at the bedside, nursing stations, and operating room and are used to study the heart over a relatively short time period.

3. **Cardiac telemetry:** This is used in the clinical setting enabling the patient to ambulate while being monitored. In cardiac telemetry, leads attached to the patient are connected to a radio transmitter, which is a small box carried by the patient. The radio transmitter sends electrical waves that represent cardiac activity to a radio transmitter connected to a video cardiac monitor located at the nurses' station and/or at a central cardiac telemetry unit.

## Waveforms and Current Flow

The lead creates the tracing by measuring the electrical activity of the heart over the lead. Each lead has two electrodes. One electrode is called the *positive* (+) pole and the other the *negative* (−) pole.

The shape of the waveform depicted in the tracing depends on placement of the lead related to the path of cardiac electrical activity.

- Electrical activity detected by the positive pole of the lead causes a positive deflection (above the isoelectric line) in the tracing.

- Electrical activity detected by the negative pole results in a negative deflection (below the isoelectric line) in the tracing.

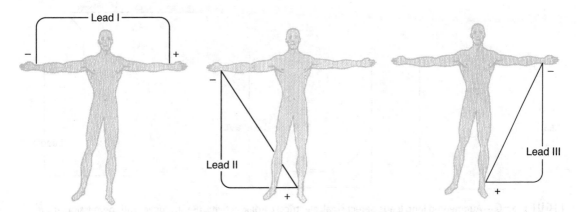

**FIGURE 3–5** · Leads are positioned on the body to form the Einthoven triangle. (Reproduced, with permission, from Keogh J, Reed D. *Schaum's Outline of ECG Interpretation*. New York: McGraw-Hill Education, 2011:48. Figure 4.1.)

The **Einthoven triangle** is used to position leads on the patient's body. This is named for Dr. Willem Einthoven, a Dutch physician and physiologist who invented the first practical ECG in 1903.

The *Einthoven triangle* (Figure 3–5) is an inverted equilateral triangle centered on the patient's chest. Corners of the triangle point to locations of where to place leads on the patient's body. There are three leads, each identified by a number and referred to commonly as the *limb leads*.

- **Lead I:** This is the top of the Einthoven triangle. The negative pole of the lead is positioned at the patient's right shoulder, and the positive pole of the lead is positioned at the patient's left shoulder. This generates a positive deflection in the tracing as current flows from right to left (negative to positive).
- **Lead II:** This is the right side of the Einthoven triangle. The negative pole of the lead is positioned at the patient's right arm (RA), and the positive pole of the lead is positioned at the patient's right leg. This generates a positive deflection in the tracing as current flows from the RA to the right leg.
- **Lead III:** This is the left side of the Einthoven triangle. The negative pole of the lead is positioned at the patient's left arm (LA), and the positive pole of the lead is positioned at the patient's left leg. This generates a positive deflection in the tracing as current flows from the LA to the left leg.

## Augmented Limb Leads

Augmented limb leads (Figure 3–6) are used to enhance tracings of small electrical waveforms of cardiac electrical activity. Augmented limb leads have one electrode, which is a positive electrode called *unipolar*. The cardiac monitor

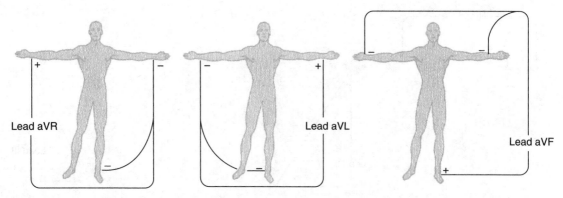

**FIGURE 3−6** · Augmented limb leads detect small electrical cardiac activity. (Reproduced, with permission, from Keogh J, Reed D. *Schaum's Outline of ECG Interpretation*. New York: McGraw-Hill Education, 2011:49. Figure 4.2.)

uses the wave detected by these leads to manipulate information from poles of the other leads, resulting in a clearer image of small waveforms.

Augmented limbs leads are as follows:

- **aVR:** Augmented voltage RA and positioned on the right arm.
- **aVL:** Augmented voltage LA and positioned on the left arm.
- **aVF:** Augmented voltage left leg (LL) and positioned on the left leg.

### Six Precordial Leads

**Six precordial leads** (Figure 3–7) are placed on the patient's chest. These are also single electrode leads, which are positive (unipolar), because of the proximity to the heart.

These leads are identified by their position on the chest. These are as follows:

- **$V_1$ and $V_2$:** Anteroseptal
- **$V_3$ and $V_4$:** Anterior
- **$V_5$ and $V_6$:** Anterolateral

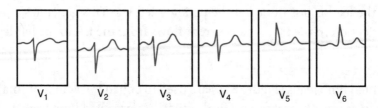

**FIGURE 3−7** · Precordial leads are positioned on the patient's chest. (Reproduced, with permission, from Keogh J, Reed D. *Schaum's Outline of ECG Interpretation*. New York: McGraw-Hill Education, 2011:49. Figure 4.3.)

## Electrodes

Electrodes must be properly placed on the patient to properly detect cardiac electrical activity. Improper placement of electrodes might cause artifacts. An *artifact* is an abnormal variation in the waveform not caused by cardiac electrical activity.

The initial step in attaching electrodes to the patient is to prepare the skin at the electrode site. This is done as follows.

- Shave the site of hair.
- Clean the site with alcohol or an acetone pad to remove oil from the skin.
- Rub (abrade) the area with a 2 × 2 gauze to ensure the skin is clean.
- Clean the site with tincture of benzoin if the patient is sweating, which is common if the patient was administered pain medication.
- Attach the lead to the electrode. It is usually uncomfortable for the patient if the lead is attached to the electrode once the electrode is positioned on the patient's skin.
- Peel back the electrode cover from the gel adhesive pad of the electrode.
- Apply the electrode to the electrode site on the patient's skin. Avoid placing electrodes over bony areas because cardiac electrical activity is better detected through tissue and fluid than bone.
- Select the lead that produces the most defined P wave, usually lead II.

## Bedside Monitors

**Bedside monitors** are used in critical care units, emergency departments, and surgical suites to monitor the patient's cardiac function. These are commonly referred to as *hardware monitors* because the leads directly connect electrodes to the cardiac monitor.

Bedside monitors provide an instant view of the patient's cardiac activity enabling health care providers to immediately intervene if the patient's cardiac function changes.

However, the patient is tethered to the bedside monitor limiting the patient's activity. Furthermore the health care team must work around the leads while caring for the patient. The patient must be placed on a portable cardiac monitor while being transported to another unit.

### Five-Lead Bedside Monitors

A five-lead bedside monitor uses five leads, each with a color-coded electrode. It is designed so that the health care team can continuously monitor any two of the five leads at the same time.

---

**NURSING ALERT**

$V_1$ should be monitored for patients with no history of dysrhythmia. Leads III and $V_3$ are monitored for ST segment monitoring when there is no ischemic indication.

---

The five leads measure voltage between the right limb lead to the feet. These are as follows:

1. LA positioned at the second intercostal space (between ribs) at the midclavicular line.

2. RA positioned at the second intercostal space at the midclavicular line.

3. LL positioned at the eighth intercostal space at the midclavicular line.

4. Right leg positioned at the eighth intercostal space at the midclavicular line.

5. Chest lead, which is one of six possible leads. These are as follows:

   i. $V_1$ positioned at the fourth intercostal space at the right sternal border.

   ii. $V_2$ positioned at the fourth intercostal space at the left sternal border.

   iii. $V_3$ positioned between the fourth and fifth intercostal space.

   iv. $V_4$ positioned at the fifth intercostal space at the left midclavicular line.

   v. $V_5$ positioned at the fifth intercostal space at the left anterior axillary line.

   vi. $V_6$ positioned at the fifth intercostal space at the midaxillary line.

## Three-Lead Bedside Monitors

A three-lead bedside monitor uses three leads, each with an electrode. One lead is negative, the other is positive, and the third is a ground. The ground lead minimizes interference from artifacts when tracing cardiac activity. The three-lead bedside monitor is typically used with portable bedside monitors to monitor leads I, II, and III.

The three leads are

1. RA positioned below the clavicle at the second intercostal space at the right midclavicular line.

2. LA positioned below the clavicle at the second intercostal space at the left midclavicular line.

3. LL positioned on the left lower rib at the eighth intercostal space at the left midclavicular line.

The lead that is monitored depends on the patient's condition.

- Premature atrial complexes, AV blocks, and sinus abnormalities can be recognized in most leads that display clear P waves. Usually lead I or II is best.
- $V_1$ and $V_6$ are best for differentiating wide QRS rhythms and monitoring for most arrhythmias. $V_1$ will help distinguish between ventricular tachycardia and supraventricular tachycardia with aberrancy.
- $V_1$ is the best lead to monitor when there is no history of arrhythmia.
- Multiple lead monitoring is better than single lead.
- ST segment monitoring:

  - Monitor leads III and $V_3$ for patients at high risk of AMI or ischemia.
  - The patient will have ST segment changes during a cardiac event. These changes are known as the *ischemic fingerprint*. If the ischemic finger print is known, then use the following leads to monitor the patient:
    - I, aVL, $V_5$, and $V_6$ reflect circumflex and the lateral wall.
    - II, III, and aVF reflect right coronary and the inferior wall.
    - $V_1$-$V_4$ reflect left anterior descending and the anterior wall.

## Telemetry Monitors

**Telemetry monitors** offer patients and health care providers more freedom than bedside monitors because the leads are connected to a wireless transmitter rather than directly to the monitor. The patient is able to move freely and the health care team has little interference from the leads while caring for the patient. However, telemetry monitors are more prone to interference, artifacts, and/or the electrodes inadvertently being removed from the patient.

- **Five-lead telemetry monitor:** This monitor uses the same electrode placement as the five-lead bedside monitor. Any of the 12 leads can be monitored as long as the $V_1$-$V_6$ leads are properly positioned on the patient's chest.
- **Three-lead telemetry monitor:** This monitor uses the same electrode placement as the three-lead bedside monitor. However, one lead at a time can be monitored.

## Troubleshooting Cardiac Monitors

Use critical thinking skills when interpreting the ECG tracing because an abnormal wave may be caused by the heart or caused by trouble with the monitor and leads, resulting in artifacts.

An **artifact** is an abnormal variation in the waveform not caused by cardiac electrical activity that might resemble an abnormal cardiac function. When noticing an abnormal cardiac tracing, verify that the cardiac monitor and leads are properly functioning.

Common causes of artifacts are

- Patient movement.
- Interference from medical equipment connected to the patient.
- Poor contact between the electrode and the patient's skin.
- A weak signal caused by a poorly functioning electrode, lead, or connector to the cardiac monitor.

### False High-Rate Alarms

Cardiac monitors usually have an alarm that sounds when the patient's heart rate increases beyond an acceptable range. This is called a **high-rate alarm**. An artifact can send a higher than normal electrical signal (high-voltage artifact) to the cardiac monitor triggering the high-rate alarm. This is called a **false high-rate alarm**.

False high-rate alarms can be caused by the following:

- Muscle movement.
- Head movement.
- Tremors in postop patient caused by shivering as a side effect of anesthesia.
- Seizure activity.
- The use of surgical clippers during an operation.

### False Low-Rate Alarms

Cardiac monitors usually have an alarm that sounds when the patient's heart rate decreases beyond an acceptable range. This is called a **low-rate alarm**. An artifact can send a lower than normal electrical signal (low-voltage artifact) to the cardiac monitor triggering the low-rate alarm. This is called a **false low-rate alarm**.

False low-rate alarms can be triggered by the following:

- Weak battery in the cardiac monitor.
- Low signal from the electrode, lead, or connect malfunction.
- Poor skin contact caused by dried gel on the electrode or sweat at the electrode site.

## Respiratory Variations

Respiratory variations can affect the cardiac electrical activity that is picked up by electrodes, resulting in a wandering isoelectric line (baseline) on the tracing.

Increased movement of the patient's abdomen with each breath taken by the patient may cause electrodes near the abdomen to move, resulting in artifacts.

Patients in respiratory distress also have exaggerated respiration that might affect the electrodes and cause the cardiac monitor to report unusual cardiac activities.

## Inspect the Cardiac Monitor

Cardiac monitors and leads can malfunction due to excessive use. Inspect the equipment and repair or replace parts that may become the source of artifacts.

Inspect for:

- Frayed wires (leads and the power cord)
- Low charge in the cardiac monitor's barriers
- Dried or cracked electrodes

If you suspect tracings while monitoring a patient, then

- Reposition electrodes until an acceptable waveform appears in the tracing.
- Monitor alternate leads. One lead might be causing the artifact. Other leads will represent actual cardiac activity.

# Reading an Electrocardiograph

The patient's cardiac function is analyzed by measuring both the height (deflection) off of the isoelectric line and the width of the wave (duration of the deflection).

The ECG graph paper is divided into a grid of small and large boxes, each a specific size, thereby making it relatively easy to measure the tracing.

- **Small box:** The **small box** is 1 mm$^2$ inside and takes 0.04 second to pass under the stylus.
- **Large box:** The **large box** comprises five small boxes. Each large box is 5 mm$^2$ and takes 0.20 second to pass under the stylus.

## Analyzing Cardiac Rhythm

Electrical activity of the patient's heart is studied by measuring the waveform tracing on the ECG graph. A minimum of 30 large boxes is required to analyze the cardiac rhythm. This is equivalent to 6 seconds of recording. Three-second marks at the top of the ECG graph paper make it easy to measure recording time.

> ### NURSING ALERT
>
> Every beat in the 6-second strip needs to be analyzed. The heart may experience intermittent changes, resulting in more than one cardiac rhythm appearing on the same strip. If this occurs, analyze each cardiac rhythm separately.

There are five characteristics of the tracing used to analyze the patient's cardiac rhythm. These are

1. **Regularity:** This is the recurrence of the same waveform. The waveform should be the same throughout the 6-second recording.

2. **Heart rate:** The **heart rate** should be between 60 and 100 beats/min.

3. **P wave:** The **P wave's** height and duration should be within normal range.

4. **PRI:** This should be within normal range (0.12-0.20 second).

5. **QRS complex:** The **QRS complex's** height and duration should be within normal range (0.04-0.10 second).

### Regularity

Cardiac electrical activity is regular if the heart functions normally. Electrical activity is the same for each heartbeat, and therefore each waveform should be the same on the ECG. This is referred to as *regularity of the tracing.*

**Regularity of the rhythm** is measured by using either an ECG caliper or an index card. An **ECG caliper** is a ruler with preset calibrations used to measure waveforms on the ECG graph. An **index card** can also be used if an ECG caliper is not available by marking the R wave on one complex and the R wave on the next complex and then using these markings to compare the R to R across the ECG strip.

Here's how to measure regularity.

1. Begin on the left side of the ECG graph paper.

2. Place the caliper on the first two R waves. Alternatively place the index card on the first two R waves and then mark both positions on the index card.

3. Move the caliper/index card to the next set of R waves. Each set of R waves should line up with the calibrations on the caliper or the markings on the index card.

4. The rhythm is regular if any irregularity that occurs is less than three small boxes.

5. Note any irregularity of more than three small boxes, since this might be clinically significant.

## Rate

The rate of the rhythm is the patient's heart rate. Before analyzing the rate, determine the regularity of the rhythm. Then decide the appropriate method to assess the rate of the tracing.

There are two methods used to measure the rate of the rhythm. The first method is used only if the rhythm is regular. The second method is used to make a quick assessment of the heart rate regardless of the regularity of the rhythm.

- *Measuring regular rhythm rate:*
  - Count the small boxes between the R waves.
  - Divide 1500 by the sum of the small boxes between the R waves to determine the rate; 1500 is the number of small boxes that passes the stylus in 1 minute.
- *Measuring irregular or regular rhythm rate:*
  - Count the number of R waves in the 6-second strip.
  - Multiply the number of R waves by 10 to arrive at the rate.
  - If the rhythm is split equally into 3-second strips, then multiply the rate by 20.

### NURSING ALERT

Measuring the distance between R waves determines the heart rate.
6 large boxes = 50 beats/min
5 large boxes = 60 beats/min
4 large boxes = 75 beats/min
3 large boxes = 100 beats/min
2 large boxes = 150 beats/min
1 large box = 300 beats/min

## P Wave

The P wave is the first waveform traced and represents the impulse at the SA node, resulting in atrial depolarization (contraction). The initial assessment of the P wave is to determine if the P wave is within normal boundaries. If it is not, then further analysis is performed.

There are four characteristics that are examined when measuring the P wave in a tracing. Further analysis is required if any of these characteristics does not appear in the tracing.

1. Are there P waves in the tracing?
   - The P wave begins when the stylus leaves the isoelectric line and ends when the stylist returns to the isoelectric line.
2. Is there one P wave for every QRS complex?
3. Is the P wave upright and rounded?
4. Is each P wave in the tracing identical to each other?

## PR Interval

The PRI is the period between the end of the P wave and the beginning of the QRS complex and represents the time the electrical impulse takes to travel to the ventricles after atrial repolarization.

Here's how to measure the PRI.

1. Count the number of small boxes from the beginning of the P wave to the beginning of the QRS complex.
2. Multiply the sum by 0.04 to derive the size of the PRI.

The normal PRI is between 0.12 and 0.20 second.

## QRS Complex

The QRS complex has three waveforms that trace the electrical impulse after leaving the AV node and travel through the bundle of His, resulting in ventricular depolarization.

Here's how to measure the QRS complex.

1. Count the number of small boxes between the beginning of the Q wave to the end of the S wave. The QRS line is thinner than the isoelectric line, which makes it easy to distinguish where one begins and the other ends.
2. Multiply the sum by 0.04 second to arrive at the measurement of the QRS complex.

The normal QRS wave is between 0.04 and 0.10 second.

# The Conduction System

The conduction system (Figure 3–8) of the heart transmits electrical impulses throughout the heart causing depolarization and repolarization of cardiac muscle, resulting in the pumping action that moves blood throughout the body. Table 3–1 contains the pathophysiological changes that might occur during depolarization/repolarization and how they appear on an ECG strip.

- **SA node:** The **SA node**, located in the upper right atrium, is the heart's intrinsic pacemaker that generates impulses that cause depolarization at a rate between 60 and 100 impulses (beats) per minute.

- **Bachmann bundles:** Impulse from the SA node is carried through interatrial pathways called the *Bachmann bundles* to the left atrium, resulting in the depolarization (contraction) of the left and right atria.
  - *ECG:* P wave is generated.

- **Internodal pathways:** These pathways carry the impulse through the right atrium to the AV node.

- **AV node:** This node is located in the right lower atrium at the interatrial septum and is the only communication pathway between the atria and the ventricles.

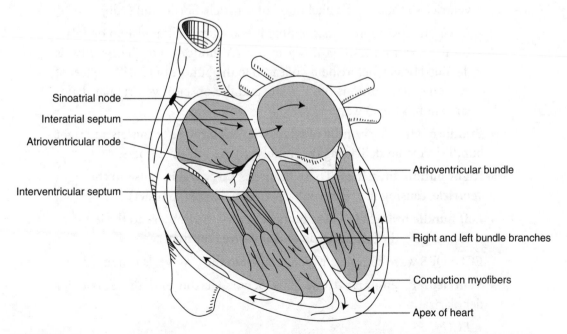

**FIGURE 3–8** • The cardiac conduction system transmits electrical impulses throughout the heart. (Reproduced, with permission, from Keogh J, Reed D. *Schaum's Outline of ECG Interpretation.* New York: McGraw-Hill Education, 2011:22. Figure 2.4.)

| TABLE 3–1 Pathophysiological Changes Seen in ECG | |
|---|---|
| Hypocalcemia | Prolonged QTI |
| Hypercalcemia | Shortened QTI |
| Hyperkalemia | Peaked T wave, PRI prolonged |
| Ischemia | T-wave inversion |
| Transmural infarct | ST elevation |
| Subendocardial injury | ST depression |
| Acute pericarditis | Diffuse ST elevation |

- *Intrinsic rate:* The AV node's intrinsic rate is 40 to 60 impulses per minute and is a backup source to generate the cardiac impulse should the SA node fail.

- *Atrial kick:* The AV node slows the impulse to the ventricles, allowing time for the atria to completely empty, which is referred to as the atrial kick.

- *Atrial fibrillation (afib):* This is the rapid depolarization and repolarization of the atrium. The AV node slows or blocks this impulse to the ventricles reducing the likelihood of ventricle fibrillation (vfib).

- *ECG:* The PRI represents the time it takes for the impulse to depolarize the atrium and then travel to the AV node where the impulse is detained briefly before being released to the bundle of His. The onset of atrial depolarization is the P wave, and the onset of ventricular depolarization is the Q wave.

- **Bundle of His:** The **bundle of His** carries the impulse to the left and right bundle branches delivering the impulse to the Purkinje fibers.

- **Right bundle branches:** These branches carry the impulse to the right ventricle, causing the right ventricle to depolarize (contract).

- **Left bundle branches:** These branches carry the impulse to the left ventricle, causing the left ventricle to depolarize (contract).

- **ECG:** QRS wave complex, which is equal to the R wave, is produced.

- **Ventricular repolarization:** This occurs at the end of ventricular depolarization.
  - *ECG:*
    - Beginning ventricular repolarization: ST segment is produced.

- Later ventricular repolarization: T wave is produced.
- Note: The U wave is produced following the T wave in 50% of patients.
- **Ventricle depolarization/repolarization:**
  - *ECG:* QTI measures the duration between depolarization and repolarization of the ventricles.

## CASE STUDY

### CASE 1

The practitioner has ordered an ECG for your patient. The ECG technician presents you with the strip shown in the figure below. Answer the following questions based on the ECG strip.

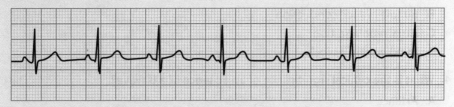

QUESTION 1. What is the regularity of the ECG tracing?
ANSWER: The rhythm is regular because the R waves of each wave line up, and there is no irregularity appearing in fewer than three small boxes.

QUESTION 2. What is the patient's heart rate?
ANSWER: The distance between R waves is approximately four large boxes, indicating that the heart rate is approximately 75 beats within, which is a normal heart rate.

QUESTION 3. What is your assessment of the P wave?
ANSWER: There is a P wave for every QRS complex. The P wave is upright and rounded, and each P wave is identical to the other P waves.

QUESTION 4. Is this a normal QRS wave?
ANSWER: There is one small box between the beginning of the Q wave and the end of the S wave. The time to complete the QRS wave is 0.04 second, which is normal. Therefore, this is a normal QRS wave.

## FINAL CHECKUP

1. **What is one of the first steps to perform before administering an ECG?**
   A. Measuring the height of the isoelectric line with either calipers or an index card.
   B. Zeroing the ECG to the normal wave form.
   C. Zeroing the ECG.
   D. Measuring the wave tracing using the ECG graph.

2. **What does the P wave measure?**
   A. Atrial depolarization.
   B. Atrial repolarization.
   C. Ventricle depolarization.
   D. Ventricle repolarization.

3. **What does a notched QRS complex indicate?**
   A. First-degree heart block.
   B. Bundle branch conduction.
   C. Atrial repolarization.
   D. Bundle branch block.

4. **What is the clinical significance of an absence of a U wave?**
   A. Artifact.
   B. None.
   C. Loose electrode lead.
   D. Fast heart rate.

5. **Which cardiac monitor is used to monitor the heart over a short time period?**
   A. A 12-lead ECG.
   B. Cardiac telemetry.
   C. An eight-lead cardiac monitor.
   D. A three-lead cardiac monitor.

6. **What do you do if you see an abnormal variation of a cardiac waveform?**
   A. Call the practitioner.
   B. Assess the electrode connections to the patient.
   C. Call the rapid response team.
   D. Ask the patient to sip water.

7. **What would you expect to be the cause of a wandering isoelectric line on the ECG tracing?**
   A. First-degree heart block.
   B. Dried gel on the electrode.

C. Respiration.

D. Second-degree heart block.

8. **What would you do if you noticed more than one cardiac rhythm appearing on the same strip?**

A. Repeat the ECG.

B. Reposition all leads.

C. Analyze each cardiac rhythm.

D. Analyze the first cardiac rhythm.

9. **What does the ST segment measure?**

A. Isoelectric line artifact.

B. Atrial repolarization.

C. The time between the end of ventricular repolarization and ventricular depolarization.

D. The time between the end of ventricular depolarization and ventricular repolarization.

10. **What does the PRI measure?**

A. The time the electrical impulse takes to travel to the ventricles after atrial repolarization.

B. The time the electrical impulse takes to travel to the atria after ventricle repolarization.

C. The time the electrical impulse takes to travel to the left atria from the right atria.

D. The time the electrical impulse takes to travel to the right atria from the left atria.

# CORRECT ANSWERS AND RATIONALES

1. C. Zeroing the ECG.
2. A. Atrial depolarization.
3. D. Bundle branch block.
4. B. None.
5. D. A three-lead cardiac monitor.
6. B. Assess the electrode connections to the patient.
7. C. Respiration.
8. C. Analyze each cardiac rhythm.
9. D. The time between the end of ventricular depolarization and ventricular repolarization.
10. A. The time the electrical impulse takes to travel to the ventricles after atrial repolarization.

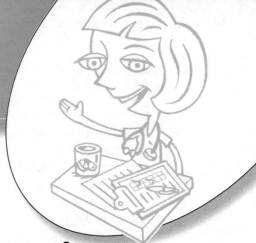

# chapter 4

# Cardiac Arrhythmias

## LEARNING OBJECTIVES

1. Arrhythmia
2. Atrial Fibrillation (AF, afib)
3. Atrial Flutter (aflutter)
4. Premature Atrial Contraction (PAC)
5. Wandering Atrial Pacemaker (WAP)
6. Paroxysmal Atrial Tachycardia (PAT, PSVT)
7. Junctional Rhythm
8. Junctional Escape Rhythm
9. Premature Junctional Contraction (PJC)
10. Accelerated Junctional Rhythm
11. Paroxysmal Junctional Tachycardia (PJT)
12. Bundle Branch Blocks
13. Premature Ventricular Contractions (PVC)
14. Ventricular Tachycardia (V-tach)
15. Ventricular Fibrillation
16. Asystole
17. Idioventricular Rhythm
18. Pacemakers

## KEY TERMS

| | |
|---|---|
| Acidosis | Multifocal Atrial Tachycardia (MAT) |
| Atrial Arrhythmias and the Electrocardiogram | Nonconducted Premature Atrial Contraction |
| Atrial Ectopic Pacemaker | Pacemaker |
| Carotid Sinus Massage | Pacemaker Mode |
| Catheter Ablation | Paroxysmal Atrial Tachycardia |
| Compensatory Pause | Permanent Pacing |
| Digitalis Glycoside | Portable Event Monitor |
| Digoxin Toxicity | Sick Sinus Syndrome |
| Electrical Cardioversion | Suppressed Automaticity |
| Epicardial Pacing | Transcutaneous Pacing |
| Holter Monitor | Transtelephonic Monitor |
| Intra-atrial Reentry | Transvenous Pacing |
| Ischemia of the Atrioventricular Node | Triggered Activity |
| Junctional Ectopic Pacemaker | Valsalva Maneuver |
| Lown Grading System | Ventricular Ectopic Pacemaker |
| Maze Procedure | Wolff-Parkinson-White Syndrome |

# Arrhythmia

All cells in the heart are capable of stimulating the heart to contract. In a regular cardiac rhythm, the **sinoatrial** (SA) node of the heart stimulates cardiac contractions. An *arrhythmia* is an irregular cardiac rhythm caused when a cardiac cell other than the SA node stimulates cardiac contractions. The SA node is called the *ectopic pacemaker*. There are three common ectopic pacemakers. These are

1. **Atrial ectopic:** Atrial ectopic pacemaker located in the atria.

2. **Junctional ectopic:** Junctional ectopic pacemaker located in the atrioventricular (AV) junction.

3. **Ventricular ectopic:** Ventricular ectopic pacemaker located in the ventricles.

## Function of the Ectopic Pacemaker

There are three ways an ectopic pacemaker works. These are

1. **Enhanced/suppressed automaticity:** The ectopic pacemaker cell creates a faster impulse than the SA node. This is referred to as *enhanced automaticity*.

The SA node gives control to the ectopic pacemaker cells, which is referred to as *suppressed automaticity. Automaticity* is the SA node's ability to spontaneously generate an impulse.

2. **Reentry:** In a normal cardiac cycle, the SA node sends an impulse to the ventricle. The SA node is located in the atria. In reentry, the impulse sent by the SA node returns back, resulting in abnormal cardiac rhythms such as atrial flutters, paroxysmal atrial tachycardia, and ventricular tachycardia. *Atrial flutter* is an abnormal rhythm in the atrium. *Paroxysmal atrial tachycardia* is a regular fast heart rhythm that begins and ends suddenly starting in the atria. *Ventricular tachycardia* is a regular fast heart rhythm that begins in the ventricle.

3. **Triggered activity (following depolarization):** The ectopic pacemaker cell sends an impulse after depolarization and before repolarization, resulting in two beats (couplets) or three beats (triplets) per cardiac cycle. This condition can occur as a result of the following:

   • Prolonged QT intervals

   • Bradycardias

   • Hypomagnesemia

   • Hypoxia

   • Digoxin toxicity

## Atrial Fibrillation

**Atrial fibrillation** (AF, afib) is when the atria quiver rather than contracting. Quivering makes it nearly impossible for the atria to pump blood into the ventricle. Normally the SA node controls the electrical impulse of the heart. In AF multiple cells in the atria send uncoordinated electrical impulses, up to 600/min, each trying to move through the AV node. The AV node controls impulses to the ventricles; however, some non-SA node electrical impulses are able to bypass the AV node and enter the ventricles, resulting in irregular contractions by the ventricles and leading to an irregular, rapid heart rate.

Some patients can live a normal life with AF; however, those patients are at risk for blood clots caused by the improper flow of blood related to disruption to atrial contractions. This can lead to stroke or kidney failure. Inconsistent atrial contractions cause the heart to weaken over time. As a result, the patient is at risk for heart failure.

## What Went Wrong?

AF is related to several underlying conditions. These are as follows:

- Hypertension
- Coronary artery disease
- Heart valve disorder
- Heart failure
- Congenital heart disease
- Cardiomyopathy
- Pulmonary embolism
- Chronic lung disease

### NURSING ALERT

Less common causes are excessive alcohol and caffeine use, stress, electrolyte imbalance, metabolic imbalances, infection, pericarditis, and hyperthyroidism. There are also cases where there is no underlying cause.

## Prognosis

AF can be controlled through treatment, although there is a tendency for AF to return even when the patient is compliant with treatment. The patient is at risk for blood clots and stroke.

## Hallmark Signs and Symptoms

Some patients may be asymptomatic. Patients who are symptomatic report

- Shortness of breath
- Dizziness
- Fainting
- Palpitations of the heart
- Chest discomfort
- Feeling tired

### NURSING ALERT

Many symptoms are related to the disruption of oxygenated blood throughout the body due to the irregular contractions of the atria.

## Common/Interpreting Test Results

AF (Figure 4–1) is diagnosed by performing one or more of the following tests:

- **Electrocardiogram (ECG):** An ECG records the electrical activities of the heart (see Chapter 3).
- **Holter monitor:** A Holter monitor records the electrical activities of the heart continuously over 3 days using electrodes that are attached to the patient during that period. The practitioner analyzes the result after the monitoring period ends.
- **Portable event monitor:** This monitor is similar to a Holter monitor but worn for a month. The patient presses a button on the portable event monitor each time he/she becomes symptomatic. The portable event monitor then records electrical activity of the heart and transmits the recording over a telephone to the practitioner who then evaluates the event.

> **NURSING ALERT**
>
> Portable event monitors are used when a patient reports irregular episodes.

- **Transtelephonic monitor:** A transtelephonic monitor is used by the patient when he/she experiences symptoms of AF. When the patient becomes symptomatic, he/she places monitoring leads or the monitor itself on to the chest. Electrical activity of the heart is then transmitted by telephone to the practitioner who then evaluates the event.

## Treatment

There are different types of treatments for AF depending on the severity of the symptoms.

- Medication:
  - **Antiarrhythmic medication:** These medications cause the heart to maintain normal sinus rhythm. These include flecainide acetate (Tambocor); propafenone (Rythmol); sotalol (Betapace); dofetilide (Tikosyn); and amiodarone (Cordarone).
  - **Digitalis glycoside:** This is a class of medication that slows the contractions of the ventricles. The most commonly used digitalis glycoside is digoxin (Lanoxin).

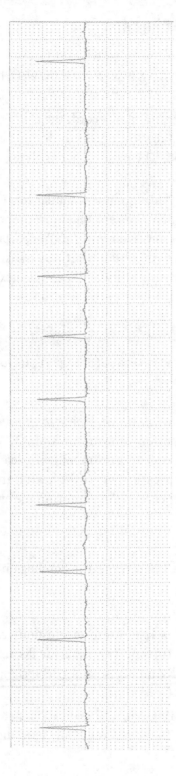

**FIGURE 4–1 •** Atrial fibrillation. (Reproduced, with permission, from Keogh J, Reed D. *Schaum's Outline of ECG Interpretation*. New York: McGraw-Hill Education, 2011:92. Figure 7.1.)

- **Beta-blockers:** This is also a class of medications that slows the contractions of the ventricles. The most commonly prescribed is metoprolol (Toprol, Lopressor).

- **Calcium channel blockers:** These medications also slow the contractions of the ventricles. The most commonly prescribed are verapamil (Calan) and diltiazem (Cardizem).

- **Anticoagulant medication:** This medication reduces the risk of formation of blood clots. Commonly prescribed anticoagulant medications are heparin, enoxaparin (Lovenox), dalteparin (Fragmin), argatroban, bivalirudin (Angiomax), fondaparinux (Arixtra), lepirudin (Refludan), warfarin (Coumadin), and dabigatran (Pradaxa).

---

**NURSING ALERT**

The patient may be required to undergo frequent blood tests to measure the partial thromboplastin time (PTT), prothrombin time (PT), and international normalized ratio (INR) depending on the anticoagulant medication that is prescribed to him/her.

---

- Procedures: There are several procedures that may be performed if medications do not reduce the symptoms of AF. These are as follows:

  - **Electrical cardioversion:** This is a procedure that delivers an electrical shock through electrodes placed on the patient's chest. The shock stops the heart for a fraction of a second. The SA node then automatically starts sending normal impulses throughout the heart. The patient is anesthetized during the procedure.

  - **Catheter ablation:** This is a procedure where tissues of the heart that cause the extra impulses are destroyed by radiofrequency energy applied to the area by a catheter that the practitioner inserts into a blood vessel. In some cases, the practitioner ablates the AV node to prevent impulses from the atria from reaching the ventricles. The patient then requires a permanent pacemaker to maintain ventricle contractions.

  - **Maze procedure:** The Maze procedure is a surgical procedure where a series of incisions are made in both atria to prevent the abnormal impulses.

- Devices:

  - **Pacemaker:** A permanent pacemaker that is implanted into the patient and sends an electrical impulse to the heart when the heart rate is critically low.

- **Lifestyle changes:** A patient diagnosed with AF might be able to improve the condition by changing behaviors. These include
  - Reduce alcohol intake.
  - Stop smoking.
  - Reduce caffeine intake.
  - Reduce intake of stimulants.

> **NURSING ALERT**
>
> Tell the patient that soft drinks, tea, and over-the-counter medication may contain alcohol, caffeine, and other stimulants.

## Nursing Diagnoses

- Impaired gas exchange
- Decreased cardiac output
- Ineffective tissue perfusion

## Nursing Interventions

- Temporarily limit the patient's activities to decrease stress on the heart.
- Monitor for:
  - Heart rate.
  - Signs of stroke related to risk for blood clots.
  - Bruising related to warfarin therapy.
- Explain to the patient:
  - He/she will recover.
  - Adjust diet related to warfarin therapy.
  - Monitor for bruising.
  - The patient may be required to undergo regular blood tests depending on the medication prescribed by the practitioner.

# Atrial Flutter

**Atrial flutter** (aflutter) is when the atria contract very rapidly—too fast to permit each impulse to move through the AV node and into the ventricles— and every second impulse is sent to the ventricles, resulting in the atria contracting twice as fast as the ventricles.

Symptoms, diagnosis, and treatment for atrial flutter are the same as for AF.

> **NURSING ALERT**
>
> You can differentiate between AF and atrial flutter by contraction of the atria. There are no contractions with AF. There are coordinated contractions between both atria in atrial flutter.

## Common/Interpreting Test Results

Atrial flutter (Figure 4–2) is detected by evaluating the ECG wave. The P wave (see Chapter 3) records activity of the atria, and the QRS complex records the activity of the ventricles. Atrial arrhythmias can be detected in the P wave.

Here are the changes.

- **Rate:** There will be more P waves than QRS complexes because there are more atrial contractions or quivers than ventricular contractions.
- **P pulmonale:** The point of the P wave is >2.5 mm, indicating an enlarged right atrium.
- **P mitrale:** The P wave is notched, indicating an enlarged left atrium.
- **Wavy baseline:** The rhythm is irregular indicating AF.
- **Sawtooth:** The sawtooth wave indicates atrial flutter.
- **Inverted P wave:** The inverted P wave indicates that the ectopic pacemaker is located in the AV junction near the AV node.
- **P wave superimposed on T wave:** The P wave superimposed on the preceding T wave indicates paroxysmal atrial tachycardia, which is a regular fast heartbeat starting in the atria that begins and ends suddenly.

> **NURSING ALERT**
>
> An increased heart rate decreases filling, causing the stroke volume to reduce the amount of blood that is ejected with each heartbeat. This results in lower cardiac output and less coronary perfusion since the heart receives its blood supply during the diastole phase. The decrease in coronary perfusion causes an increased heart rate to supply coronary muscles with oxygen. Eventually the myocardium outstrips the supply of oxygenated blood, resulting in the patient becoming symptomatic.

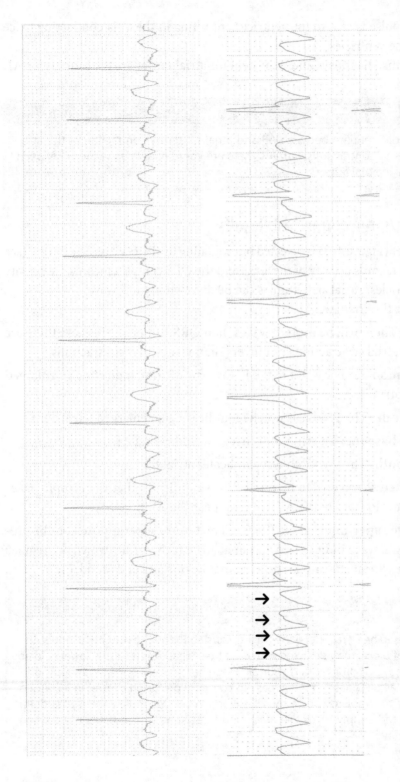

**FIGURE 4–2** • Atrial flutter. (A: Reproduced, with permission, from Keogh J, Reed D. *Schaum's Outline of ECG Interpretation.* New York: McGraw-Hill Education, 2011:93, Figure 7.2.; B: Reproduced, with permission, from Keogh J, Reed D. *Schaum's Outline of ECG Interpretation.* New York: McGraw-Hill Education, 2011:106. Figure 7.10.)

## Nursing Diagnoses

- Impaired gas exchange
- Decreased cardiac output
- Ineffective tissue perfusion

## Nursing Interventions

- Temporarily limit the patient's activities to decrease stress on the heart.
- Monitor for:
  - Heart rate.
  - Signs of stroke related to risk for blood clots.
  - Bruising related to warfarin therapy.
- Explain to the patient:
  - He/she will recover.
  - Adjust diet related to warfarin therapy.
  - Monitor for bruising.
  - The patient may be required to undergo regular blood tests depending on the medication prescribed by the practitioner.

# Premature Atrial Contraction

*Premature atrial contraction* (PAC) is a premature contraction of the atrium caused by a premature impulse before the SA node impulse by one or more atrial ectopic pacemaker cells. As a result, there is disruption to normal sinus rhythm. When the premature impulse reaches the AV node, the impulse continues along the same path as the impulse from the SA node would follow.

There is also a **nonconducted PAC**. A nonconducted PAC occurs when the impulse from the PAC is not passed along to the ventricles by the AV node.

## What Went Wrong?

PAC is related to several underlying conditions. These are as follows:

- Enlarged left/right atrium
- Hypertension
- Stress

- Heart valve disorder
- Postmyocardial infarction
- Stimulants
- Caffeine
- Tobacco
- Alcohol
- Digitalis toxicity
- Epinephrine
- Norepinephrine
- Hypoxia (lower oxygen in the blood)
- Abnormal blood level of magnesium
- Abnormal blood level of potassium

## Prognosis

PACs self-resolve by age 30 unless there is an underlying structural cardiac problem.

## Hallmark Signs and Symptoms

Symptoms result when the PAC occurs early in the cardiac cycle, and the patient has no effective heartbeat. Patients report:

- Skipped heartbeat.
- Palpitations.
- The heart has stopped.

### NURSING ALERT

Symptoms of PACs are virtually the same as for premature ventricular contractions (PVCs) (see Premature Ventricular Contractions).

## Common/Interpreting Test Results

PAC is diagnosed by performing one or more of the following tests:

- **ECG:** An ECG records the electrical activities of the heart (see Chapter 3).
- **Holter monitor:** (see Nursing Diagnoses under "Atrial Flutter")

- **Portable event monitor:** (see Nursing Diagnoses under "Atrial Flutter")
- **Transtelephonic monitor:** (see Nursing Diagnoses under "Atrial Flutter")

PAC (Figure 4–3) affects the P wave (see Chapter 3); however, the P wave may be difficult to detect because it is hidden in the preceding T wave, causing the T wave to appear distorted. Two telltale signs of a PAC are an abnormal P wave and a distorted T wave. The QRS complex might also be notched or wider than normal.

Other changes to the ECG are as follows:

- **Bigeminal:** Every other beat is a PAC.
- **Trigeminal:** Every third beat is a PAC.
- **Quadrigeminal:** Every fourth beat is a PAC.
- **Couplet:** There is a pair of PACs.
- **Premature atrial tachycardia (PAT):** PAT is when there is more than three series of PACs. This implies the sudden start and breaks occur by the atrial ectopic pacemaker.

The nonconducted PAC (Figure 4–4) is identified on the ECG as a P wave without a QRS complex, similar to the wave pattern of a cardiac arrest or cardiac block.

---

**NURSING ALERT**

An atrial contraction can appear later in the cardiac cycle. This is called an *atrial escape beat*.

---

## Treatment

Treatment of PAC is focused on alleviating the symptoms by using medications.

- Medication:
  - **Beta-blockers:** Beta-blockers are a class of medications that slow the contractions of the ventricles. The most commonly prescribed is metoprolol (Toprol, Lopressor).
  - **Calcium channel blockers:** These medications also slow the contractions of the ventricles. The most commonly prescribed are verapamil (Calan) and diltiazem (Cardizem).

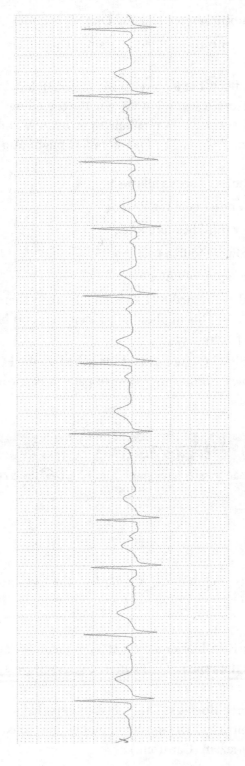

**FIGURE 4–3** • Premature atrial contractions. (Reproduced, with permission, from Keogh J, Reed D. *Schaum's Outline of ECG Interpretation*. New York: McGraw-Hill Education, 2011:95. Figure 7.3.)

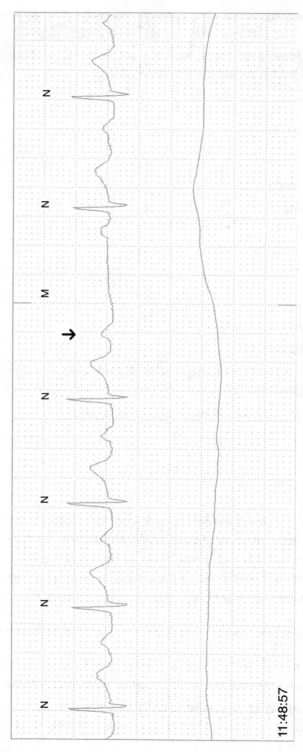

11:48:57

**FIGURE 4–4 ·** Noncoducted premature atrial contraction. (Reproduced, with permission, from Keogh J, Reed D. *Schaum's Outline of ECG Interpretation.* New York: McGraw-Hill Education, 2011:99. Figure 7.6.)

**NURSING ALERT**

The patient should avoid soft drinks, tea, and over-the-counter medication, which may contain alcohol, caffeine, and other stimulants.

## Nursing Diagnoses

- Anxiety
- Ineffective coping
- Impaired comfort

## Nursing Interventions

- Monitor for:
  - Anxiety
  - Hypertension
- Explain to the patient:
  - Assure the patient that there is generally no reason for concern, if he/she is healthy.
  - To decrease intake of caffeine, tobacco, or alcohol.
  - To reduce levels of exercise, if the patient is overexercising.

# Wandering Atrial Pacemaker

*Wandering atrial pacemaker* (WAP) occurs when the electrical impulse shifts between the SA node, atria, or the AV node, and returns back as a result of stimulation of the vagal nerve. Stimulation of the vagal nerve decreases the heart rate. As a result the AV node or the atria take over the pacemaking role. Normal heart rate returns when the vagal nerve is no longer stimulated.

## What Went Wrong?

WAP occurs in normal sleep. There is not one set of conditions that cause a WAP. However, patients who are predisposed to WAP are those with

- **Multifocal atrial tachycardia (MAT):** This is a heart rate >100/min caused by an atrial pacemaker. If the heart rate falls to 100 or less, it becomes a WAP.

- **Chronic obstructive pulmonary disease (COPD):** COPD patients have increased vagal tone due to respiratory strain.

In addition, WAP occurs as a result of:

- Medication (digitalis)
- Cardiac sinus disorder
- Heart disease
- Strain related to respiratory effort
- Lifting heavy weights

## Prognosis

Normal rhythm returns for most patients without treatment.

## Hallmark Signs and Symptoms

Patients diagnosed with a WAP are asymptomatic.

## Common/Interpreting Test Results

A WAP is diagnosed by performing an ECG. WAP (Figure 4–5) affects the P wave as the pacemaker wanders around the atria. The PR interval (PRI) is shorter when the pacemaker site is close to the AV node.

## Treatment

No treatment is usually necessary for a WAP because the condition is transitory and the heart returns to normal rhythm. However, WAP may be resolved by treating the underlying cause of the disorder.

## Nursing Diagnoses

- Risk for ineffective coping
- Anxiety
- Deficient knowledge

## Nursing Interventions

- Monitor the patient for signs and symptoms of other arrhythmias or an underlying cardiac disorder.

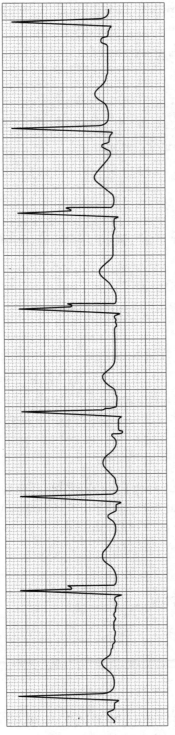

**FIGURE 4–5** • Wandering atrial pacemaker. (Reproduced, with permission, from Keogh J, Reed D. *Schaum's Outline of ECG Interpretation.* New York: McGraw-Hill Education, 2011:102. Figure 7-8.)

- Explain to the patient:
  - To report any symptoms to the practitioner.
  - No treatment is necessary.
  - The condition is transitory and the patient's heart will return to a normal rhythm without interventions.

# Paroxysmal Atrial Tachycardia

*Paroxysmal atrial tachycardia* (PAT), also known as a *paroxysmal supraventricular tachycardia* (PSVT), is a sudden increase in heart rate that suddenly returns to a normal heart rate. The increase is from 130 to 230 beats/min.

PAT can occur in patients who have healthy or diseased hearts. Some patients may tolerate PAT, while other patients may experience palpitations. PAT is not life-threatening, except in patients diagnosed with Wolff-Parkinson-White syndrome. *Wolff-Parkinson-White syndrome* is a heart disorder where there is an abnormal extra electrical pathway in the heart.

> **NURSING ALERT**
>
> PAT is the most common form of tachycardia in infants and children.

## What Went Wrong?

PAT is caused by an irritable ectopic atrial pacemaker. Irritation can be caused by one or more of the following:

- **Atrial automaticity:** Increases in the atrial pacemaker activity can result in increased cardiac rhythm.
- **Intra-atrial reentry:** In a normal cardiac cycle, impulses from the SA node terminate at the ventricles. However, impulses from the atrial pacemaker circulate within the atria.
- Caffeine.
- Stress.
- Alcohol.
- Drug toxicity (digoxin).
- COPD.
- Pericarditis (inflamed pericardium).

## Prognosis

Patients with a structurally normal heart can expect to return to activities of daily living following treatment. The prognosis for a patient who has an underlying structural heart disorder depends on resolving the underlying disorder. A few patients are at risk for sudden death.

## Hallmark Signs and Symptoms

In PAT, less time is spent filling the heart with blood, resulting in decreased oxygen in the blood. Compounding the problem is that the heart beats fast, increasing the consumption of oxygen.

Symptoms of PAT are as follows:

- Chest pain (angina)
- Shortness of breath
- Increased anxiety
- Altered mental status
- Light-headedness
- Palpitations
- Dizziness

## Common/Interpreting Test Results

PAT is diagnosed by performing an ECG. PAT (Figure 4–6) is detected by evaluating the ECG wave. PAT affects the P wave and has the following characteristics:

- **P wave:** Difficult to assess because the P wave is hidden by the T wave. When cardiac rhythm slows, there is one P wave for every QRS complex unless there is an underlying AV block.
- **PRI:** The PRI is not measurable because of distortion of the P wave.

## Treatment

PAT is focused on alleviating the symptoms by using medications.

- Medication:
  - **Antiarrhythmic medication:** These medications cause the heart to maintain normal sinus rhythm. These include flecainide acetate (Tambocor); propafenone (Rhythmol); sotalol (Betapace); dofetilide (Tikosyn); and amiodarone (Cordarone).

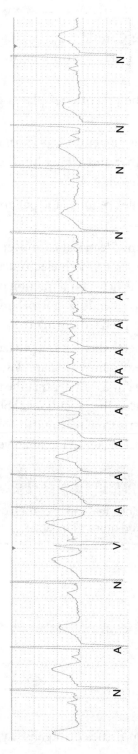

**FIGURE 4–6** • Paroxysmal atrial tachycardia. (Reproduced, with permission, from Keogh J, Reed D. *Schaum's Outline of ECG Interpretation.* New York: McGraw-Hill Education, 2011:103. Figure 7.9.)

- Procedure:
  - **Carotid sinus massage:** Carotid sinus massage is a procedure where the practitioner applies gentle pressure on the patient's neck over the carotid artery.
  - **Pressure on eyelids:** The practitioner places gentle pressure over the patient's closed eyelids.
  - **Valsalva maneuver:** This maneuver is performed by pressing both nostrils of the patient together and asking him/her to exhale through the nose, as if blowing a balloon.
  - **Dive reflex:** The dive reflex requires the patient's face or entire body to be placed in cool water.
  - **Electrical cardioversion:** Electrical cardioversion is a procedure that delivers an electrical shock through electrodes placed on the patient's chest. The shock stops the heart for a fraction of a second. The SA node then automatically starts sending normal impulses throughout the heart. The patient is anesthetized during the procedure.
  - **Catheter ablation:** Catheter ablation is a procedure where tissues of the heart, which cause the extra impulses, are destroyed by radiofrequency energy applied to the area by a catheter that the practitioner inserts into a blood vessel. In some cases, the practitioner ablates the AV node to prevent impulses from the atria from reaching the ventricles. The patient then requires a permanent pacemaker to maintain ventricular contractions.

## NURSING ALERT

The patient should avoid soft drinks, tea, and over-the-counter medication, which may contain alcohol, caffeine, and other stimulants.

## Nursing Diagnoses

- Anxiety
- Impaired comfort
- Impaired gas exchange

## Nursing Interventions

- Monitor for signs of:
  - Decreased blood flow to tissues or organs (hypoperfusion) because of decreased cardiac output.

- Decreased pulse pressure.
- Cool extremities.
- Altered mental state.
- Rapid resting heart rate.
- Alternating breathing between deep and shallow.
- Prepare for synchronized cardioversion, if patient is unstable.
- Assess for life-threatening arrhythmias.
- Assess for signs of drug toxicity and withhold if the patient is toxic; that is, seizures, respiratory arrest, and arrhythmias.
- Limit patient's activities to reduce cardiac workload.
- Explain to the patient:
  - The importance of regular examinations to ascertain for any changes in rhythm.
  - To call the physician if the patient feels light-headed or dizzy, as this can be a symptom of a change in rhythm.
  - To avoid ethanol, caffeine, and nicotine, as they can trigger an arrhythmia.

# Junctional Rhythm

The heart rate is set by impulses generated by the SA node that contract the atria, move through the bundle of His, and then move along the Purkinje fibers to the ventricles. If the impulse from the SA node slows or is blocked, the ectopic pacemaker near the AV node takes over, resulting in a **junctional rhythm**. The atria may contract before, during, or after the ventricles using a pathway other than the SA node pathway.

If conduction of impulses from the SA node is slowed or blocked, the ectopic pacemaker near the AV node takes over as the heart's pacemaker, resulting in a junctional rhythm. The atria may contract before, during, or after the ventricles; however, this occurs using an alternative pathway to the SA node pathway.

## What Went Wrong?

A junctional rhythm begins by an ectopic pacemaker located either in the AV node or in the AV junction when the rate of impulses from the SA node falls below the rate of the AV node. When the impulse originates in junctional tissue, the atrial depolarization is retrograde. *Retrograde* is when the impulse flows backward through the atria.

## Prognosis

A patient can return to normal activities of daily living following treatment of junctional rhythm if he/she is asymptomatic. The patient may experience increased vagal tone.

## Hallmark Signs and Symptoms

Junctional rhythms are characterized by the following:

- **Junctional beat:** Less than three impulses generated by the AV node or by the AV junction.
- **Junctional rhythm:** Three or more impulses generated by the AV node or by the AV junction.

Common junctional rhythms are as follows:

- Junctional escape beat
- Accelerated junctional
- Junctional tachycardia
- Premature junctional contraction

### NURSING ALERT

The ectopic pacemaker's site near the AV node is referred to as the *AV junction*.

## Common/Interpreting Test Results

Junctional rhythms (Figure 4–7) affect the P wave because there is retrograde depolarization of the atria. The P wave will be negative in lead II. The characteristic of the P wave is determined by the ectopic pacemaker closest to the AV node. The ECG has the following characteristics:

- **Atria depolarization occurs first:** The P wave comes before the QRS complex.
- **Atria and ventricles depolarized simultaneously:** The P wave is buried in the QRS complex.
- **Atria depolarization occurs after ventricular depolarization:** The P wave is after the QRS complex.
- **PRI:** <0.10 second because the impulse from the ectopic pacemaker site is close to the AV node.

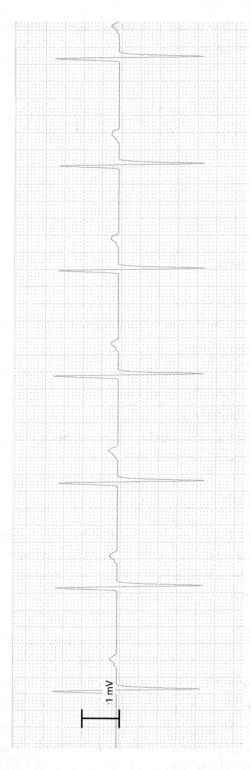

**FIGURE 4–7** • Junctional rhythm rate of 50. (Reproduced, with permission, from Keogh J, Reed D. *Schaum's Outline of ECG Interpretation*. New York: McGraw-Hill Education, 2011:117. Figure 8.1.)

- **QRS complex:** Narrow because ventricles are depolarized through the normal conduction pathways.

## Treatment

If the patient is asymptomatic, no treatment is necessary. If the patient is symptomatic, he/she may require a permanent pacemaker or may undergo radiofrequency ablation.

## Nursing Diagnoses

- Anxiety
- Impaired comfort
- Impaired gas exchange

## Nursing Interventions

- Monitor the patient for signs and symptoms of other arrhythmias or an underlying cardiac disorder.
- Explain to the patient:
  - To report any symptoms to the practitioner.
  - No treatment is necessary.
  - The condition is transitory and the patient's heart will return to a normal rhythm without interventions.

# Junctional Escape Rhythm

A *junctional escape rhythm* occurs when the SA node is suppressed to a level where the ectopic pacemaker at the AV junction takes over as the primary cardiac pacemaker. This may also occur when the impulse from the SA node doesn't reach the AV junction within 1.5 seconds.

## What Went Wrong?

Common causes of a junctional escape rhythm are as follows:

- **Sick sinus syndrome:** This is a malfunction of the SA node.
- **Digoxin toxicity:** Digoxin toxicity can depress the SA node.
- **Ischemia of the AV node:** Pathway to the AV node is narrowed or blocked. This occurs with acute inferior infarction involving the posterior descending artery, which is the origin of the AV nodal artery branch.

- **Postcardiac surgery:** The patient may experience cardiac inflammation following surgery.
- **Acute inflammation:** Acute inflammation, such as acute rheumatic fever and Lyme disease, involves the cardiac conduction system.
- **Medication:** Medication that causes sinus bradycardia such as beta-blockers, calcium channel blockers, and antiarrhythmic agents slows impulse generation by the SA node below the threshold when the AV node naturally takes over as the primary cardiac pacemaker.
- **Isoproterenol (Isuprel) infusion:** Isoproterenol is a bronchodilator prescribed to relieve bronchospasm. Infusion of isoproterenol may lead to an abnormally slow heart rate.

## Prognosis

A patient can return to normal activities of daily living following treatment of junctional escape rhythm.

## Hallmark Signs and Symptoms

In junctional escape rhythm, the patient may experience abnormal slowing of the heart (bradycardia) that can result in poor oxygenation of the blood.

Symptoms of junctional escape rhythm are as follows:

- Fatigue
- Poor exercise tolerance
- Difficulty breathing (dyspnea)
- Light-headedness
- Palpitations
- Dizziness
- Fainting (syncope)

## Common/Interpreting Test Results

Junctional escape rhythm is diagnosed by performing an ECG. A junctional escape rhythm (Figure 4–8) affects the P wave, the PRI, and the heart rate and rhythm. Junctional escape rhythm has the following ECG characteristics:

- **P wave:** Inverted in lead II. P wave occurs before or after the QRS complex, or the P wave may not be present.
- **PRI:** <0.10 second.

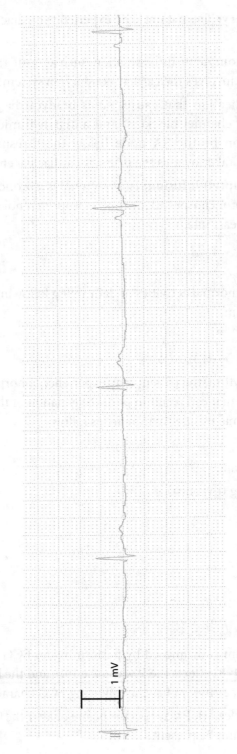

**FIGURE 4–8** • Junctional escape rhythm converting to sinus bradycardia. (Reproduced, with permission, from Keogh J, Reed D. *Schaum's Outline of ECG Interpretation*. New York: McGraw-Hill Education, 2011:118. Figure 8.2.)

1 mV

- **Heart rate:** Between 40 and 60 beats/min.
- **Rhythm:** Regular if there is an escape beat; irregular if there is an escape rhythm.

## Treatment

The treatment of junctional escape rhythm depends on if the patient is symptomatic and the underlying cause.

- **Increased vagal tone:** This decreases the heart rate. If the junctional escape rhythm is the result of increased vagal tone and the patient is asymptomatic, then no treatment is warranted.
- **Loss of atrial kick:** The atrial kick is the starting force by the atrial contraction that occurs before the ventricles contract. If the junctional escape rhythm is the result of loss of atrial kick leading to decreased cardiac function, then increase cardiac output and treat the underlying cause of the junctional escape rhythm.
- **Sick sinus syndrome:** This is a malfunction of the SA node. If the junctional escape rhythm is the result of sick sinus syndrome or AV block(s), then the patient requires insertion of a permanent pacemaker.
- **Digoxin toxicity:** If the junctional escape rhythm is the result of digoxin toxicity, then administer digoxin immune fab (Digibind).

## Nursing Diagnoses

- Anxiety
- Ineffective peripheral tissue perfusion
- Impaired gas exchange

## Nursing Interventions

- Monitor for signs of:
  - Decreased blood flow to tissues or organs (hypoperfusion) because of decreased cardiac output.
  - Decreased pulse pressure.
  - Cool extremities.
  - Altered mental state.
  - Rapid resting heart rate.
  - Alternating breathing between deep and shallow.

- Prepare for synchronized cardioversion, if patient is unstable.
- Assess for life-threatening arrhythmias.
- Assess for signs of drug toxicity and withhold if the patient is toxic; that is, seizures, respiratory arrest, and arrhythmias.
- Limit patient's activities to reduce cardiac workload.
- Explain to the patient:
  - The importance of regular examinations to ascertain for any changes in rhythm.
  - To call the physician if the patient feels light-headed or dizzy, as this can be a symptom of a change in rhythm.
  - To avoid ethanol, caffeine, and nicotine, as they can trigger an arrhythmia.

# Premature Junctional Contraction

*Premature junctional contraction* (PJC) is an impulse from the ectopic pacemaker site near the AV node that occurs early in the cardiac cycle. PJCs are a sign that the patient may be developing a junctional rhythm.

## What Went Wrong?

Common causes of a PJC are as follows:

- Digitalis toxicity.
- Enhanced automaticity of the AV node.
- Coronary artery disease (CAD).
- Heart failure.
- Cardiac valve disease.
- Irritated myocardium related to decreased oxygenation (hypoxemia).

## Prognosis

The patient may experience palpitations occasionally but should return to normal activities of daily living with ongoing treatment.

## Hallmark Signs and Symptoms

The patient is typically asymptomatic and does not become symptomatic unless the PJC leads to a junctional rhythm.

## Common/Interpreting Test Results

PJC is diagnosed by performing an ECG.

A PJC (Figure 4–9) affects the P wave, the PRI, and the heart rate and rhythm and has the following ECG characteristics:

- **P wave:** Inverted in lead II. P wave occurs just before or after the QRS complex or is not present at all.
- **PRI:** <0.10 second.
- **QRS complex:** Appears premature but normal.
- Rhythm
  - **Couplets:** Two sequential PJCs
  - **Triplets:** Three sequential PJCs
  - **Junctional rhythm:** More than three sequential PJCs
- Distinguish from a PAC
  - PAC is more common than a PJC.
  - **P wave:** Consider PJC if the P wave
    - Is not obvious
    - Is inverted
    - Is after the QRS

## Treatment

There is no treatment required for PJC.

## Nursing Diagnoses

- Anxiety
- Knowledge deficit
- Risk for ineffective activity planning

## Nursing Interventions

- Monitor the patient for signs and symptoms of other arrhythmias or an underlying cardiac disorder.
- Explain to the patient:
  - To report any symptoms to the practitioner.

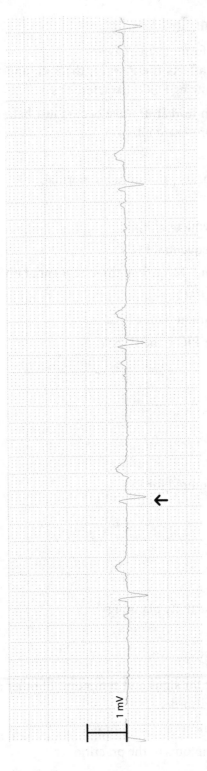

**FIGURE 4–9 •** Premature junctional escape. (Reproduced, with permission, from Keogh J, Reed D. *Schaum's Outline of ECG Interpretation*. New York: McGraw-Hill Education, 2011:120. Figure 8.3.)

- No treatment is necessary.
- The condition is transitory and the patient's heart will return to a normal rhythm without interventions.

# Accelerated Junctional Rhythm

An accelerated junctional rhythm is similar to a junctional escape rhythm except the cardiac rate is between 60 and 100 beats/min. A junctional escape rhythm has a cardiac rate of between 40 and 60 beats/min.

## What Went Wrong?

Common causes of an accelerated junctional rhythm are as follows:

- **Digoxin toxicity:** Digoxin toxicity slows conduction through the AV node, causing the AV node to assume role of the pacemaker.
- **Ischemia of the AV node:** Pathway to the AV node is narrowed or blocked. This occurs with acute inferior infarction involving the posterior descending artery, which is the origin of the AV nodal artery branch.
- **Postcardiac surgery:** The patient may experience cardiac inflammation following surgery.
- **Acute inflammation:** Acute inflammation, such as acute rheumatic fever and Lyme disease, involves the cardiac conduction system.
- **Medication:** Medication that causes sinus bradycardia, such as beta-blockers, calcium channel blockers, and antiarrhythmic agents, slows impulse generation by the SA node below the threshold when the AV node naturally takes over as the primary cardiac pacemaker.
- **Isoproterenol (Isuprel) infusion:** Isoproterenol is a bronchodilator prescribed to relieve bronchospasm. Infusion of isoproterenol may lead to an abnormally slow heart rate.
- **Anoxia:** Anoxia is the total depletion of oxygen that can increase the adrenergic tone or makes it less likely to respond to catecholamines such as norepinephrine.
- **Acidosis:** Acidosis is a condition of having excessive acid in the body fluid, which can increase the adrenergic tone or make it less likely to respond to catecholamines such as norepinephrine.
- Heart failure.

## Prognosis

A patient can return to normal activities of daily living following treatment of accelerated junctional rhythm.

## Hallmark Signs and Symptoms

In accelerated junctional rhythm, the patient may be asymptomatic; however, abnormal slowing of the heart (bradycardia) can result in poor oxygenation of the blood.

Symptoms of accelerated junctional rhythm are as follows:

- Fatigue
- Poor exercise tolerance
- Difficulty breathing (dyspnea)
- Light-headedness
- Palpitations
- Dizziness
- Fainting (syncope)

## Common/Interpreting Test Results

Accelerated junctional rhythm is diagnosed by performing an ECG.

Accelerated junctional rhythm (Figure 4–10) affects the P wave and the PRI and has the following ECG characteristics:

- **P wave:** Inverted in lead II. P wave occurs before or after the QRS complex or the P wave may not be present.
- **PRI:** <0.10 second.
- **Heart rate:** Between 40 and 60 beats/min.
- **Rhythm:** Regular.

## Treatment

The treatment of an accelerated junctional rhythm depends on if the patient is symptomatic and the underlying cause.

- No treatment is necessary if the cardiac rate of the accelerated junctional rhythm is the same as the rate of impulses from the SA node. There is adequate perfusion, and the patient is asymptomatic.

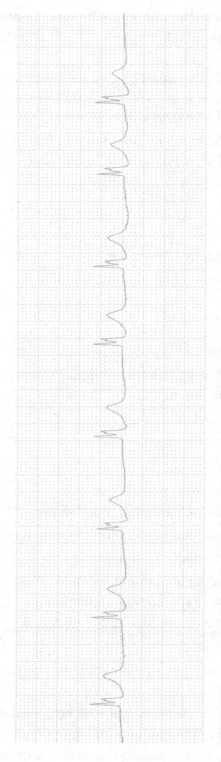

**FIGURE 4–10** • Accelerated junctional rhythm. (Reproduced, with permission, from Keogh J, Reed D. *Schaum's Outline of ECG Interpretation*. New York: McGraw-Hill Education, 2011:122. Figure 8.4.)

- **Medication:** Review the patient's medications to determine if one or more medications might be the cause of accelerated junctional rhythm.
- **Pacemaker:** Assess if the patient's decreased cardiac function is caused by the loss of an atrial kick. A pacemaker may be indicated to restore AV synchronization and the atrial kick.
- **Digoxin toxicity:** Administer digoxin immune fab (Digibind) if the accelerated junctional rhythm is caused by digoxin toxicity.

## Nursing Diagnoses

- Anxiety
- Ineffective peripheral tissue perfusion
- Impaired gas exchange

## Nursing Interventions

- Monitor for signs of:
  - Decreased blood flow to tissues or organs (hypoperfusion) because of decreased cardiac output.
  - Decreased pulse pressure.
  - Cool extremities.
  - Altered mental state.
  - Rapid resting heart rate.
  - Alternating breathing between deep and shallow.
- Prepare for synchronized cardioversion, if patient is unstable.
- Assess for life-threatening arrhythmias.
- Assess for signs of drug toxicity and withhold if the patient is toxic; that is, seizures, respiratory arrest, and arrhythmias.
- Limit patient's activities to reduce cardiac workload.
- Explain to the patient:
  - The importance of regular examinations to ascertain for any changes in rhythm.
  - To call the physician if the patient feels light-headed or dizzy, as this can be a symptom of a change in rhythm.
  - To avoid ethanol, caffeine, and nicotine, as they can trigger an arrhythmia.

# Paroxysmal Junctional Tachycardia

*Paroxysmal junctional tachycardia* (PJT) occurs when an ectopic pacemaker located near the AV junction becomes the primary cardiac pacemaker and sends impulses at a rate greater than 100 impulses per minute. PJT can occur at any age but has been seen in younger people who do not have a diagnosis of heart disease. The patient may decompensate quickly because the fast heart rate results in increased consumption of oxygen, and the patient loses 30% of the cardiac stroke volume because the atrial kick is lost.

## What Went Wrong?

Common causes of PJT are as follows:

- **Digoxin toxicity:** This slows conduction through the AV node, causing the AV node to assume role of the pacemaker.
- **Postcardiac surgery:** The patient may experience cardiac inflammation following surgery.
- **Acute inflammation:** Acute inflammation, such as acute rheumatic fever and Lyme disease, involves the cardiac conduction system.
- **Medication:** Medication that causes sinus bradycardia, such as beta-blockers, calcium channel blockers, and antiarrhythmic agents, slows impulse generation by the SA node below the threshold when the AV node naturally takes over as the primary cardiac pacemaker.
- **Ischemia of the AV node:** Pathway to the AV node is narrowed or blocked. This occurs with acute inferior infarction involving the posterior descending artery, which is the origin of the AV nodal artery branch.

## Prognosis

The patient will live a healthy life without restriction. Patients who experience episodes of PJT will require medication and may require cardioversion and will expect to have a fair to good outcome.

## Hallmark Signs and Symptoms

In PJT, the patient may be asymptomatic unless the patient has an underlying heart disease.

Symptoms of PJT are as follows:

- Light-headedness
- Palpitations

- Dizziness
- Fainting (syncope)
- Chest discomfort

## Common/Interpreting Test Results

PJT is diagnosed by performing an ECG.

PJT (Figure 4–11) affects the P wave and the PRI and has the following ECG characteristics:

- **P wave:** Inverted in lead II. P wave occurs before or after the QRS complex, or the P wave may not be present.
- **PRI:** <0.10 second.
- **Heart rate:** >100 beats/min.
- **Rhythm:** Regular.
- Distinguish between PJT and PAT:
    - PAT is more common than PJT.
    - If a definite determination cannot be made, then the patient has supraventricular tachycardia (SVT).
    - Administer adenosine to slow down the heart enough to differentiate a PJT from a PAT.
    - P wave:
        - **PJT:** Hidden in the QRS complex
        - **PAT:** Hidden in preceding T wave

## Treatment

The treatment of a PJT depends on if the patient is symptomatic and the underlying cause.

- **Beta-blockers:** Beta-blockers are a class of medications that slow the contractions of the ventricles. The most commonly prescribed is metoprolol (Toprol, Lopressor).
- **Calcium channel blocker:** These medications also slow the contractions of the ventricles. The most commonly prescribed are verapamil (Calan) and diltiazem (Cardizem).

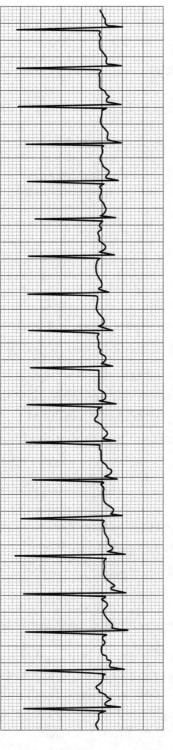

**FIGURE 4–11 •** Paroxysmal junctional tachycardia. (Reproduced, with permission, from Keogh J, Reed D. *Schaum's Outline of ECG Interpretation*. New York: McGraw-Hill Education, 2011:124. Figure 8.5.)

## Nursing Diagnoses

- Impaired gas exchange
- Decreased cardiac output
- Anxiety

## Nursing Interventions

- Monitor for signs of:
  - Decreased blood flow to tissues or organs (hypoperfusion) because of decreased cardiac output.
  - Decreased pulse pressure.
  - Cool extremities.
  - Altered mental state.
  - Rapid resting heart rate.
  - Alternating breathing between deep and shallow.
- Prepare for synchronized cardioversion, if patient is unstable.
- Assess for life-threatening arrhythmias.
- Assess for signs of drug toxicity and withhold if the patient is toxic; that is, seizures, respiratory arrest, and arrhythmias.
- Limit patient's activities to reduce cardiac workload.
- Explain to the patient:
  - The importance of regular examinations to ascertain for any changes in rhythm.
  - To call the physician if the patient feels light-headed or dizzy, as this can be a symptom of a change in rhythm.
  - To avoid ethanol, caffeine, and nicotine, as they can trigger an arrhythmia.

# Bundle Branch Blocks

The bundle of His conducts impulses that regulate the heartbeat from the right atrium to the left and right ventricles. The bundle of His causes contraction (depolarization) of both ventricles. The bundle branch block delays or blocks impulses through the bundle of His, resulting in contraction of one ventricle before the other ventricle. This causes ventricular arrhythmias.

## What Went Wrong?

Common causes of bundle branch block are as follows:

- Left bundle branch block:
  - Congestive heart failure
  - Hypertension
  - Cardiomyopathy
- Right bundle branch block:
  - Congenital heart defect
  - Myocardial infarction (MI)
  - Hypertension
  - Scar tissue from cardiac surgery
  - Cardiac infection

## Prognosis

Most patients are asymptomatic and can live a normal life without treatment. Patients who are symptomatic will require ongoing medication and possibly a pacemaker depending on the underlying condition that is causing the bundle branch block. The patient is at risk for a slow heart rate that can lead to cardiac disorders and sudden cardiac death.

## Hallmark Signs and Symptoms

In bundle branch block the patient may be asymptomatic.

Symptoms of bundle branch block are as follows:

- Light-headedness
- Slow heart rate
- Fainting (syncope)

## Common/Interpreting Test Results

Bundle branch block is diagnosed by performing an ECG. Bundle branch block affects the QRS complex. There is a notched QRS complex. The heart rate is usually the impulse of the underlying impulse.

## Treatment

Most patients are asymptomatic and require no treatment. The focus of treatment for patients who are symptomatic is treating the underlying cause of bundle branch block. The practitioner may implant a pacemaker if the bundle branch block results in frequent fainting episodes.

## Nursing Diagnoses

- Impaired gas exchange
- Decreased cardiac output
- Ineffective tissue perfusion

## Nursing Interventions

- Monitor the patient for signs and symptoms of other arrhythmias or an underlying cardiac disorder.
- Explain to the patient:
  - To report any symptoms to the practitioner.
  - No treatment is necessary.
  - The condition is transitory and the patient's heart will return to a normal rhythm without interventions.

# Premature Ventricular Contractions

*Premature ventricular contractions* (PVCs) are extra beats that originate either in the right or left ventricles early in the cardiac cycle. This is caused by an ectopic impulse site located below the bundle of His.

Premature beats are graded using the **Lown Grading System** where the higher the grade, the more serious the condition. The grading scale is

- Grade 0 = No premature beats
- Grade 1 = Occasional (<30/h)
- Grade 2 = Frequent (>30/h)
- Grade 3 = Multiform
- Grade 4 = Repetitive (A = couplets, B = salvos of = or >3)
- Grade 5 = R-on-T pattern

## Premature Ventricular Contraction Pauses

A pause follows a PVC. The pause can be

- **Compensatory (typical):** A compensatory pause occurs because the SA node is not depolarized by the PVC. This is characterized as
  - The time between the R wave that occurs before and after the PVC is equal to the R-R interval of the underlying regular rhythm.
- **Noncompensatory:** A noncompensatory pause occurs because the PVC depolarizes the SA node. This is characterized as
  - The time between the R wave that occurs before and after the PVC is not equal to the R-R interval of the underlying regular rhythm.

## Premature Ventricular Contraction Naming Conventions

A PVC (Figure 4–12) is identified by the frequency of the PVC. Here are terms used to identify a PVC:

- **Rare PVC:** Less than six PVCs per minute.
- **Frequent PVC:** Six or more PVCs per minute.
- **Bigeminy:** PVC occurs with every other contraction.
- **Trigeminy:** PVC occurs with every third contraction.
- **Quadrigeminy:** PVC occurs with every fourth contraction.
- **Couplet (paired):** PVC occurs back to back.
- **Triplet:** PVC occurs in a set of three.
- **Ventricular tachycardia (burst of V-tach, run of V-tach, paroxysmal):** (see Figure 10–3) PVC occurring in a set greater than three.

## Premature Ventricular Contractions Focal

A PVC (see Figure 4–12) is also described as to the foci (number) of the ectopic impulse site that is causing the PVC. These are called

- **Unifocal:** There is one ectopic impulse site that is causing the PVC. Each PVC looks the same on the ECG.
- **Multifocal:** There are multiple ectopic impulse sites causing the PVC. PVCs look different on the ECG because each might be caused by a different ectopic site.

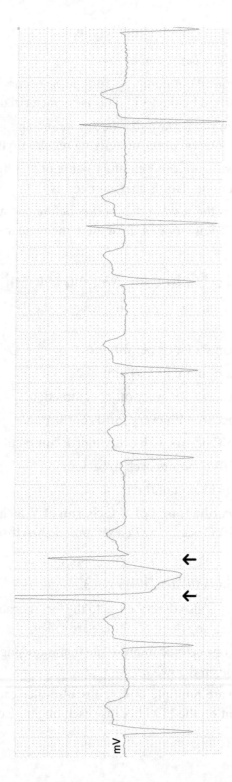

**FIGURE 4–12 ·** Premature ventricular contractions. (Reproduced, with permission, from Keogh J, Reed D. *Schaum's Outline of ECG Interpretation.* New York: McGraw-Hill Education, 2011:146. Figure 10.2.)

## Premature Ventricular Contractions and R-on-T Phenomenon

The R-on-T phenomenon is when the PVC (grade V PVC) occurs during the relative refractory period. It is at this time when the ventricles are recovering from contraction, and this is represented on the ECG as the T wave.

When the ventricular ectopic site sends an impulse (represented as the R wave on the ECG), the ventricles are stimulated to contract, although the ventricles still haven't recovered from the previous contraction stimulated by the underlying rhythm. This is depicted on the ECG as a ventricular rhythm beginning from the middle of the T wave.

This is the most vulnerable time for the ventricles and can lead to tachycardia (rhythm greater than 100 beats/min) or ventricular fibrillation, which is the fluttering of the ventricles leading to cardiac arrest.

## What Went Wrong?

There are four common causes of PVCs. These are as follows:

1. Cardiac disease:
   - Acute MI
   - Cardiac ischemia
   - Myocarditis (inflammation of the cardiac tissue and cells)
   - Cardiomyopathies
   - Myocardial contusion
   - Valve disease, especially mitral valve
2. Medications:
   - Tricyclic antidepressants' (such as amitriptyline or nortriptyline) interactions with quinidines
   - Digoxin at toxic levels
   - Sympathomimetics, epinephrine
   - Aminophylline
   - Caffeine
3. Hormones:
   - Increased catecholamines through emotional stress or use of drugs (cocaine, amphetamines, alcohol, tobacco)
4. Medical conditions:
   - Hypokalemia

- Hypomagnesemia
- Hypoxia
- Hypercapnia

## Prognosis

PVCs occur infrequently and therefore do not disrupt the patient's activities of daily living. However, frequent PVCs coupled with underlying heart disease place the patient at a higher risk of death.

## Hallmark Signs and Symptoms

The patient may report one or more of the following symptoms:
- The patient is aware of his/her heartbeat.
- Dizziness.
- Shortness of breath.
- Palpitations.
- Occasional forceful beats.

## Common/Interpreting Test Results

PVCs are diagnosed by performing an ECG.
   PVCs (Figure 4–13) have the following characteristics on an ECG:
- **QRS complex:** Wide, >0.12 second. Takes on a bizarre and abnormal appearance compared with the underlying rhythm.
- **Underlying rhythm:** Regular except for interruptions of PVC and subsequent pause, which makes the rhythm irregular.
- **P wave:** No P wave is associated with the PVC.
- **PRI:** No PRI.
- **T wave:** Opposite deflection from the main deflection. Repolarization is abnormal.

## Treatment

Treatment of PVCs depends on a number of factors.
- **Grade 1 PVC:** No treatment is necessary if the patient is relatively healthy.

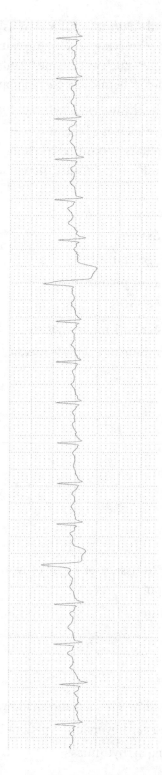

**FIGURE 4–13** • Normal sinus rhythm with unifocal premature ventricular contraction. (Reproduced, with permission, from Keogh J, Reed D. *Schaum's Outline of ECG Interpretation.* New York: McGraw-Hill Education, 2011:145. Figure 10.1.)

- **Grade 2 PVC:** Occasional <30/min unifocal; if asymptomatic no treatment is necessary, consider treating underlying causes such as electrolyte imbalances, avoiding triggers such as caffeine. Digibind for digoxin toxicity, 12-lead ECG to rule out ischemic disease (angioplasty may be needed).
- **Grade 3 PVC:** Frequent 0.30/min; see treatment for grade 2 PVC.
- **Grade 4/5 PVC:** Repetitive such as a bigeminy pattern; grade 5 is an R-on-T phenomenon. The patient is administered antiarrhythmic medications such as amiodarone and lidocaine because there is a higher mortality rate for this condition.
- Reverse the underlying cause:
  - **Hypoxia:** Administer oxygen.
  - **Heart failure:** Encourage diuresis.
  - **Hypokalemia:** Administer potassium.
  - **Hypomagnesemia:** Administer magnesium.
  - **Myocarditis:** Administer anti-inflammatory medication.
  - **Drug-induced:** Discontinue or decrease medication.

## Nursing Diagnoses

- Anxiety
- Risk for falls
- Decreased cardiac output

## Nursing Interventions

- Monitor for signs of:
  - Decreased blood flow to tissues or organs (hypoperfusion) because of decreased cardiac output.
  - Decreased pulse pressure.
  - Cool extremities.
  - Altered mental state.
  - Rapid resting heart rate.
  - Alternating breathing between deep and shallow.
- Prepare for synchronized cardioversion, if patient is unstable.
- Assess for life-threatening arrhythmias.

- Assess for signs of drug toxicity and withhold if the patient is toxic; that is, seizures, respiratory arrest, and arrhythmias.
- Limit patient's activities to reduce cardiac workload.
- Explain to the patient:
  - The importance of regular examinations to ascertain for any changes in rhythm.
  - To call the physician if the patient feels light-headed or dizzy, as this can be a symptom of a change in rhythm.
  - To avoid ethanol, caffeine, and nicotine, as they can trigger an arrhythmia.

# Ventricular Tachycardia

*Ventricular tachycardia* (V-tach) (Figure 4–14) is an impulse rate of 120 beats/min or greater that is generated from one or multiple ectopic sites in the ventricles. Monomorphic ventricular tachycardia is from one ectopic site, and polymorphic ventricular tachycardia is from multiple ectopic sites.

## What Went Wrong?

There are a number of causes of V-tach including

- Heart failure
- Mitral valve disorder
- Scar tissue from MI
- **Electrolyte imbalance:** Hypokalemia, hypomagnesemia, and hypocalcemia can result in V-tach.
- Medication:
  - **Antiarrhythmic:** Quinidine (quinidine gluconate, quinidine sulfate); procainamide (Pronestyl); dofetilide (Tikosyn)
  - **Psychotropic:** Tricyclic antidepressant
  - **Antiemetics:** Prochlorperazine (Compro, Procomp); promethazine (Promethegan)
  - Cocaine
  - Methamphetamines
- Procedure:
  - Catheter insertion into the pulmonary artery and into the right ventricle.

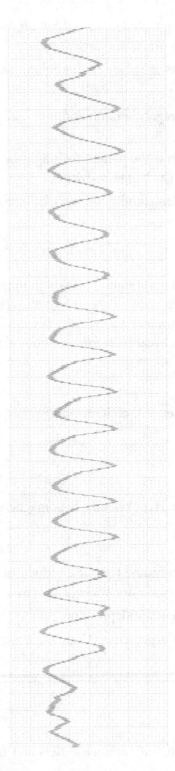

**FIGURE 4–14 •** Ventricular tachycardia. (Reproduced, with permission, from Keogh J, Reed D. *Schaum's Outline of ECG Interpretation*. New York: McGraw-Hill Education, 2011:150. Figure 10.4.)

## Prognosis

Prognosis depends on the duration of the arrhythmia and prompt response. Recurrent V-tach signals a poor prognosis.

## Hallmark Signs and Symptoms

The patient may report one or more of the following symptoms:

- The patient is aware of his/her heartbeat.
- Dizziness.
- Shortness of breath.
- Chest pain (angina).
- Palpitations.
- Weak pulse or no pulse.

## Common/Interpreting Test Results

V-tach (Figure 4–15) is diagnosed by performing an ECG.
V-tach is identified on an ECG by the following characteristics:

- **P wave:** The P wave is hidden within the QRS complex and might be occasionally seen between QRS complexes.
- **PRI:** Not measurable.
- **QRS complex:** Wide, distorted, and bizarre.
- **Rhythm:** Regular but can be irregular.
- Torsades de pointes wave form R-on-T phenomenon as a result hypomagnesemia and prolonged QT intervals.

## Treatment

V-tach is treated depending on the characteristics of the condition. Treatment is as follows:

- Stable monomorphic V-tach
  - Administer antiarrhythmics such as amiodarone, lidocaine, and procainamide.
  - Cardioversion or defibrillation.
  - Rebalance electrolytes (potassium, magnesium, calcium).
- Unstable monomorphic V-tach caused by hemodynamic instability
  - Cardioversion or defibrillation

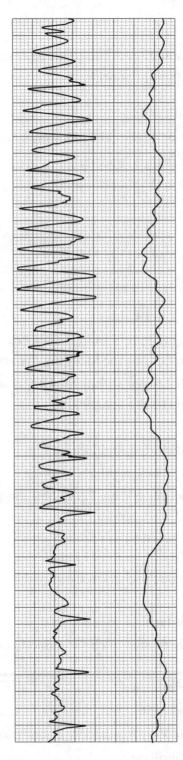

**FIGURE 4–15** • Polymorphic ventricular tachycardia or torsades de pointes. (Reproduced, with permission, from Keogh J, Reed D. *Schaum's Outline of ECG Interpretation*. New York: McGraw-Hill Education, 2011:152. Figure 10.5.)

- Chronic or recurrent V-tach
  - Administer antiarrhythmic.
  - Radiofrequency ablation (destroying the ectopic site).
  - Implant an automatic implantable cardiac defibrillator (AICD).
  - Electrophysiology studies (EP) done in the EP laboratory with the electrophysiologist. Patient susceptibility to these lethal rhythms is tested in a controlled environment.
- Polymorphic V-tach (torsades de pointes) (see Figure 4–15)
  - Rebalance electrolytes (potassium, magnesium, calcium)
  - Defibrillation

## Nursing Diagnoses

- Impaired gas exchange
- Decreased cardiac output
- Ineffective tissue perfusion

## Nursing Interventions

- Begin cardiopulmonary resuscitation (CPR) if pulse is absent.
- Prepare to administer medication per physician's order or protocol.
- Explain to the patient:
  - Necessity of follow-up.
  - To call the physician if the patient experiences dizziness.
  - The importance of regular examinations.

# Ventricular Fibrillation

*Ventricular fibrillation* is the quivering of the ventricles, resulting in a rhythm that cannot support perfusion of blood vessels and is the primary cause of sudden cardiac death. The patient is hemodynamically unstable. There is no cardiac output. The patient is pulseless without blood pressure, unresponsive, and death is imminent because ventricular fibrillation progresses to ventricular standstill or asystole.

## What Went Wrong?

Ventricular fibrillation can be caused by a number of conditions. The most common are as follows:

- Structural heart disease
  - Myocardial ischemia or infarction, resulting from coronary artery disease.
  - Dilated and hypertrophic cardiomyopathies are the second most important cardiac cause of sudden death.
  - Aortic stenosis.
  - Aortic dissection.
  - Pericardial tamponade.
  - Congenital heart disease.
  - Myocarditis.
- Nonstructural heart condition
  - Heart block.
  - Pre-excitation where ventricles become depolarized too soon.
  - Long QT syndrome where there is a delayed repolarization of the heart.
  - Short QT syndrome: A QT interval <300 milliseconds, doesn't change with heart rate, and the heart has no structural defects.
  - Electrocution.
  - Medication-induced QT prolongation with torsades de pointes, such as drug–drug interaction between quinidines and tricyclic antidepressants.
  - Brugada syndrome: Inherited syndrome that is responsible for sudden cardiac death. Only detected with a 12-lead ECG. Diagnosis is difficult, usually after the patient dies unexpectedly from cardiac arrest.
  - Can be an adverse effect of inserting a catheter into the pulmonary artery such as placement of a pacemaker.
- Hypoxia
  - Aspiration
  - Sleep apnea
  - Primary pulmonary hypertension
  - Pulmonary embolism
  - Tension pneumothorax

- Metabolic imbalance
  - Electrolyte disturbances and acidosis
- Toxins
  - Cocaine toxicity
  - Digoxin toxicity
  - Sepsis
- Neurological conditions
  - Seizure
  - Cerebrovascular accident such as a hemorrhage or ischemic stroke
  - Drowning followed by rewarming of the body

## Prognosis

Prognosis depends on how long it takes to establish a beating heart.

## Hallmark Signs and Symptoms

The patient symptoms are as follows:

- No pulse.
- Breathing is stopped (apnea).
- No palpable blood pressure.

## Common/Interpreting Test Results

Ventricular fibrillation is diagnosed by performing an ECG.

Ventricular fibrillation (Figure 4–16) is identified on an ECG by the following characteristics:

- **P wave:** None
- **QRS complex:** None
- **PRI:** Not measurable
- **Wave:**
  - Fine wave (see Figure 4–16) requires antiarrhythmic medication before defibrillation as it is of longer duration.
  - Coarse wave (see Figure 10–7) is likely to respond to defibrillation because it is a new onset.

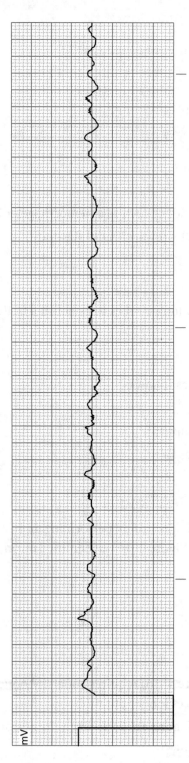

**FIGURE 4–16** • Fine ventricular fibrillation. (Reproduced, with permission, from Keogh J, Reed D. *Schaum's Outline of ECG Interpretation.* New York: McGraw-Hill Education, 2011:154. Figure 10.6.)

## Treatment

The treatment for ventricular fibrillation depends on if the ventricular fibrillation is witnessed.

- If witnessed:
  - Defibrillation is administered to the patient followed by CPR. Defibrillation can be administered using:
    - **Automated external defibrillator (AED):** Start CPR, attach the AED, and follow instructions announced by the AED.
    - **Monophasic defibrillator:** Set the defibrillator to 360 J and administer one shock. Continue CPR for 2 minutes and then repeat defibrillation.
    - **Biphasic defibrillator:** Set the defibrillator to 200 J and administer one shock. Continue CPR for 2 minutes and then repeat defibrillation.
  - Obtain IV access and intubate to open an airway after the initial shock. Continue CPR during IV access and intubation. Don't interrupt compressions to check the patient's pulse if the clinical picture doesn't improve.
- If not witnessed or the patient is in ventricular fibrillation for a few minutes:
  - Provide 2 minutes of CPR and then defibrillate since defibrillation is more effective after the heart receives circulated blood as a result of CPR.
  - Administer antiarrhythmic medication:
    - **Amiodarone:** 300 mg IV/IO repeat once at 150 mg IV. If rhythm converts consider 1 mg/min IV drip over 6 hours and then 0.5 mg/min over 18 hours; maximum dose of 2.2 g in 24 hours. Amiodarone slows the conduction through accessory pathways and slows heart rate to allow for full repolarization.
    - **Lidocaine:** 1 to 1.5 mg/kg IV/IO, repeat every 5 to 10 minutes at 0.5 mg/kg to 0.75 mg/kg; maximum dose 3 mg/kg. If rhythm converts consider 1 to 4 mg/min IV maintenance drip of class IB antiarrhythmic that increases electrical stimulation threshold of the ventricle, resulting in suppression of the automaticity of conduction.
  - Administer vasopressors and anticholinergic medication:
    - **Epinephrine:** (1:10,000) 1 mg IV/IO repeat every 3 to 5 minutes. Its action is to increase peripheral resistance via α-receptor-dependent vasoconstriction and to increase cardiac output via its binding to β-receptors.
    - **Vasopressin:** 40 units IV/IO once, can be used as an alternative to the first or second dose of epinephrine. As an alternate to epinephrine,

vasopressin causes peripheral vasoconstriction that ultimately helps increase blood pressure.

- Continue with 2 minutes of CPR followed by defibrillation and medication while reversing the underlying cause of ventricular fibrillation.
- The decision to stop resuscitative efforts is made by the patient's family, the patient's living will, and/or the patient's physician.

## Nursing Diagnoses

- Impaired gas exchange
- Decreased cardiac output
- Ineffective tissue perfusion

## Nursing Interventions

- Begin CPR (place on monitor, BP, P, R, pulse oximetry).
- Perform defibrillation, if certified.
- Prepare to administer medications per physician's order or protocol.
- Explain to the patient:
  - Patient is more than likely noncoherent. Speak to family.
  - Call the physician, nurse practitioner, or physician's assistant if the patient experiences dizziness.
  - The importance of regular examinations after rhythm has been stabilized.

# Asystole

*Asystole* is a condition when there is no ventricular depolarization, resulting in absent perfusion of the vital organs. The patient is unresponsive, not breathing, and has no pulse or blood pressure. There is poor prognosis since survival rate is less than 2%.

## What Went Wrong?

Asystole is commonly caused by the following conditions:

- Hyperkalemia.
- Hypothermia.

- Acidosis.
- Stroke.
- Pulmonary embolus (saddle embolus).
- Drug overdose (narcotics) that suppresses respiration leading to hypoxemia.
- MI complicated by ventricular fibrillation or V-tach that deteriorates to asystole.
- Proximal occlusion of the right coronary artery, causing the SA and AV node to infarct.
- An infarct that creates a block affecting both bundle branches.
- Indirect lightning strike.

## Prognosis

Prognosis is poor unless the heart can be restarted. The longer asystole continues, the more tissue is lost.

## Hallmark Signs and Symptoms

The patient's symptoms are as follows:

- No pulse.
- Breathing is stopped (apnea).
- No palpable blood pressure.
- Cyanosis.

## Common/Interpreting Test Results

Asystole is diagnosed by performing an ECG.

Asystole (Figure 4–17) is identified on an ECG by the following characteristics:

- **P wave:** Absent (flat line) but may be present if the patient was in AV block such as Mobitz II or third-degree block.
- **QRS complex:** None.
- **PRI:** Not measurable.

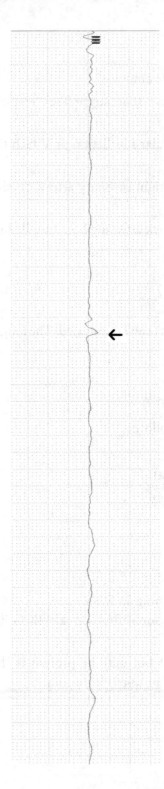

**FIGURE 4–17 •** Asystole with agonal beat. (Reproduced, with permission, from Keogh J, Reed D. Schaum's Outline of ECG Interpretation. New York: McGraw-Hill Education, 2011:159. Figure 10.8.)

## Treatment

Treatment for asystole is CPR and administering rescue medications and transcutaneous pacing. Rescue medications are as follows:

- **Epinephrine:** (1:10,000) 1 mg IV/IO, repeat every 3 to 5 minutes.
- **Vasopressin:** 40 units IV/IO once, can be used as an alternative to the first or second dose of epinephrine.
- **Atropine:** 0.03 mg/kg (dosing not to be less than 0.1 mg, due to paradoxical bradycardia) IV/IO every 3 to 5 minutes to a total dose of 3 mg. Blocks vagal causes, resulting in increased conduction through the AV node.

## Nursing Diagnoses

- Impaired gas exchange
- Decreased cardiac output
- Ineffective tissue perfusion

## Nursing Interventions

- Begin CPR.
- Prepare to administer medication per physician's order or protocol.
- Explain to the patient:
  - If asystole exists, patient is not conscious. Talk to family members if they are present. Refer to basic life support (BLS) protocol.

# Idioventricular Rhythm

An *idioventricular rhythm* is a rhythm that begins in the ventricles when the SA node does not stimulate the ventricles because the heart rate has slowed between 30 and 40 beats/min. An **accelerated idioventricular rhythm** (AIVR) can occur, resulting in a rate between 41 and 100 beats/min, which is slower than V-tach.

## What Went Wrong?

An idioventricular rhythm can be caused by the following:

- Myocardial ischemia or infarct especially following an inferior MI that affects the SA node.

- Digoxin toxicity.
- Hypokalemia.
- Reperfusion rhythm that occurs after blood returns to an area of the heart that lacks blood flow due to an ischemia or infarction.

## Prognosis

Idioventricular rhythm is usually a transient rhythm and rarely causes symptoms. Patients who report symptoms will undergo further assessment to determine the underlying cause of idioventricular rhythm.

## Hallmark Signs and Symptoms

Patients may be asymptomatic. The patients who are symptomatic report symptoms of:

- Light-headedness
- Slow heart rate
- Fainting (syncope)

## Common/Interpreting Test Results

Idioventricular rhythm is diagnosed by performing an ECG.

Idioventricular rhythm (Figure 4–18) is identified on an ECG by the following characteristics:

- **P wave:** Absent.
- **QRS complex:** Wide, >0.10 second, and bizarre in appearance.
- **PRI:** Not measurable.
- **Rhythm:** Regular.
- **Rate:** 50 to 120 beats/min.

## Treatment

No treatment is necessary for an idioventricular rhythm as long as the rate is adequate to perfuse the circulatory system because suppressing the ventricular rhythm might lead to a worse rhythm that reduces perfusion.

## Nursing Diagnoses

- Impaired gas exchange

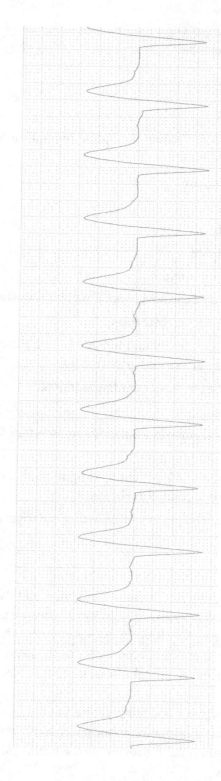

**FIGURE 4–18** • Accelerated idioventricular rhythm. (Reproduced, with permission, from Keogh J, Reed D. *Schaum's Outline of ECG Interpretation*. New York: McGraw-Hill Education, 2011:162. Figure 10.10.)

- Risk for falls
- Risk for activity intolerance

## Nursing Interventions

- Monitor for signs of:
  - Decreased blood flow to tissues or organs (hypoperfusion) because of decreased cardiac output.
  - Decreased pulse pressure.
  - Cool extremities.
  - Altered mental state.
  - Rapid resting heart rate.
  - Alternating breathing between deep and shallow.
- Prepare for synchronized cardioversion, if patient is unstable.
- Assess for life-threatening arrhythmias.
- Assess for signs of drug toxicity and withhold if the patient is toxic; that is, seizures, respiratory arrest, and arrhythmias.
- Limit patient's activities to reduce cardiac workload.
- Explain to the patient:
  - The importance of regular examinations to ascertain for any changes in rhythm.
  - To call the physician if the patient feels light-headed or dizzy, as this can be a symptom of a change in rhythm.
  - To avoid ethanol, caffeine, and nicotine, as they can trigger an arrhythmia.

# Pacemakers

A *pacemaker* is a battery-operated electronic device that monitors cardiac activity. The pacemaker sends a pulse of electricity to the heart, causing cardiac muscles to contract and reestablish normal sinus rhythm when an abnormal rhythm is detected. The pacemaker is connected to the heart by one or more electrodes. An *electrode* is an electrical connector that is placed directly into the cardiac muscle.

Newer pacemakers monitor blood temperature, breathing, and cardiac electrical activity and store this information in the pacemaker's memory. Data can then be transferred to a computer for review by the health care provider.

The health care provider can program the pacemaker to modify the data monitored by the pacemaker and the response of the pacemaker to abnormal cardiac conditions. The health care provider can adjust:

- Sensitivity of the impulse in millivolts
- When to send the impulse

There are two categories of pacemakers:

1. **Internal:** The pacemaker is implanted into the patient's chest.
2. **External:** The pacemaker is outside the patient's body.

There are four types of external pacemakers:

1. **Transcutaneous (TCP):** Pads containing electrodes are placed on the patient's chest. The pads are connected via wires to the pacemaker.
2. **Tranvenous:** Electrodes/wires are placed into a vein and into either the right atrium or right ventricle. The wires are connected to the pacemaker. This is used until an internal pacemaker is implanted.
3. **Transthoracic (percussive):** This is a mechanical pacing method where a closed fist strikes the left lower edge of the sternum and is used as a life-saving method.
4. **Epicardial:** Electrodes are placed on the outer wall of the ventricle (epicardium) during open-heart surgery. The electrodes are connected via wires to the pacemaker.

## Pacemaker Function

A pacemaker can send an impulse to the heart either on a fixed rate or demand rate depending on the patient's condition and the health care provider's treatment plan for the patient.

- **Fixed rate:** At the fixed rate setting, the pacemaker delivers an impulse to the heart at a set rate regardless of the patient's condition. The pacemaker does not monitor the patient's cardiac activity before, during, or after sending the impulse to the heart. The pacemaker competes with the patient's own heart rate. This increases the risk of the R-on-T phenomenon. Fixed rate is commonly used in transcutaneous pacing in emergency conditions.
- **Demand rate:** At the demand rate setting, the pacemaker senses the patient's cardiac rhythm and delivers an impulse when the pacemaker senses no intrinsic activity. For example, a pacemaker-generated impulse

is sent if the patient's natural heart rate falls below 50 beats/min. Demand rate is commonly used in an internal pacemaker.

- Types of demand rate pacemaker
  - **Single chamber:** The pacemaker senses and paces the atria or ventricular.
  - **Dual chamber:** The pacemaker is able to sense and pace both the atria and ventricles, thereby simulating the natural AV synchronization. This preserves the atrial kick.

## Pacemaker Modes

A *pacemaker mode* defines how the pacemaker is functioning. The pacemaker mode is defined by up to five letters; however, usually the first three letters describe the mode. Here is how to decode the pacemaker modes:

- The first letter defines the chamber paced.
  - *A:* Atria
  - *V:* Ventricle
  - *D:* Dual, for both atria and ventricles
- The second letter defines the chamber being paced.
  - *A:* Atria
  - *V:* Ventricles
  - *D:* Dual, for both atria and ventricles
  - *O:* None sensed
    - *O* is used when pacing is not dependent on sensing electrical activity.
- The third letter is the pacemaker's programmed response to the sensing
  - *I:* The pacemaker is inhibited.
  - *T:* The pacemaker is triggered to respond.
  - *D:* Any electrical activity by the atria or ventricles will inhibit the pacemaker; however, if the pacemaker senses any atrial activity then a V-paced beat will be triggered.
  - *O:* None.
- The fourth letter is the programmability and rate response of the pacemaker
  - *P:* Simple programmability
  - *M:* Multiprogrammability

- *C:* Communication
- *R:* Rate-response ("physiologic") pacing
- *O:* No programmability or rate modulation
- The fifth letter relates to the antitachyarrythmia function
  - *P:* Pacing (antitachyarrhythmia)
  - *S:* Shock
  - *D:* Dual (pacing + shock)

# Transcutaneous Pacing

*Transcutaneous pacing* is an external pacemaker because the pacemaker electrodes are located outside the patient's body. Transcutaneous pacing is used as a temporary solution to maintain a sinus rhythm until transvenous pacing is implemented or transcutaneous pacing is no longer indicated.

Electrodes are placed on the anterior and posterior chest walls. The pacemaker then sends an impulse over wires to the electrodes. The impulse is conducted through the chest wall to the myocardium stimulating the heart.

Transcutaneous pacing is the initial pacing method in cardiac emergencies and is in standby mode if a patient is at risk of decompensation, such as experiencing progressively longer pauses in cardiac rhythm or having a risk of progressing to a higher degree of heart block.

## When to Use Transcutaneous Pacing

Transcutaneous pacing is used when a patient

- Is experiencing hemodynamically unstable bradycardia and doesn't respond to atropine.
- Has a type II second-degree AV block.
- Has new-onset bundle branch block related to an acute MI.
- Has a bundle branch block with a first-degree AV block.
  - **QRS complex:** Wide
  - **T wave:** Tall and broad

When using transcutaneous pacing

- The patient should be sedated if he/she is conscious since transcutaneous pacing is painful.
- Use large electrode pads to reduce the risk of burning the skin.

- The amount of milliamperes (mA) required to capture (contract the heart) varies, depending on the patient. Lower milliamperes are required for cachectic or skinny patients. Higher milliamperes are required for obese patients or patients with large muscle mass.

- Apply the minimum amount of milliamperes and increase the amount until the patient responds to pacing.

- Continue to monitor the patient to assess the clinical response to pacing. The patient's blood pressure and mentation should improve.

- Start at the pacing rate that produces improved clinical status of the patient. This decreases myocardial oxygen consumption ($MVO_2$) and prevents further myocardial damage.

Transcutaneous pacing is not used in bradycardia secondary to the following conditions because the heart cannot contract.

- **Ischemia:** Injured muscles may not be able to contract; sodium potassium pump is not working.

- **Hypoxia:** Oxygen is not available for metabolism and energy production, and patient becomes acidotic.

- Pulseless electrical activity (PEA).

## Transvenous Pacing

*Transvenous pacing* is inserting electrodes through a vein into the right atrium, right ventricle, or both. An impulse is delivered if the heart has profound bradycardia. Transvenous pacing is used if the patient does not respond to transcutaneous pacing. Transvenous pacing is used as a temporary solution to the patient's cardiac conduction problem until the health care provider is able to implant a permanent pacemaker.

Transvenous pacing is a less invasive procedure than an implanted pacemaker because the pacemaker's electrodes are passed through a vein. Transvenous pacing requires less milliamperes to contract cardiac muscle than other external pacing methods because the electrodes are directly connected to the endocardium.

Transvenous pacing is used when the patient requires demand rate pacing to treat symptomatic bradycardia or complete heart block with slow ventricular response. However, transvenous pacing is not useful when there are no cardiac contractions or contractions are impaired, resulting from a drug overdose, hypoxemia, or acidosis.

# Epicardial Pacing

*Epicardial pacing* is used during open-heart surgery to maintain or reestablish cardiac rhythm. Electrodes are placed on the atria and the ventricles, enabling dual-chamber sensing and pacing. Wires connected to electrodes exit the chest wall and connect via cable to the external pacemaker. As with transvenous pacing, epicardial pacing requires less milliamperes to contract cardiac muscle than other external pacemakers because electrodes connect directly the endocardium.

The epicardial pacemaker is able to sense intrinsic activity and provides a demand rate impulse as required by the patient's condition.

Epicardial pacing is used for emergency pacing when the patient has symptomatic bradycardia and heart block. The health care provider may place the epicardial pacemaker on standby at a lower than intrinsic rate if the patient is likely to become symptomatic. The health care provider may use epicardial pacing to improve the patient's cardiac output by manipulating his/her heart rate.

# Permanent Pacing

*Permanent pacing* occurs when a pacemaker is implanted in the patient's chest. The health care provider weighs the benefits and risks of the implant.

A permanent pacemaker is implanted by an electrophysiologist in the electrophysiology laboratory (EP lab) under local anesthetic and/or conscious sedation. A pulse generator is placed beneath the skin on the nondominant side of the patient. This reduces interference with the patient's normal activities. Electrodes of the permanent pacemaker are placed through the subclavian or cephalic vein into the atria and/or ventricle using a fluoroscopy to guide placement.

Once in place, the health care provider can initiate single or dual-chamber pacing or AV synchronous pacing. Biventricular pacing reduces ventricular remodeling that can result from single ventricular pacing and can improve cardiac function in patients who have congestive heart failure. In biventricular pacing one electrode is inserted into the right ventricle against the septum and another electrode is inserted in the lateral wall of the left ventricle.

Permanent pacemakers are powered by a battery that lasts between 5 and 12 years. The patient and the health care provider monitor the battery condition regularly.

**NURSING ALERT**

Not all patients who have a temporary pacemaker require a permanent pacemaker.

## Capture vs Failure to Capture

A pacemaker sends an impulse to the heart when a cardiac event is detected such as a profound slow heartbeat. This is referred to as a *capture* because the impulse causes the heart to contract and a QRS complex appears on the ECG (Figure 4–19).

Failure to capture occurs when the impulse fails to cause the heart to contract. The ECG shows the pacemaker impulse but no QRS complex. Failure to capture can be caused by the following:

- The pacemaker fails to sense intrinsic cardiac activity in demand pacing and is unable to deliver the impulse appropriately.
- The impulse occurs during the absolute refractory period or the wrong point in the cardiac cycle.
- High pacing thresholds caused by:
  - Acidosis/alkalosis
  - Hyperkalemia
  - Broken wires
  - Pacemaker box failure
  - Bad connection to an external pulse generator
  - Battery failure
  - An inflammatory reaction or fibrosis at the electrode-myocardium interface
  - Remedy:
    - Increase the milliamperes and check all connections.
    - Have the bedside monitor and transcutaneous pacing on standby in case complete failure to capture occurs.

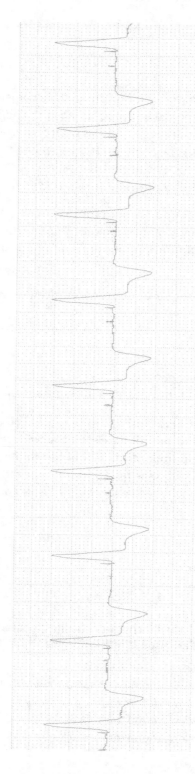

**FIGURE 4–19 ∙** Capture one QRS for every pacemaker spike; 100% AV pacing and sensing appropriately. (Reproduced, with permission, from Keogh J, Reed D. *Schaum's Outline of ECG Interpretation.* New York: McGraw-Hill Education, 2011:173. Figure 11.1.)

## CASE STUDY

### CASE 1

A 53-year-old construction worker is brought to the emergency department by paramedics. The patient reported a strange feeling in his chest while at the work site. He denies any chest pains but reports his heart feels like it is pounding. He says he actually felt his heartbeat and his heart stop and start. He says that at times he felt a little dizzy but never fainted. The patient reports feeling this way a few days out of the month. Why would the practitioner do the following?

QUESTION 1. Ask the patient, do you drink coffee or alcohol or smoke?
ANSWER: The patient's symptoms may indicate PACs or PVCs. Both disorders can be caused by the intake of relatively high amounts of caffeine and alcohol and heavy use of tobacco.

QUESTION 2. Ask the patient, have you ever been diagnosed with a heart disorder?
ANSWER: PAC can be caused by a heart valve disorder, enlarged atrium, or scar tissue related to a previous MI.

QUESTION 3. Order an electrolyte panel?
ANSWER: Abnormal levels of magnesium and potassium can cause PACs.

QUESTION 4. Order a Holter monitor?
ANSWER: The Holter monitor records the electrical activities of the heart continuously over 3 days using electrodes that are attached to the patient during that period. The practitioner analyzes the result after the monitoring period ends. The Holter monitor may be able to record electrical activities of the patient's heart during an episode.

## FINAL CHECKUP

1. **Why might paroxysmal atrial tachycardia be life-threatening to some patients diagnosed with Wolff-Parkinson-White syndrome?**

    A. The heart rate decreases to critical levels.
    B. Wolff-Parkinson-White syndrome is a heart disorder where there is an abnormal extra electrical pathway in the heart.
    C. The pacemaker wanders around the atria.
    D. The pacemaker wanders around the ventricles.

2. **A 53-year-old woman is diagnosed with PAC. Why does the practitioner tell the patient to press her nostrils together and exhale through her nose?**

   A. This is the dive reflex used as a nonmedication treatment of PAC.

   B. This is the carotid sinus massage used as a nonmedication treatment of PAC.

   C. This is the Valsalva maneuver used as a nonmedication treatment of PAC.

   D. This treatment increases blood flow to the heart.

3. **A 67-year-old woman is diagnosed with an irregular heartbeat. The practitioner suggests that the patient undergo catheter ablation. She asks how this procedures works. What is the best response?**

   A. Catheter ablation is a procedure that delivers an electrical shock through electrodes placed on the patient's chest. The shock stops the heart for a fraction of a second. The SA node then automatically starts sending normal impulses throughout the heart. The patient is anesthetized during the procedure.

   B. Catheter ablation is a procedure that creates an ectopic pacemaker.

   C. Catheter ablation is a procedure where tissues of the heart that cause the extra impulses are destroyed by radiofrequency energy applied to the area by a catheter that the practitioner inserts into a blood vessel. In some cases, the practitioner ablates the AV node to prevent impulses from the atria from reaching the ventricles. The patient then requires a permanent pacemaker to maintain ventricular contractions.

   D. Catheter ablation is open-heart surgery during which part of the heart is removed and replaced with an internal pacemaker.

4. **How can digoxin toxicity cause accelerated junctional rhythm?**

   A. Digoxin toxicity slows conduction through the AV node, causing the AV node to assume role of the pacemaker.

   B. Digoxin toxicity increases conduction through the AV node, causing the AV node to assume role of the pacemaker.

   C. Digoxin toxicity interferes with operations of the internal pacemaker.

   D. Digoxin toxicity stimulates the SA node.

5. **Which of the following is the most serious conduction of a premature heartbeat according to the Lown Grading System?**

   A. Grade 4

   B. Grade 5

   C. Grade 6

   D. Grade 7

6. **What is the difference between unifocal and multifocal PVCs on an ECG?**

   A. Each unifocal PVC looks the same. Each multifocal PVC looks different.

   B. Each unifocal PVC looks different. Each multifocal PVC looks the same.

C. Each unifocal PVC has a different P wave. Each multifocal PVC has multiple P waves.

D. There is no noticeable different on the ECG.

7. **What treatment would you expect the practitioner to order for grade 1 PVC?**

A. 24-hour monitoring in the cardiac care unit.

B. Treat the underlying causes of the PVC.

C. Administer lidocaine and amiodarone.

D. No treatment.

8. **A 34-year-old man is transported to the emergency department feeling dizzy. He tells you that he is being treated for ventricular fibrillation by his primary practitioner. The patient tells you that the primary practitioner told him to take himself to the hospital any time he had symptoms of a ventricular fibrillation episode. What is the best response?**

A. Immediately place the patient on a heart monitor and begin lidocaine intravenously.

B. Prepare to give amiodarone 300 mg intravenously.

C. Ask the patient if he was prescribed warfarin and the last time he had a PT/INR performed.

D. Rush the patient into the ED and get the crash cart.

9. **Why would a practitioner prescribed metoprolol for a patient diagnosed with PJT?**

A. Metoprolol is a beta-blocker that slows contraction of the ventricles.

B. Metoprolol is a beta-blocker that increases contraction of the ventricles.

C. Metoprolol is a calcium channel blocker that slows contraction of the ventricles.

D. Metoprolol is a calcium channel blocker that increases contraction of the ventricles.

10. **A 41-year-old man reports that he has a strange heartbeat because the practitioner told him he has sick sinus syndrome. What is sick sinus syndrome?**

A. Sick sinus syndrome is a decrease in the heart rate due to increased pressure in the sinus cavity.

B. Sick sinus syndrome is a condition that prevents the patient from performing the Valsalva maneuver.

C. Sick sinus syndrome is malfunction of the AV node.

D. Sick sinus syndrome is malfunction of the SA node.

# CORRECT ANSWERS AND RATIONALES

1. B. Wolff-Parkinson-White syndrome is a heart disorder where there is an abnormal extra electrical pathway in the heart.
2. C. This is the Valsalva maneuver used as a nonmedication treatment of PAC.
3. C. Catheter ablation is a procedure where tissues of the heart that cause the extra impulses are destroyed by radiofrequency energy applied to the area by a catheter that the practitioner inserts into a blood vessel. In some cases, the practitioner ablates the AV node to prevent impulses from the atria from reaching the ventricles. The patient then requires a permanent pacemaker to maintain ventricular contractions.
4. A. Digoxin toxicity slows conduction through the AV node, causing the AV node to assume role of the pacemaker.
5. B. Grade 5.
6. A. Each unifocal PVC looks the same. Each multifocal PVC looks different.
7. D. No treatment.
8. C. Ask the patient if he was prescribed warfarin and the last time he had a PT/INR performed.
9. A. Metoprolol is a beta-blocker that slows contraction of the ventricles.
10. D. Sick sinus syndrome is malfunction of the SA node.

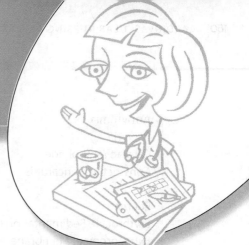

# Cardiac Inflammatory Disorders

## KEY TERMS

| | |
|---|---|
| Arrhythmia | Fungi |
| Bacteria | Heart Failure |
| Cardiac Tamponade | Intra-Aortic Balloon Pump |
| Constrictive Pericarditis | Myocardium |
| Dyspnea | Parasites |
| Edema | Petechiae |
| Erythrocyte Sedimentation Rate (ESR) | Stroke |
| Extracorporeal Membrane Oxygenation (ECMO) | Viruses |

# Myocarditis

**Myocarditis** is an inflammation of the middle layer of the heart wall called the *myocardium*. Inflammation is the immune response to a localized infection cause by a microorganism; however, the immune response typically continues after the infection resolves. The extended immune response may impair cardiac contractions, resulting in decreased flow of the blood throughout the body and increased risk of blood clots because of accumulated blood.

A patient may recover; however, some patients may experience damage to the myocardium, which can lead to the following:

- **Heart failure:** Heart failure occurs when the heart is unable to pump blood throughout the body efficiently.

- **Stroke:** A stroke occurs when a blood clot blocks the flow of blood through a blood vessel, resulting in necrosis of tissues that are supplied blood from the blocked blood vessel.

- **Heart attack:** A heart attack (myocardial infarction) occurs when coronary arteries are blocked, preventing blood to flow to cardiac tissue leading to the death of the tissue. Blockage is likely caused by a blood clot.

- **Arrhythmia:** Inflammation can negatively impact the sinoatrial (SA) node, atrioventricular (AV) node, and impulse conduction through the heart muscle, resulting in irregular contractions that can lead to sudden death.

## What Went Wrong?

The cause of myocarditis isn't known; however, the following microorganisms are suspected of causing myocarditis.

- **Viruses:** Viruses are the microorganisms most commonly associated with myocarditis. These include the following:
  - **Coxsackie virus B** (symptoms similar to the flu)
  - **Adenovirus** (symptoms similar to the common cold)
  - **Parvovirus B19** (causes fifth disease, which is a contagious viral infection in school-age children that occurs in the winter and spring, characterized by sudden bright red cheeks)
  - **Echoviruses** (causes gastrointestinal infections)
  - **Epstein-Barr virus** (causes mononucleosis)
  - **Rubella** (German measles)
  - **Human immunodeficiency virus** (HIV)
- **Bacteria:** There are many bacteria that can cause myocarditis. Following are the most common:
  - *Staphylococcus:* These species cause abscess and boils and can result in bacteremia (sepsis) if the bacteria enters the bloodstream.
  - *Streptococcus:* There are two groups: Group A causes sore throat, cellulitis, and scarlet fever. Group B causes unary tract disease, blood infection, and pneumonia.
  - *Corynebacterium diphtheriae:* These bacteria cause diphtheria.
  - *Borrelia burgdorferi:* These bacteria cause Lyme disease.
- **Parasites:** A parasite is an organism that lives in a person using the person's nutrients to survive. There are many parasites that can cause myocarditis. The most common of these are the following:
  - *Trypanosoma cruzi:* This is transmitted by an insect bite and causes the tropical disease/sleeping sickness.
  - *Toxoplasma gondii:* The most common parasite found in cat feces and contaminated food or water that causes flu-like symptoms.
- **Fungi:** Fungi are microorganisms that reproduce through tiny spores in the air, entering body through the lungs or on the skin. Some fungi can cause myocarditis. These include the following:
  - *Candida* (yeast infection)

- *Aspergillus* (molds)
- *Histoplasma* (found in bird droppings)

> **NURSING ALERT**
>
> Myocarditis can also be caused by other diseases such as Wegener granulomatosis and lupus, which are rare inflammatory disorders. Allergic reactions and toxic reactions to medications and street drugs can also result in myocarditis.

## Prognosis

Outcomes vary depending on the etiology. Improvement depends on the stresses caused by the underlying disease. Some cases resolve spontaneously; others develop dilated cardiomyopathy, such as congestive heart failure.

## Hallmark Signs and Symptoms

The patient may be asymptomatic except for symptoms of a viral infection (ie, headache, body ache, fever, and joint pain). The heart may or may not be affected. The symptoms resolve within 10 days, and there are no adverse effects on the heart.

The patient may experience symptoms in more serious cases of myocarditis. Symptoms include the following:

- **Arrhythmia:** Abnormal heartbeat due to inflammation affecting the conduction paths in the heart.
- **Shortness of breath (dyspnea):** Shortness of breath at rest or during physical activity is caused by decreased oxygenation of the blood resulting from arrhythmia.
- **Swelling of extremities:** Swelling (edema) is caused by fluid retention related to decreased or insufficient cardiac contractions.
- **Chest pain:** Chest pain may be related to insufficient oxygen supplied to the heart related to decreased or insufficient cardiac contractions.
- **Fatigue:** The patient may report being tired. This is caused by low oxygen levels in the blood related to decreased or insufficient cardiac contractions.

> **NURSING ALERT**
>
> Children can develop myocarditis and display symptoms similar to adults in addition to fainting and a bluish/gray coloration of the skin related to decreased or insufficient cardiac contractions.

## Common/Interpreting Test Results

When the patient is symptomatic, arrhythmia is initially detected by listening to the patient's heartbeat. If arrhythmia is suspected, then the following tests are performed:

- **Electrocardiogram (ECG):** The ECG (see Chapter 3) measures impulse condition of the heart and will depict the arrhythmia.

- **Echocardiogram:** A device called a *transducer* sends sound waves through the chest wall. The heart deflects sound waves back to the transducer, which sends a corresponding image of the heart on a screen. A trained practitioner can visualize the structure and function of the heart.

- **Chest X-ray:** A chest X-ray shows the size and shape of the heart.

- **Blood test:** A complete blood count (CBC) and cardiac enzymes test are ordered. The CBC test will indicate if there is any inflammation and the likelihood of what might be causing the inflammation. The cardiac enzymes blood test will indicate if there is damage to cardiac tissues. Erythrocyte sedimentation rate will assess the inflammation.

## Treatment

Treatment focuses on resolving the underlying cause of the inflammation (ie, virus, bacteria, parasite, fungi). Medication is prescribed to treat the arrhythmia and symptoms that results from the inflammation. Commonly prescribed medications are as follows:

- **Diuretics:** A diuretic (furosemide [Lasix]) reduces fluid retention by excreting excess fluids.

- **Beta-blockers:** Beta-blockers are also a class of medications that slow the contractions of the ventricles. The most commonly prescribed is metoprolol (Toprol, Lopressor).

- **Angiotensin-converting enzyme (ACE) inhibitors:** ACE inhibitors prevent the production of the angiotensin II enzyme that causes blood vessels to constrict. As a result, blood vessels relax (dilate) easing the flow of blood throughout the body. Commonly prescribed ACE inhibitors are enalapril (Vasotec), captopril (Capoten), lisinopril (Zestril, Prinivil), and ramipril (Altace).

- **Angiotensin II receptor blockers (ARBs):** ARBs block the angiotensin II enzyme from working (see ACE inhibitors). Commonly prescribed ARBs are losartan (Cozaar), eprosartan (Teveten), and candesartan (Atacand).

- **Anticoagulant medication:** Anticoagulant medicines reduce the risk of formation of blood clots. Commonly prescribed anticoagulant medications are heparin, enoxaparin (Lovenox), dalteparin (Fragmin), argatroban, bivalirudin (Angiomax), fondaparinux (Arixtra), lepirudin (Refludan), warfarin (Coumadin), and dabigatran (Pradaxa).

> **NURSING ALERT**
>
> Practitioners may prescribe the following medications that contain both ARBs and diuretics: irbesartan and hydrochlorothiazide (Avalide) and losartan and hydrochlorothiazide (Hyzzar)

In severe cases, the following treatment is common:

- **Intravenous (IV) medications:** Medications that would have been prescribed by mouth are given directly into the patient's veins to increase the therapeutic effect of the medicine.

- **Extracorporeal membrane oxygenation (ECMO):** Blood is removed from the patient's body and placed through a device that removes carbon dioxide and adds oxygen to the blood. The blood is then returned to the patient.

- **Intra-aortic balloon pump:** A balloon is inserted into the aorta and is then inflated and deflated to increase blood flow throughout the body.

- **Heart transplant:** The patient's heart is removed and replaced with a donor heart.

## Nursing Diagnoses

- Hyperthermia
- Decreased cardiac output
- Activity intolerance

## Nursing Interventions

- Temporarily limit the patient's activities to decrease stress on the heart.
- Provide bedside commode.
- Monitor for the following:
  - Difficulty breathing (dyspnea) because of fluid overload.
  - Heart rate more than 100 beats per minute (tachycardia) because infection or inflammation may increase the heart rate.

- No competitive sports.
- Return to normal activities slowly once physician approves.

# Pericarditis

Pericarditis is the inflammation of the fluid sac that contains the heart called the *pericardium*. The increase of blood by the inflammation process causes the pericardium to swell, resulting in layers of the pericardium rubbing together causing irritation.

Pericarditis can result in the following complications:

- **Cardiac tamponade:** The inner layer of the pericardium is lubricated with fluid, preventing the heart from rubbing against the pericardium. Too much fluid in the pericardium is called *cardiac tamponade* and can lead to the increased pressure on the heart that prevents the heart from filling with blood properly. As a result, there is a drop in cardiac output leading to a critical drop in blood pressure.

- **Constrictive pericarditis**: Tissues in the pericardium can become damaged from chronic pericarditis, resulting in scar tissues replacing tissues in the pericardium. Scar tissue is a nonfunctioning tissue that causes the pericardium to thicken and lose elasticity, increasing pressure on the heart and decreasing cardiac function.

## What Went Wrong?

The underlying cause of pericarditis is not known; however, the following situations may lead to pericarditis:

- **Heart attack:** Irritation of the heart muscle may cause a delayed irritation of the pericardium, which is referred to as Dressler syndrome. Dressler syndrome is caused by an autoimmune response where the inflammatory process starts to attack the patient's own tissues in the heart and pericardium.

- **Cardiac surgery:** Dressler syndrome (see heart attack) may occur following cardiac surgery.

- **Viral infection**

- **Trauma**

- **Systemic inflammatory disorder:** Inflammatory disorders such as rheumatoid arthritis and lupus affect the entire body and can involve the pericardium.

## Prognosis

Outcome of acute pericarditis is often self-limited, resolving in 2 to 6 weeks. Patients are typically treated with nonsteroidal anti-inflammatory drugs (NSAIDs) to decrease the inflammation of the pericardium.

## Hallmark Signs and Symptoms

Commonly reported symptoms of pericarditis are as follows:

- **Sharp, cutting pain over the center or left side of the chest:** The pain may radiate to the back, neck, and shoulder blades and become worse when the patient inhales and lies supine. Pain lessens when the patient sits upright. The pain is caused by layers of the pericardium rubbing against each other. The pain is similar to the pain reported during a heart attack.
- **Palpitations:** The heart rate increases to compensate for the decreased oxygenation caused by excess fluid in the pericardium interfering with cardiac output.
- **Shortness of breath when reclining:** Additional pressure is placed on the heart when the patient reclines, increasing the impact excess fluid in the pericardium has on cardiac output and resulting in fluid backing up in the lungs.
- **Weakness:** Weakness is due to the decrease in oxygen in the blood caused by decreased cardiac output.
- **Swelling:** Swelling is commonly seen in the leg and abdomen caused by pooling of blood due to decreased ability of the heart to pump blood.
- **Low-grade fever:** The low-grade fever is caused by inflammation in the pericardium.
- **Dry cough:** Dry cough is the result of fluid backed up due to decreased cardiac output.

### NURSING ALERT

Suspect acute pericarditis if symptoms develop suddenly. Acute pericarditis resolves quickly. Suspect chronic pericarditis if symptoms develop gradually and last for 6 weeks.

## Common/Interpreting Test Results

The initial diagnosis is to rule out a heart attack since pain from pericarditis can be similar to pain associated with a heart attack. You may be able to hear a pericardial friction rub using the stethoscope. The following tests are performed to confirm the diagnosis:

- **ECG:** The ECG (see Chapter 4) measures impulse conditions of the heart and will indicate a heart attack.

- **Echocardiogram:** A transducer sends sound waves through the chest wall. The heart deflects sound waves back to the transducer, which sends a corresponding image of the heart on a screen. A trained practitioner can visualize the structure and function of the heart. This may show fluid accumulation in the pericardium.

- **Chest X-ray:** A chest X-ray shows the size and shape of the heart and may show an enlarged heart if excess fluid is in the pericardium.

- **Computed tomography (CT):** A CT scan provides highly detailed images of the heart and is likely to show thickening of the pericardium or other likely causes of the pain.

- **Cardiac magnetic resonance imaging (MRI):** The MRI presents the practitioner with cross-sectional images of the heart that can show changes in the heart and the pericardium.

- **Blood tests:**

  - *CBC:* High white blood cell count indicates the inflammatory response.

  - *Cardiac enzymes:* Cardiac enzymes indicate if there is damage to cardiac tissues as a result of a heart attack.

  - *Erythrocyte sedimentation rate:* This test is done to assess inflammation.

## Treatment

Many acute pericarditis cases are self-resolving. In some cases the practitioner may prescribe the following medications or perform the following procedures:

- Medications:

  - **Anti-inflammatory:** Anti-inflammatory medications reduce the body's inflammation responses. These include prednisone, methyl-prednisolone (Medrol), and ibuprofen (Motrin, Advil).

- **Antigout:** Antigout medication such as colchicine (Colcrys) reduces inflammation throughout the body and can be effective for pericarditis. However, these medications are not prescribed for patients who have kidney or liver disease.
- Procedures:
  - **Pericardiocentesis:** Pericardiocentesis is a procedure that drains fluid from the pericardium. A catheter is inserted through the chest wall and into the pericardium guided by the echocardiogram. Fluid is then drained over several days in the hospital.
  - **Pericardiectomy:** Pericardiectomy is the surgical removal of the pericardium. This procedure is common for patients diagnosed with constrictive pericarditis.

## Nursing Diagnoses

- Acute pain
- Decreased cardiac output
- Risk for activity intolerance

## Nursing Interventions

- Place the patient in full Fowler's position to ease breathing.
- Explain to the patient:
  - He/she will recover.
  - Slowly resume daily activities.
  - Plan for rest periods during the day due to fatigue.
  - Perform coughing and deep breathing exercises—patient may have been avoiding deep breathing due to discomfort.

# Endocarditis

Endocarditis is an infection of the inner lining of the heart called the *endocardium*. Endocarditis is less common in patients who do not have a history of cardiac defects. Patients who have the following conditions are at a high risk for endocarditis:

- **Congenital heart defects:** A congenital heart defect is a malformation of the heart at birth.

- **Artificial heart valve:** Microorganisms have a tendency to grow on prosthetic heart valves.

- **Damaged heart valves:** Heart valves that are scarred or damaged by infections, such as rheumatic fever, make the patient prone to endocarditis.

- **Previous episodes of endocarditis:** Endocarditis can damage cardiac valves and cardiac tissue, exposing the patient to future infection.

- **IV street drug use:** The use of contaminated needles exposes the patient's blood to bacterial infection that can result in endocarditis.

Patients diagnosed with endocarditis are exposed to the following complications:

- **Systematic infection:** Microorganisms that cause endocarditis can travel through the bloodstream and infect other parts of the patient's body.

- **Stroke:** The microorganism that clumps together at a site in the heart can break loose and float in the bloodstream possibly blocking a blood vessel and leading to tissue necrosis in the brain.

- **Heart failure:** Growth of the microorganism in the heart can damage the endocardium, decreasing the heart's ability to pump blood and eventually leading to heart failure.

## What Went Wrong?

Endocarditis occurs when a microorganism that causes disease (pathogen), commonly bacteria or fungi, enters the patient's bloodstream and is distributed throughout the body and passes through the heart where the pathogen attaches to the endocardium causing an inflammatory reaction. Pathogens are more likely to adhere to damaged heart valves or artificial heart valves than to healthy heart valves.

The pathogen is usually one of many common pathogens that enter the body regularly and are destroyed by the patient's immune system before or after they enter the bloodstream.

However, the pathogen is likely to survive in the bloodstream in patients with a compromised immune system. Those patients require prophylactic antibiotics before any routine care, such as dental treatment, that might expose blood to bacteria.

## Prognosis

The prognosis depends on both the organism (as some are more virulent than others) and the degree of damage to the heart. Myocarditis may recur.

## Hallmark Signs and Symptoms

Symptoms of endocarditis include the following:

- **Fatigue:** Weakness is due to the decrease in oxygen in the blood caused by decreased cardiac output.
- **Swelling:** Swelling is commonly seen in the leg and abdomen caused by pooling of blood due to decreased ability of the heart to pump blood.
- **Dry cough:** Dry cough is the result of fluid backed up due to decreased cardiac output.
- **Osler node:** These are red, tender spots on the skin of the hands and feet caused by deposits of immune complex.
- **Fever:** Fever is the body's immune response to the microorganism.
- **Chills:** Chills are the result of muscles expanding and contracting to generate heat as part of the immune response to combat the microorganism.
- **Shortness of breath:** This is caused by fluid backing up in the lungs as a result of decreased cardiac output.
- **Petechiae:** Petechiae are tiny blood vessels that burst and bleed into the skin and appear as tiny purple or red spots on the skin, inside the mouth, or on the whites of the eyes.
- **Hematuria:** Blood in the urine (hematuria) is caused by infection.
- **Tender spleen:** Tenderness may be caused by an enlarged spleen. The spleen is part of the lymph system and produces white blood cells that engulf microorganisms. An enlarged spleen indicates that the spleen is working to produce white blood cells to combat the infection and remove microorganisms from the blood.

## Common/Interpreting Test Results

Endocarditis appears as a heart murmur. A heart murmur is an extra heart sound such as the sound of blood rushing through the heart. If this is a new or changed heart murmur and the patient is symptomatic, the following tests are ordered:

- Blood tests:
  - **CBC:** A high white blood cell count indicates the presence of the inflammatory response. Decreased red blood cell count indicates anemia, which occurs in endocarditis.

- **Erythrocyte sedimentation rate:** To assess inflammation.
- **Culture and sensitivity:** The laboratory will grow the microorganism found in blood (culture) in a petri dish and then determine which medications can be used to kill the microorganism (sensitivity).
- **ECG:** The ECG (see Chapter 4) measures impulse condition of the heart and will indicate abnormal conduction of the impulse throughout the heart.
- **Transesophageal echocardiogram:** A transducer is passed into the patient's esophagus and sends sound waves to the heart. The heart deflects sound waves back to the transducer, which sends a corresponding image of the heart to a screen. A trained practitioner can visualize the structure and function of the heart. This may show fluid accumulation in the pericardium.
- **Chest X-ray:** A chest X-ray shows the size and shape of the heart and may show an enlarged heart. The X-ray will also indicate if the infection has affected the patient's lungs.

## Treatment

Based on the results of the culture and sensitivity blood test, the practitioner will order medication that will kill the pathogen. Medication is typically given intravenously in high doses in a health care facility.

After each round of medication, the practitioner is likely to order a CBC to assess if there is a decrease in the inflammation response, indicating that the pathogen is destroyed. It can take between 2 and 6 weeks to resolve the endocarditis. Early treatment is given inpatient in the hospital. Once symptoms stabilize, treatment can move to outpatient weekly visits.

---

**NURSING ALERT**

A second culture and sensitivity test may not be ordered because test results are typically not available for several weeks, and during that period the patient may show signs that the endocarditis has resolved.

---

The pathogen may cause permeant damage to heart valves requiring surgery to repair or replace the valve.

## Nursing Diagnoses

- Decreased cardiac output
- Risk for injury
- Activity intolerance

## Nursing Interventions

- Monitor for signs of heart failure because of increased stress on heart due to altered valve function.
  - Breathing difficulties (dyspnea).
  - Heart rate more than 100 beats/min (tachycardia).
  - Crackles in lungs.
  - Neck vein distention.
  - Edema, usually of extremities; may also be of sacrum in bed-bound patients.
  - Weight gain.
- Monitor for embolism—a piece of vegetation from valve may have broken off into circulation.
  - Blood in the urine (hematuria).
  - Pain with each breath due to pulmonary embolism.
- Monitor renal function:
  - Increased blood urea nitrogen (BUN).
  - Increased creatinine clearance.
  - Decreased urine output.
- Prophylactic antibiotics are required before, during, and after medical procedures that expose the patient's blood to microorganisms—otherwise it is easy for microorganisms to enter the bloodstream and colonize the heart valves.
- Explain to the patient:
  - Need to complete antibiotic course.
  - Can have a relapse.
  - Call the physician, nurse practitioner, or physician assistant if the patient develops fever, chills, or night sweats.

## CASE STUDY

### CASE 1

A 58-year-old man is taken to the emergency department reporting sharp piercing pain in his chest. He reports that the pain moves to his back and shoulder blades. He states that the pain is worse when lying down on his back. Furthermore, he tells you that he has difficulty breathing when reclining. The practitioner suspects pericarditis and tells the patient that he has ordered several tests. Based on the test results, the practitioner tells the patient that he may have cardiac tamponade and may have to undergo pericardiocentesis. Here are questions asked by the patient. What is your best response?

QUESTION 1. What is cardiac tamponade?
ANSWER: The heart is contained in a sac called the *pericardium*. Cardiac tamponade is a condition where too much fluid fills the pericardium.

QUESTION 2. Why is the pain worse when lying on my back?
ANSWER: Fluid in the pericardium is pressed against your heart when lying on your back, causing you severe pain.

QUESTION 3. What is pericarditis?
ANSWER: Pericarditis is an inflammation of the fluid sac that contains the heart called the *pericardium*. The increase of blood by the inflammation process causes the pericardium to swell, resulting in layers of the pericardium rubbing together, which causes irritation.

QUESTION 4. What is pericardiocentesis?
ANSWER: Pericardiocentesis is a procedure that drains fluid from the pericardium. A catheter is inserted through the chest wall and into the pericardium guided by an echocardiogram. Fluid is then drained.

## FINAL CHECKUP

1. **Why would a patient with a history of endocarditis be prescribed antibiotics before receiving dental treatment?**

    A. Bacteria in the mouth and gums could enter the bloodstream and infect the patient's heart.

    B. The patient may still have the bacteria that cause endocarditis and the bacteria may be transmitted to the dentist.

    C. The bacteria are dormant and the procedure may reactivate the bacteria.

    D. The patient does not need to take antibiotics before receiving dental treatment.

2. **Why does a patient who is diagnosed with pericarditis report sharp, cutting pain over the chest?**

    A. The patient is experiencing a heart attack.
    B. This is a side effect of the medication prescribed to treat pericarditis.
    C. The pain is due to layers of the pericardium rubbing against each other.
    D. The pain is due to layers of the pericardium rubbing against the heart.

3. **What causes constriction in constrictive pericarditis?**

    A. Coronary blood vessels narrow because of plaque.
    B. Coronary blood vessels narrow because of a clot.
    C. Tissues in the pericardium can become damaged from chronic pericarditis, resulting in scar tissues replacing tissues in the pericardium.
    D. The pericardium loses lubrication.

4. **Why is a patient diagnosed with myocarditis prescribed Lopressor?**

    A. Lopressor is a beta-blocker that slows the contractions of the ventricles.
    B. Lopressor is an ACE inhibitor that prevents blood vessels from narrowing.
    C. Lopressor reduces fluid retention.
    D. Lopressor increases blood pressure.

5. **Why might a patient diagnosed with myocarditis be at risk for heart failure?**

    A. Inflammation of the outer layer of the heart reduces the ability of the heart to contract, preventing the heart from efficiently pumping blood.
    B. Myocarditis can weaken the heart, preventing the heart from efficiently pumping blood throughout the body.
    C. Inflammation causes layers of the myocardium to rub together, decreasing the pumping action of the heart.
    D. Heart failure is a possible side effect of beta-blockers but has a lower probability of occurrence.

6. **Why would a patient diagnosed with myocarditis experience arrhythmia?**

    A. ACE inhibitors prescribed to treat myocarditis may cause arrhythmia.
    B. Inflammation disrupts the conduction paths in the heart.
    C. Rubbing of layers of the myocardium causes extra impulses that contract the heart.
    D. Rubbing of layers of the myocardium causes extra irritation that contracts the heart.

7. **Why would a patient diagnosed with pericarditis experience swelling of the legs?**

   A. Swelling is a sign that fluid is backed up in the lungs.

   B. Fluid retained by the abdomen prevents the heart from contracting normally, resulting in decreased cardiac output.

   C. Swelling is due to fluid retention caused by Lasix, prescribed to increase cardiac output.

   D. Swelling is commonly seen in the leg and abdomen caused by pooling of blood due to decreased ability of the heart to pump blood.

8. **How can endocarditis lead to a stroke?**

   A. A patient diagnosed with endocarditis is not at risk for a stroke.

   B. The use of IV street drugs can cause a stroke in a patient diagnosed with endocarditis.

   C. The microorganism that clumps together at a site in the heart can break loose and float in the bloodstream, possibly blocking a blood vessel and leading to tissue necrosis in the brain.

   D. The stroke is caused by constrictive endocarditis.

9. **What is the purpose of implanting an intra-aortic balloon pump in a patient diagnosed with myocarditis?**

   A. A balloon is inserted into the aorta and is then inflated and deflated to increase blood flow throughout the body.

   B. The balloon is inflated to block return blood flow.

   C. The balloon filters clots from the blood to prevent a stroke.

   D. A balloon is inserted into the aorta and is then inflated and deflated to decrease blood flow throughout the body.

10. **Upon assessing a new patient you notice Osler nodes. What would you suspect?**

    A. A stroke or heart attack is imminent.

    B. The patient requires a workup for myocarditis.

    C. The patient requires a workup for pericarditis.

    D. The patient requires a workup for endocarditis.

# CORRECT ANSWERS AND RATIONALES

1. A. Bacteria in the mouth and gums could enter the bloodstream and infect the patient's heart.
2. C. The pain is due to layers of the pericardium rubbing against each other.
3. C. Tissues in the pericardium can become damaged from chronic pericarditis, resulting in scar tissues replacing tissues in the pericardium.

4. A. Lopressor is a beta-blocker that slows the contractions of the ventricles.

5. B. Myocarditis can weaken the heart, preventing the heart from efficiently pumping blood throughout the body.

6. B. Inflammation disrupts the conduction paths in the heart.

7. D. Swelling is commonly seen in the leg and abdomen caused by pooling of blood due to decreased ability of the heart to pump blood.

8. C. The microorganism that clumps together at a site in the heart can break loose and float in the bloodstream, possibly blocking a blood vessel and leading to tissue necrosis in the brain.

9. A. A balloon is inserted into the aorta and is then inflated and deflated to increase blood flow throughout the body.

10. D. The patient requires a workup for endocarditis.

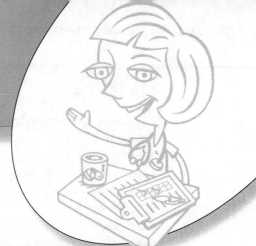

# chapter 6

# Cardiac Valve Disorders

## LEARNING OBJECTIVES

1. Valve Disorder
2. Mitral Insufficiency (MI)
3. Mitral Valve Prolapse (MVP)
4. Mitral Stenosis
5. Mitral Valve Regurgitation (MVR)
6. Tricuspid Insufficiency
7. Tricuspid (Atrioventricular) Valve Stenosis
8. Tricuspid (Atrioventricular) Valve Regurgitation (TR)
9. Pulmonary Valve Stenosis
10. Pulmonary Valve Regurgitation
11. Aortic Valve Stenosis (AS)
12. Aortic Valve Regurgitation (Incompetence)
13. Aortic Insufficiency
14. Papillary (Chordae) Muscle Rupture

## KEY TERMS

Angiotensin-Converting Enzyme
   Inhibitors
Annuloplasty
Antiarrhythmic Medications
Atrial Fibrillation
Beta-Blockers
Calcification
Calcium Channel Blocker
Carcinoid Syndrome
Cardiac Catheterization
Cardiac Valve Disorder
Cardiomyopathy
Commissurotomy

Congenital Cardiac Valve Disorder
Connective Tissue Disease
Diuretic
Echocardiograph
Infective Endocarditis
Leaky Valve
Pulsating Neck Veins
Rheumatic Fever
Torn Chordae
Valvular Insufficiency
Valvular Stenosis
Valvuloplasty
Vasodilator

# Valve Disorder

There are four chambers of the heart—right atrium, right ventricle, left atrium, and left ventricle (see Chapter 1). The right atrium receives deoxygenated blood from the circulatory system and sends deoxygenated blood to the right ventricle. The right ventricle sends deoxygenated blood to the lungs. The left atrium receives oxygenated blood from the lungs and sends oxygenated blood to the left ventricle. The left ventricle sends oxygenated blood to the circulatory system.

Each chamber of the heart has a one-way valve that allows blood to flow in one direction. The valve also prevents blood from flowing backward. These valves are the tricuspid valve, pulmonary valve, mitral valve, and aortic valve. The tricuspid valve allows blood to flow from the right atrium into the right ventricle. The pulmonary valve allows blood to flow from the right ventricle to the pulmonary artery. The mitral valve allows blood to flow from the left atrium to the left ventricle. The aortic valve allows blood to flow from the left ventricle to the aorta.

A *cardiac valve disorder* is a condition when a valve malfunctions. There are two underlying causes of cardiac valve disorder:

- **Valvular stenosis:** This occurs when the tissue in the valve become stiff, resulting in narrowing of the valve opening, reducing blood flow through the valve. Mild stiffness does not affect cardiac function. An adequate amount of blood flows through the heart without causing symptoms. However, severe stiffness reduces blood flow, resulting in inadequate blood flow throughout the body.

- **Valvular insufficiency:** This occurs when the valve does not completely close, resulting in blood flowing back into the previous chamber of the heart (**regurgitates**). Valvular insufficiency is commonly referred to as *incompetence* or simply a *leaky valve*.

There are three causes of cardiac valve disorders. These are

- **Congenital cardiac valve disorder:** This disorder occurs when the valves develop abnormally before birth. Typically the valve is of inappropriate size for the heart; the valve is not properly attached to the heart; or the valve is malformed.

- **Acquired cardiac valve disorder:** This disorder occurs when the valve malfunctions as a result of an infection.

- **Unknown:** The cause of some cardiac valve disorders is unknown.

# Mitral Insufficiency

*Mitral insufficiency* (MI) is the most common form of valvular heart disease. Patients who have MI may or may not experience symptoms depending on the phase of the disease; those who have chronic MI compensate for the disorder and may appear asymptomatic and can tolerate normal exercise.

## What Went Wrong?

Leakage of the mitral valve causes blood to flow back from the left ventricle to the left atrium. As a result, blood might flow back into the lungs. Mitral regurgitation is due to an incompetent valve, damage from rheumatic fever, coronary artery disease (CAD), or endocarditis.

## Prognosis

The prognosis may be chronic, with stabilization of symptoms, or acute (usually after myocardial infarction), leading to valve replacement.

## Hallmark Signs and Symptoms

- Orthopnea due to the pressure rising into the atria, causing backflow into the lungs.

- Fatigue because of an ineffective heart.
- Systolic murmur at the apex, $S_3$ gallop.
- Left ventricular hypertrophy—the size of the ventricle can reflect the amount of regurgitation.

## Common/Interpreting Test Results

- Echocardiogram shows the underlying etiology of the insufficiency.
- Cardiac catheterization depicts the flow through the mitral valve and can measure amount of regurgitation as well as pressures in the chambers.

## Treatment

Patients with chronic, stable disease may be managed for years without symptoms, or their symptoms may be under control with medication. Others may require surgery, depending on the symptoms. Ventricular damage may occur before symptoms present, so frequent monitoring is indicated.

- Administer vasodilators to reduce flow by lowering systemic vascular resistance.
- Administer anticoagulant medication following surgery to prevent thrombus around the aortic valve.
  - Heparin
  - Warfarin (Coumadin)
  - Dalteparin (Fragmin)
  - Enoxaparin (Lovenox)
- Mitral valve repair or replacement.

## Nursing Diagnoses

- Anxiety
- Decreased cardiac output
- Activity intolerance

## Nursing Interventions

- Place patient in a high Fowler's position to facilitate breathing.

- Monitor for
  - Pulmonary edema because of fluid overload.
  - Thrombus because of a prosthetic valve.
  - Arrhythmias because the heart may be irritable during and after surgery.
- Intake and output to monitor fluid balance.
- Weigh the patient daily to check fluid overload.
- Explain to the patient
  - Schedule rest periods during the day.
  - Restrict to low-salt and low-fat diets.

## Mitral Valve Prolapse

The mitral valve has two raised areas (cusps) that help control blood flow between the left atrium and the left ventricle by preventing blood from flowing back from the left ventricle to the left atrium.

Mitral valve prolapse (MVP) occurs when the mitral valve loses support and flops (fails) into the left atrium when the heart contracts. As a result, the valve stretches, leading to leaks.

## What Went Wrong?

MVP can be caused by damage to the mitral valve tissue or abnormal development of the mitral valve. There is also a genetic predisposition to MVP. In addition, MVP can be caused by the following:

- **Connective tissue disease:** This is a condition caused by cartilage that is malformed.
- **Torn chordae:** The chordae is a cord-like tendon that connects the papillary muscles to the mitral valve. This can be torn.
- **CAD**
- **Heart attack (myocardial infarction):** A heart attack may cause tissue damage around the mitral valve such as a torn chordae that can weaken the mitral valve, resulting in prolapse.
- **Cardiomyopathy:** This is an abnormality of the heart muscle that causes the mitral valve to weaken.

## Prognosis

Most patients with MVP are unaware they have it until symptoms start occurring. Often it is an incidental finding on an echocardiogram. A large majority of patients require no treatment other than endocarditis prophylaxis during dental and unsterile procedures. Some patients experience symptom progression, developing arrhythmias and requiring medications. Severe MVP may require mitral valve repair or replacement.

> **NURSING ALERT**
>
> MVP is classified based on thickness and displacement; symmetric or asymmetric tips of the leaflet; and whether or not leaflet tip turns outward (flail) or inward (nonflail).

## Hallmark Signs and Symptoms

Patients diagnosed with MVP experience no symptoms. Rarely patients are symptomatic. Those who do experience symptoms report

- **Palpitations:** Increase in the heart rate is the result of compensation of the heart for the reduced blood flow through the mitral valve.
- **Fatigue:** Fatigue is caused by decreased circulation of oxygenated blood.
- **Chest pains:** These are associated with increased activity of the heart related to the narrowing of the mitral valve.
- **Shortness of breath when lying flat (orthopnea) or during activity:** Abnormal opening of the mitral valve increases pressure that backs up blood into the lungs. Lying down causes increased pressure on the lungs.
- **Dizziness:** This is related to decreased circulation of oxygenated blood.
- **Late systolic murmur:** A murmur is an extra heart sound caused by actions of the prolapsed mitral valve.

## Common/Interpreting Test Results

When the patient is symptomatic, a late systolic murmur is initially detected when listening to the patient's heart. If MVP is suspected, then the following test is performed:

- **Echocardiograph:** This provides a two- and three-dimensional look at the functioning heart. The mitral valve leaflets are measured for thickness and displacement.

> **NURSING ALERT**
>
> Surgical repair of the mitral valve is preferred over replacing the mitral valve since repairing has fewer side effects.

## Treatment

No treatment is necessary if the patient is asymptomatic. If the patient is symptomatic, then the following treatment may be necessary:

- **Beta-blockers:** These are a class of medications that slow the contractions of the ventricles and are prescribed if the patient reports palpitations and chest pains. The most commonly prescribed is metoprolol (Toprol, Lopressor).
- **Surgical repair:** Surgical repair of the mitral valve is performed when the patient experiences severe symptoms.

> **NURSING ALERT**
>
> A patient diagnosed with MVP should take antibiotic prophylaxis before a procedure such as dental treatment because he/she is at a higher risk for infective endocarditis.

## Nursing Diagnoses

- Anxiety
- Decreased cardiac output
- Activity intolerance

## Nursing Interventions

- Place patient in a high Fowler's position to facilitate breathing.
- After surgery, monitor for
  - Pulmonary edema to look for blood flowing back into lungs.
  - Heart failure to assess for a poorly functioning heart.
  - Thrombus because of a prosthetic valve.
  - Arrhythmias because the heart may be irritated after surgery.
  - Arterial blood gas (ABG) to check for adequate oxygenation and acid-base balance.
- Weigh the patient daily to assess for fluid overload.

- Explain to the patient
  - Proper recovery from major surgery.
  - Schedule rest periods during the day.
  - Restrict to low-sodium and low-fat diets.

# Mitral Stenosis

Mitral stenosis is the narrowing (stenosis) of the opening of the mitral valve. Stenosis reduces blood flow into the left ventricle, causing a buildup of blood in the lungs and throughout the body, leading to swelling of the ankles and feet and difficulty breathing.

Decreased blood flow from the left atrium into the left ventricle causes the heart to work harder, leading to an irregular heartbeat (arrhythmia) that may increase the risk of blood pooling, leading to blood clots.

## What Went Wrong?

Scaring of the mitral valve from rheumatic fever is the most common cause of mitral stenosis. Other less common causes are as follows:

- **Congenital heart defects:** A congenital heart defect is a malformation of the heart at birth.
- **Calcification of the mitral valve:** Increased calcium in the blood forms deposits on the mitral valve, causing it to narrow.
- **Infective endocarditis:** Endocarditis is an infection of the inner lining of the heart called the *endocardium* and can cause tissue damage to the mitral valve.

## Prognosis

Mitral valve stenosis may be asymptomatic for years, never needing attention. However, eventually symptoms may occur and progress, necessitating intervention. Medication may be enough, or surgical intervention may be necessary.

## Hallmark Signs and Symptoms

The patient is typically asymptomatic in the early stage of mitral stenosis. In later stages the patient may report the following symptoms:

- **Palpitations:** Increase in the heart rate is the result of compensation of the heart for the reduced blood flow through the mitral valve.

- **Chest pains:** These are associated with increased activity of the heart related to the narrowing of the mitral valve.
- **Shortness of breath when lying flat (orthopnea) or during activity:** Narrowing of the mitral valve increases pressure that backs up blood into the lungs. Lying down causes increased pressure on the lungs.
- **Edema:** Decreased circulation of blood flow to the left ventricle causes heart failure, resulting in swelling usually in the legs.
- **Atrial fibrillation:** This is caused by the atrium's inability to contract properly due to the narrowing of the mitral valve.
- **Risk for blood clots (thromboembolism):** Decreased ability of blood to flow properly through mitral valve results in pooling of blood in the atrium, increasing the risk of blood clots.
- **Fatigue:** Fatigue is caused by decreased circulation of oxygenated blood.
- **Coughing with blood-tinged sputum:** Narrowing of the mitral valve increases pressure that backs up blood into the lungs, resulting in coughing and blood-tinged sputum.

## Common/Interpreting Test Results

When the patient is symptomatic, arrhythmia is initially detected when listening to the patient's heart. If arrhythmia is suspected, then the following tests are performed:

- **Chest X-ray:** A chest X-ray shows the size and shape of the heart. An enlarged heart is a complication of mitral stenosis.
- **Electrocardiogram (ECG):** The ECG (see Chapter 4) measures impulse condition of the heart and will indicate atrial fibrillation.
- **Transthoracic echocardiogram:** A device called a *transducer* sends sound waves through the chest wall. The heart deflects sound waves back to the transducer, which sends a corresponding image of the heart on a screen. A trained practitioner can visualize the structure and function of the heart.
- **Transesophageal echocardiogram:** A transducer is passed into the patient's esophagus, which sends sound waves to the heart. The image is similar to transthoracic echocardiogram.
- **Cardiac catheterization:** This is a procedure that involves passing a thin flexible tube called a *catheter* through blood vessels either in the groin or arm or into the heart. Dye is injected through the catheter, making the heart visible on an X-ray.

## Treatment

No treatment is provided unless the patient is symptomatic. The following medications are administered to reduce the workload of the heart and help return the heart to normal rhythm, which reduces symptoms.

- **Diuretics:** A diuretic (furosemide [Lasix]) reduces fluid retention by excreting excess fluids.

- **Anticoagulant medication:** This medication reduces the risk of formation of blood clots. Commonly prescribed anticoagulant medications are heparin, enoxaparin (Lovenox), dalteparin (Fragmin), argatroban, bivalirudin (Angiomax), fondaparinux (Arixtra), lepirudin (Refludan), warfarin (Coumadin), and dabigatran (Pradaxa).

- **Beta-blockers:** These are a class of medications that slow the contractions of the ventricles. The most commonly prescribed is metoprolol (Toprol, Lopressor).

- **Calcium channel blocker:** This medication also slows the contractions of the ventricles. The most commonly prescribed are verapamil (Calan) and diltiazem (Cardizem).

- **Antiarrhythmic medication:** These medications cause the heart to maintain normal sinus rhythm. These include flecainide acetate (Tambocor), propafenone (Rhythmol), sotalol (Betapace), dofetilide (Tikosyn), and amiodarone (Cordarone).

Nonsurgical procedures and surgical procedures can be used to reduce the stenosis.

- **Valvuloplasty:** This is a nonsurgical procedure where a balloon-tipped catheter is inserted into a blood vessel in the patient's groin or arm and is moved into the mitral valve. The balloon is then inflated, widening the mitral valve. The balloon is then deflated and removed.

- **Commissurotomy:** This is an open-heart surgery during which the mitral valve is cleared of scar tissue or calcium deposits, increasing blood flow through the mitral valve.

- **Mitral valve replacement:** The mitral valve is surgically removed and replaced by either a mechanical device or tissues from a pig, cow, or deceased human donor. Mechanical mitral valves carry an ongoing risk for blood clots.

### NURSING ALERT

Commissurotomy may have to be repeated if mitral valve stenosis reoccurs.

## Nursing Diagnoses

- Anxiety
- Decreased cardiac output
- Activity intolerance

## Nursing Interventions

- Place patient in a high Fowler's position to ease breathing.
- Monitor for
  - Pulmonary edema caused by a complication of surgery.
  - Thrombus because of a prosthetic valve.
  - Arrhythmias because of an irritated heart; patient may feel palpitations, anxiety.
  - ABG to monitor for oxygenation, acidosis, and alkalosis.
- Weigh the patient daily to determine fluid balance.
- Explain to the patient
  - Be aware of signs and symptoms and to report changes in condition.
  - Schedule rest periods during the day.
  - Restrict to low-sodium and low-fat diets.

# Mitral Valve Regurgitation

Mitral valve regurgitation (MVR) occurs when the mitral valve does not close tightly, resulting in blood flowing backward (retrograde) from the left ventricle to the left atrium. Depending on the severity of the leak, blood flow may be interrupted slightly; in severe leaks, blood flow is disrupted sufficiently to cause the patient to feel tired and cause fluid buildup in the lungs (acute pulmonary edema), resulting in shortness of breath and swelling in the legs.

## What Went Wrong?

MVR can be caused by a congenital defect in the mitral valve at birth. This is referred to as *primary mitral regurgitation* because there is no underlying cause of the leak. Secondary MVR has an underlying cause for the leak, which could be a congenital defect of the left ventricle or one of the following:

- **MVP:** This (see Mitral Valve Prolapse) occurs when the mitral valve loses support and flops (fails) into the left atrium when the heart contracts.
- **Torn chordae:** The chordae is a cord-like tendon that connects the papillary muscles to the mitral valve. This can be torn.
- **Infective endocarditis:** Endocarditis is an infection of the inner lining of the heart called the *endocardium* and can cause tissue damage to the mitral valve.
- **Rheumatic fever:** Rheumatic fever is the result of untreated strep throat that can leave scar tissues on the mitral valve.
- **Heart attack:** A heart attack can cause tissue damage to the mitral valve.
- **Cardiomyopathy:** This is an abnormality of the heart muscle as a result of years of high blood pressure and conditions that make the heart work hard, resulting in an enlarged left ventricle that stretches tissues around the mitral valve.

## Prognosis

MVR can lead to irreversible damage to the heart if not corrected by surgery. The patient's heart can weaken and may develop heart failure, atrial fibrillation, and endocarditis.

## Hallmark Signs and Symptoms

The patient may be asymptomatic if the leak is mild and not realize the leak exists. Symptoms can develop quickly. In more severe leaks, the patient will report the following:

- **Palpitations:** Increase in the heart rate is the result of compensation of the heart for the blood flowing backward through the mitral valve.
- **Shortness of breath when lying flat (orthopnea) or during activity:** The backward blood flow through the mitral valve increases pressure that backs up blood into the lungs. Lying down causes increased pressure on the lungs.
- **Edema:** Decreased circulation of blood flow to the left ventricle causes heart failure, resulting in swelling usually in the legs.
- **Fatigue:** Fatigue is caused by decreased circulation of oxygenated blood.
- **Coughing at night:** Backflow of blood through mitral valve increases pressure that backs up blood into the lungs, resulting in coughing.

## Common/Interpreting Test Results

When the patient is symptomatic, heart murmur (abnormal sound) is initially detected when listening to the patient's heart. If heart murmur is suspected, then the following tests are performed:

- **Chest X-ray:** A chest X-ray shows the size and shape of the heart. An enlarged heart is a complication of mitral stenosis.

- **ECG:** The ECG (see Chapter 4) measures impulse condition of the heart and will indicate atrial fibrillation.

- **Transthoracic echocardiogram:** A device called a *transducer* sends sound waves through the chest wall. The heart deflects sound waves back to the transducer, which sends a corresponding image of the heart on a screen. A trained practitioner can visualize the structure and function of the heart.

- **Transesophageal echocardiogram:** A transducer is passed into the patient's esophagus, which sends sound waves to the heart. The image is similar to a transthoracic echocardiogram.

- **Cardiac catheterization:** This is a procedure that involves passing a thin flexible tube called a *catheter* through blood vessels either in the groin or arm or into the heart. Dye is injected through the catheter, making the heart visible on an X-ray.

## Treatment

No treatment is provided if the patient is asymptomatic. If the patient is symptomatic, he/she is prescribed medication to reduce the symptoms and the risk of complications from MVR. A patient with severe symptoms may undergo corrective surgery.

- **Diuretics:** A diuretic (furosemide [Lasix]) reduces fluid retention by excreting excess fluids.

- **Anticoagulant medication:** This medication reduces the risk of formation of blood clots. Commonly prescribed anticoagulant medications are heparin, enoxaparin (Lovenox), dalteparin (Fragmin), argatroban, bivalirudin (Angiomax), fondaparinux (Arixtra), lepirudin (Refludan), warfarin (Coumadin), and dabigatran (Pradaxa).

- **Surgical repair:** Surgical repair of the mitral valve is performed to tighten or replace the ring around the valve (**annuloplasty**) or to reconnect torn cords or remove excess tissue.

- **Mitral valve replacement:** The mitral valve is surgically removed and replaced by either a mechanical device or tissues from a pig, cow, or deceased human donor. Mechanical mitral valves carry an ongoing risk for blood clots.

## Nursing Diagnoses

- Anxiety
- Decreased cardiac output
- Activity intolerance

## Nursing Interventions

- Place patient in a high Fowler's position to facilitate breathing.
- After surgery, monitor for
  - Pulmonary edema to look for blood flowing back into lungs.
  - Heart failure to assess for a poorly functioning heart.
  - Thrombus because of a prosthetic valve.
  - Arrhythmias because the heart may be irritated after surgery.
  - ABG to check for adequate oxygenation and acid-base balance.
- Weigh the patient daily to assess for fluid overload.
- Explain to the patient
  - Proper recovery from major surgery.
  - Schedule rest periods during the day.
  - Restrict to low-sodium and low-fat diets.

# Tricuspid Insufficiency

Tricuspid insufficiency is a congenital disorder that leads to the dilation of the right ventricle, preventing the muscles and valves of the tricuspid to close properly. Tricuspid insufficiency can also be secondary to other disorders.

## What Went Wrong?

Leakage in the tricuspid valve causes a backflow from the right ventricle to the right atrium. This results in increased pressure in the atrium and higher resistance to blood flowing from veins, resulting in enlargement of the right atrium. This may occur from an anatomic problem, but usually occurs from right ventricular over-load (in turn caused by left ventricular overload). It may also occur due to an inferior myocardial infarction or damage from endocarditis.

## Prognosis

If the underlying problem can be resolved, the insufficiency may subside. If resolution does not occur, tricuspid valve repair or replacement may be necessary.

## Hallmark Signs and Symptoms

- Difficulty breathing (dyspnea) due to backflow into the lungs.
- Fatigue because the heart is working inefficiently.
- Jugular venous distention due to overload in the right atrium.
- Hepatic congestion from backflow.
- $S_3$ murmur upon inspiration.

## Common/Interpreting Test Results

- X-ray shows enlarged right ventricle and right atrium because of volume overload.
- Echocardiogram depicts prolapsed tricuspid valve and enlarged right side of the heart.
- ECG depicts enlarged right ventricle and right atrium, characterized by broad P and QRS waves.

## Treatment

- Correct any underlying heart disease to reduce pressure on the right atrium, ventricle, and thus, the valve.
- Administer anticoagulant medication following surgery to prevent throm-bus around the tricuspid valve.
  - Heparin
  - Warfarin (Coumadin)
  - Dalteparin (Fragmin)
  - Enoxaparin (Lovenox)
- Tricuspid valve repair or replacement.

## Nursing Diagnoses

- Anxiety
- Decreased cardiac output
- Activity intolerance

## Nursing Interventions

- Place patient in a high Fowler's position to facilitate breathing.
- Monitor for
  - Pulmonary edema because backflow to the lungs may occur.
  - Heart failure to assess cardiac function.
  - Thrombus because of a prosthetic valve.
  - Arrhythmias because the heart may be irritable.
  - ABG to assess for adequate oxygenation and acid-base balance.
- Weigh the patient daily to look for fluid overload.
- Explain to the patient
  - Symptoms to look for.
  - Schedule rest periods during the day.
  - Restrict to low-sodium and low-fat diets.

# Tricuspid (Atrioventricular) Valve Stenosis

Tricuspid valve stenosis is the narrowing of the tricuspid valve as a result of thickening or stiffness that prevents the valve from completely opening. The stenosis reduces blood flow from the right atrium to the right ventricle, disrupting normal blood flow, which can lead to the patient reporting symptoms.

## What Went Wrong?

The cause of tricuspid valve stenosis is usually an underlying condition (secondary), although congenital abnormalities (primary) are less common. Common causes of tricuspid valve stenosis are as follows:

- **Infective endocarditis:** Endocarditis is an infection of the inner lining of the heart called the *endocardium* and can cause tissue damage to the mitral valve.

- **Rheumatic fever:** Rheumatic fever is the result of untreated strep throat that can leave scar tissue on the mitral valve.
- **Cardiomyopathy:** This is an abnormality of the heart muscle as a result of years of high blood pressure and conditions that make the heart work hard, resulting in an enlarged left ventricle that stretches tissues around the mitral valve.

## Prognosis

Untreated tricuspid valve stenosis can lead to an enlarged right atrium that can alter pressure and blood flow to the heart. The patient's symptoms should decrease after treatment; however, the patient should be monitored regularly for cardiac disorders.

> **NURSING ALERT**
>
> A patient diagnosed with tricuspid valve stenosis is at risk for endocarditis and requires prophylactic antibiotic treatment before any routine medical or dental procedure.

## Hallmark Signs and Symptoms

The patient may be asymptomatic if the stenosis is mild and may not realize that the condition exists. In more severe narrowing, the patient will report

- **Fatigue:** Fatigue is caused by decreased circulation of oxygenated blood.
- **Shortness of breath when lying flat (orthopnea) or during activity:** The backward blood flow through the tricuspid valve increases pressure that backs up blood into the lungs. Lying down causes increased pressure on the lungs.
- **Edema:** Decreased circulation of blood flow to the right ventricle causes heart failure, resulting in swelling usually in the legs.
- **Rapid weight gain:** Decreased circulation can result in fluid retention, leading to rapid weight gain.
- **Fluttering feeling in the neck:** Fluttering is caused by irregular heart rate as a result of disruption of blood flow.
- **Atrial fibrillation:** This is caused by the atrium's inability to contract properly due to the narrowing of the tricuspid valve.

- **Risk for blood clots (thromboembolism):** Decreased ability of blood to flow properly through tricuspid valve results in pooling of blood, increasing the risk of blood clots.
- **Palpitations:** Increase in the heart rate is the result of compensation of the heart for the reduced blood flow through the mitral valve.

## Common/Interpreting Test Results

When the patient is symptomatic, arrhythmia is initially detected when listening to the patient's heart. If arrhythmia is suspected, then the following tests are performed:

- **Chest X-ray:** A chest X-ray shows the size and shape of the heart. An enlarged heart is a complication of mitral stenosis.
- **ECG:** The ECG (see Chapter 4) measures impulse condition of the heart and will indicate atrial fibrillation.
- **Transthoracic echocardiogram:** A device called a *transducer* sends sound waves through the chest wall. The heart deflects sound waves back to the transducer, which send a corresponding image of the heart on a screen. A trained practitioner can visualize the structure and function of the heart.
- **Transesophageal echocardiogram:** A transducer is passed into the patient's esophagus, which sends sound waves to the heart. The image is similar to transthoracic echocardiogram.
- **Cardiac catheterization:** This is a procedure that involves passing a thin flexible tube called a *catheter* through blood vessels either in the groin or arm or into the heart. Dye is injected through the catheter, making the heart visible on an X-ray.

## Treatment

No treatment is necessary if the patient is asymptomatic. If the patient is symptomatic, medications are prescribed to lessen the symptoms. If the patient has severe symptoms, then surgical intervention is necessary.

- **Diuretics:** A diuretic (furosemide [Lasix]) reduces fluid retention by excreting excess fluids.
- **Anticoagulant medication:** This medication reduces the risk of formation of blood clots. Commonly prescribed anticoagulant medications are heparin, enoxaparin (Lovenox), dalteparin (Fragmin), argatroban,

bivalirudin (Angiomax), fondaparinux (Arixtra), lepirudin (Refludan), warfarin (Coumadin), and dabigatran (Pradaxa).

- **Beta-blockers:** These are a class of medications that slow the contractions of the ventricles. The most commonly prescribed is metoprolol (Toprol, Lopressor).

- **Calcium channel blocker:** This medication also slows the contractions of the ventricles. The most commonly prescribed are verapamil (Calan) and diltiazem (Cardizem).

- **Antiarrhythmic medication:** These medications cause the heart to maintain normal sinus rhythm. These include flecainide acetate (Tambocor), propafenone (Rhythmol), sotalol (Betapace), dofetilide (Tikosyn), and amiodarone (Cordarone).

- **Angiotensin-converting enzyme (ACE) inhibitors:** ACE inhibitors prevent the production of the angiotensin II enzyme that causes blood vessels to narrow. As a result, blood vessels relax (dilate) easing the flow of blood throughout the body. Commonly prescribed ACE inhibitors are enalapril (Vasotec), captopril (Capoten), lisinopril (Zestril, Prinivil), and ramipril (Altace).

- **Vasodilators:** This is a class of medication that causes blood vessels to widen. The commonly prescribed vasodilator is sodium nitroprusside (Nitropress).

- **Valvuloplasty:** This is a nonsurgical procedure where a balloon-tipped catheter is inserted into a blood vessel in the patient's groin or arm and is moved into the tricuspid valve. The balloon is then inflated, widening the tricuspid valve. The balloon is then deflated and removed.

- **Commissurotomy:** This is an open-heart surgery during which the tricuspid valve is cleared of scar tissue or calcium deposits, increasing blood flow through the tricuspid valve.

- **Tricuspid valve replacement:** The tricuspid valve is surgically removed and replaced by either a mechanical device or tissues from a pig, cow, or deceased human donor. Mechanical tricuspid valves carry an ongoing risk for blood clots.

## Nursing Diagnoses

- Anxiety
- Decreased cardiac output
- Activity intolerance

## Nursing Interventions

- Place patient in a high Fowler's position to facilitate breathing.
- After surgery, monitor for
  - Pulmonary edema to look for blood flowing back into lungs.
  - Heart failure to assess for a poorly functioning heart.
  - Thrombus because of a prosthetic valve.
  - Arrhythmias because the heart may be irritated after surgery.
  - ABG to check for adequate oxygenation and acid-base balance.
- Weigh the patient daily to assess for fluid overload.
- Explain to the patient
  - Proper recovery from major surgery.
  - Schedule rest periods during the day.
  - Restrict to low-sodium and low-fat diets.

# Tricuspid (Atrioventricular) Valve Regurgitation

Tricuspid valve regurgitation (TR) occurs when blood flows back from the right ventricle into the right atrium when the former contracts. The backflow, called *retrograde,* is the result of incomplete closure of the tricuspid valve, which is seen in late stages of right-sided heart failure. Right-sided heart failure occurs following left-sided heart failure that causes increased blood pressure in the lungs, leading to damage to the right side of the heart.

## What Went Wrong?

The most common cause of TR is an enlarged right ventricle as a result of left-sided heart failure. The right ventricle supplies blood to the lungs; however, blood pressure increases during left-sided heart failure, resulting in increased resistance to blood flow into the lungs, causing the right ventricles to compensate. The overworked right ventricles increase in size, resulting in distortion around the tricuspid valve. Other causes of tricuspid valve regurgitation are as follows:

- **Infective endocarditis:** Endocarditis is an infection of the inner lining of the heart called the endocardium and can cause tissue damage to the tricuspid valve.

- **Cardiomyopathy:** This is an abnormality of the heart muscle as a result of years of high blood pressure and conditions that make the heart work hard, resulting in an enlarged left ventricle that stretches tissues around the tricuspid valve.

- **Congenital heart defects:** A congenital heart defect is a malformation of the heart at birth. Ebstein anomaly is a congenital defect of the tricuspid valve.

## Prognosis

If treated, the prognosis is good. However, the patient may experience pulmonary hypertension and cardiac dilation as a result of untreated TR. The patient may be at risk for ascites, embolization, and cardiac cirrhosis.

## Hallmark Signs and Symptoms

Patients who are diagnosed with TR report the following symptoms:

- **Edema:** Decreased circulation of blood flow to the right ventricle causes heart failure, resulting in swelling usually in the legs and abdomen.

- **Fatigue:** Fatigue is caused by decreased circulation of oxygenated blood.

- **Pulsating neck veins:** These are caused by increased blood pressure because of the disruption of blood flow related to the underlying cause of TR.

- **Decreased urination:** Decreased urination is caused by disruption of blood flow that reduces adequate blood flow to the kidneys.

## Common/Interpreting Test Results

Some patients are asymptomatic. In symptomatic patients, the physical assessment may reveal an enlarged liver or an enlarged spleen, and a pulse over the liver, indicating increased blood pressure along with a heart murmur. The following tests will likely be ordered if these signs are present.

- **Chest X-ray:** A chest X-ray shows the size and shape of the heart. An enlarged heart is a complication of mitral stenosis.

- **ECG:** The ECG (see Chapter 4) measures impulse condition of the heart and will indicate atrial fibrillation.

- **Transthoracic echocardiogram:** A device called a *transducer* sends sound waves through the chest wall. The heart deflects sound waves back to the transducer, which sends a corresponding image of the heart on a screen. A trained practitioner can visualize the structure and function of the heart.

- **Transesophageal echocardiogram:** A transducer is passed into the patient's esophagus, which sends sound waves to the heart. The image is similar to transthoracic echocardiogram.
- **Cardiac catheterization:** This is a procedure that involves passing a thin flexible tube called a *catheter* through blood vessels either in the groin or arm or into the heart. Dye is injected through the catheter, making the heart visible on an X-ray.

## Treatment

Treatment of TR focuses on treating symptoms with medication. In severe cases, surgical intervention is necessary.

- **Diuretics:** A diuretic (furosemide [Lasix]) reduces fluid retention by excreting increased fluids.
- **Beta-blockers:** These are a class of medications that slow the contractions of the ventricles. The most commonly prescribed is metoprolol (Toprol, Lopressor).
- **Calcium channel blocker:** This medication also slows the contractions of the ventricles. The most commonly prescribed are verapamil (Calan) and diltiazem (Cardizem).
- **Surgical repair:** Surgical repair of the tricuspid valve is performed to tighten or replace the ring around the valve (**annuloplasty**) or to reconnect torn cords or remove excess tissue.
- **Tricuspid valve replacement:** The tricuspid valve is surgically removed and replaced by either a mechanical device or tissues from a pig, cow, or deceased human donor. Mechanical tricuspid valves carry an ongoing risk for blood clots.

## Nursing Diagnoses

- Anxiety
- Decreased cardiac output
- Activity intolerance

## Nursing Interventions

- Place patient in a high Fowler's position to facilitate breathing.
- After surgery, monitor for
  - Pulmonary edema to look for blood flowing back into lungs.
  - Heart failure to assess for a poorly functioning heart.
  - Thrombus because of a prosthetic valve.
  - Arrhythmias because the heart may be irritated after surgery.
  - ABG to check for adequate oxygenation and acid-base balance.
- Weigh the patient daily to assess for fluid overload.
- Explain to the patient
  - Proper recovery from major surgery.
  - Schedule rest periods during the day.
  - Restrict to low-sodium and low-fat diets.

# Pulmonary Valve Stenosis

Pulmonary valve stenosis is the narrowing of the pulmonary valve, decreasing blood flow from the right ventricle to the pulmonary artery. The pulmonary artery carries deoxygenated blood from the right ventricle to the lungs. Pulmonary valve stenosis typically is diagnosed in childhood as a result of congenital defect.

## What Went Wrong?

Pulmonary valve stenosis is commonly caused by congenital abnormal development of the pulmonary valve. The result is thick leaflets in the pulmonary valve or leaflets that do not separate during development. Other causes are as follows:

- **Rheumatic fever:** Rheumatic fever is the result of untreated strep throat that can leave scar tissue on the pulmonary valve.
- **Carcinoid syndrome:** Carcinoid syndrome is the release of serotonin from carcinoid tumors in the digestive system. Serotonin can cause narrowing of the pulmonary valve.

## Prognosis

The prognosis for a patient who is treated for pulmonary valve stenosis is good. If the patient has severe pulmonary valve stenosis, the patient may be at risk for arrhythmia, heart failure, infection, and cardiomyopathy.

## Hallmark Signs and Symptoms

The patient may be asymptomatic and not realize there is pulmonary valve stenosis. As symptoms materialize, the patient reports:

- **Fatigue:** Fatigue is caused by decreased circulation of oxygenated blood.
- **Palpitations:** Increase in the heart rate is the result of compensation of the heart for the reduced blood flow through the pulmonary valve.
- **Shortness of breath during activity:** There is a decrease in oxygenated blood resulting from the pulmonary valve stenosis.
- **Chest pains:** These are associated with increased activity of the heart related to the narrowing of the pulmonary valve.
- **Fainting (syncope):** Decreased circulation of oxygenated blood can cause temporary loss of consciousness.

## Common/Interpreting Test Results

When the patient is symptomatic, heart murmur (abnormal sound) is initially detected when listening to the patient's heart. The murmur appears in the upper left area of the chest. If heart murmur is suspected, then the following tests are performed:

- **Chest X-ray:** A chest X-ray shows the size and shape of the heart. An enlarged heart is a complication of mitral stenosis.
- **ECG:** The ECG (see Chapter 4) measures impulse condition of the heart.
- **Transthoracic echocardiogram:** A device called a *transducer* sends sound waves through the chest wall. The heart deflects sound waves back to the transducer, which send a corresponding image of the heart on a screen. A trained practitioner can visualize the structure and function of the heart.
- **Transesophageal echocardiogram:** A transducer is passed into the patient's esophagus, which sends sound waves to the heart. The image is similar to transthoracic echocardiogram.

- **Cardiac catheterization:** This is a procedure that involves passing a thin flexible tube called a *catheter* through blood vessels either in the groin or arm or into the heart. Dye is injected through the catheter, making the heart visible on an X-ray.

## Treatment

No treatment is provided unless the patient is symptomatic. Treatment is

- **Valvuloplasty:** This is a nonsurgical procedure where a balloon-tipped catheter is inserted into a blood vessel in the patient's groin or arm and is moved into the pulmonary valve. The balloon is then inflated, widening the pulmonary valve. The balloon is then deflated and removed.
- **Pulmonary valve replacement:** The pulmonary valve is surgically removed and replaced by either a mechanical device or tissues from a pig, cow, or deceased human donor. Mechanical pulmonary valves carry an ongoing risk for blood clots.

## Nursing Diagnoses

- Anxiety
- Decreased cardiac output
- Activity intolerance

## Nursing Interventions

- Place patient in a high Fowler's position to facilitate breathing.
- After surgery, monitor for
  - Pulmonary edema to look for blood flowing back into lungs.
  - Heart failure to assess for a poorly functioning heart.
  - Thrombus because of a prosthetic valve.
  - Arrhythmias because the heart may be irritated after surgery.
  - ABG to check for adequate oxygenation and acid-base balance.
- Weigh the patient daily to assess for fluid overload.
- Explain to the patient
  - Proper recovery from major surgery.
  - Schedule rest periods during the day.
  - Restrict to low-sodium and low-fat diets.

# Pulmonary Valve Regurgitation

Pulmonary valve regurgitation is the backflow of blood from the pulmonary artery into the right ventricle because pressure is higher in the pulmonary artery than in the right ventricle. Volume of blood in the right ventricle increases, leading to right ventricle failure. A small amount of blood may flow backward into the right ventricle without causing any symptoms.

## What Went Wrong?

Pulmonary valve regurgitation is commonly caused by congenital abnormal development of the pulmonary valve. The result is malformation of the pulmonary valve preventing a secure seal. Other causes are as follows:

- **Rheumatic fever:** Rheumatic fever is the result of untreated strep throat that can leave scar tissues on the pulmonary valve, preventing a good seal.
- **Infective endocarditis:** Endocarditis is an infection of the inner lining of the heart called the *endocardium* and can cause tissue damage to the pulmonary valve.
- **Pulmonary hypertension:** Pulmonary hypertension is increased pressure in the pulmonary arteries caused by blood in the lungs (pulmonary emboli), chronic obstructive pulmonary disease (COPD), or connective tissue disorder.
- **Carcinoid syndrome:** Carcinoid syndrome is the release of serotonin from carcinoid tumors in the digestive system. Serotonin can cause leakage of the pulmonary valve.

## Prognosis

Prognosis is good if the patient undergoes treatment. In severe cases, the patient may be at risk for heart failure, pulmonary hypertension, and an enlarged heart.

## Hallmark Signs and Symptoms

The patient may be asymptomatic expect for symptoms of a viral infection (ie, headache, body ache).

- **Shortness of breath during activity:** The backward blood flow through the pulmonary valve decreases the amount of blood that can be oxygenated by the lungs.

- **Rapid breathing:** There is an increase in carbon dioxide in the blood (respiratory acidosis). The body compensates by increasing breathing to expel carbon dioxide.

- **Fatigue:** Fatigue is caused by decreased circulation of oxygenated blood.

- **Arrhythmia:** Arrhythmia is an irregular heartbeat caused by disruption of oxygenated blood flow.

## Common/Interpreting Test Results

When the patient is symptomatic, the following tests are performed:

- **Chest X-ray:** A chest X-ray shows the size and shape of the heart.

- **ECG:** The ECG (see Chapter 4) measures impulse condition of the heart.

- **Transthoracic echocardiogram:** A device called a *transducer* sends sound waves through the chest wall. The heart deflects sound waves back to the transducer, which sends a corresponding image of the heart on a screen. A trained practitioner can visualize the structure and function of the heart.

- **Transesophageal echocardiogram:** A transducer is passed into the patient's esophagus, which sends sound waves to the heart. The image is similar to transthoracic echocardiogram.

- **Cardiac catheterization:** This is a procedure that involves passing a thin flexible tube called a *catheter* through blood vessels either in the groin or arm or into the heart. Dye is injected through the catheter, making the heart visible on an X-ray.

## Treatment

Treatment focuses on resolving the underlying cause of pulmonary valve regurgitation.

- **Beta-blockers:** These are a class of medications that slow the contractions of the ventricles. The most commonly prescribed is metoprolol (Toprol, Lopressor).

- **Calcium channel blocker:** This medication also slows the contractions of the ventricles. The most commonly prescribed are verapamil (Calan) and diltiazem (Cardizem).

- **Antiarrhythmic medication:** These medications cause the heart to maintain normal sinus rhythm. These include flecainide acetate (Tambocor), propafenone (Rhythmol), sotalol (Betapace), dofetilide (Tikosyn), and amiodarone (Cordarone).

- **Pulmonary valve replacement:** The pulmonary valve is surgically removed and replaced by either a mechanical device or tissues from a pig, cow, or deceased human donor. Mechanical pulmonary valves carry an ongoing risk for blood clots.

> **NURSING ALERT**
>
> Pulmonary valve replacement is rarely performed.

## Nursing Diagnoses

- Anxiety
- Decreased cardiac output
- Activity intolerance

## Nursing Interventions

- Place patient in a high Fowler's position to facilitate breathing.
- After surgery, monitor for
  - Pulmonary edema to look for blood flowing back into lungs.
  - Heart failure to assess for a poorly functioning heart.
  - Thrombus because of a prosthetic valve.
  - Arrhythmias because the heart may be irritated after surgery.
  - ABG to check for adequate oxygenation and acid-base balance.
- Weigh the patient daily to assess for fluid overload.
- Explain to the patient:
  - Proper recovery from major surgery.
  - Schedule rest periods during the day.
  - Restrict to low-sodium and low-fat diets.

# Aortic Valve Stenosis

Aortic valve stenosis (AS) is the narrowing of the aortic valve that decreases blood flow between the left ventricle and the aorta. The aortic valve opens when pressure in the left ventricle rises above pressure in the aorta, causing blood to enter the aorta and the circulatory system. Narrowing of the aortic valve prevents the aortic valve from completely opening, resulting in ejection of blood flow into the aorta; as a result, the left ventricle works harder to pump blood, leading to a weakened left ventricle and heart failure.

## What Went Wrong?

Aortic valve stenosis can be caused by the following:

- **Congenital heart defects:** A congenital heart defect is a malformation of the aortic valve at birth.
- **Calcification of the aortic valve:** Increased calcium in the blood forms deposits on the aortic valve, causing the aortic valve to narrow. This occurs with adults over 65 years of age.
- **Rheumatic fever:** Rheumatic fever is the result of untreated strep throat that can leave scar tissue on the aortic valve.

## Prognosis

Prognosis is good for a patient who undergoes treatment. If left untreated, the patient may be at risk for angina, fainting, heart failure, arrhythmias, and cardiac arrest.

## Hallmark Signs and Symptoms

Symptoms occur gradually and may not be associated with AS. A patient diagnosed with AS will report the following symptoms:

- **Fatigue:** Fatigue is caused by decreased circulation of oxygenated blood.
- **Shortness of breath during activity:** The backward blood flow through the aortic valve decreases the amount of blood that can be oxygenated by the lungs.
- **Chest pains:** These are associated with increased activity of the heart related to the narrowing of the aortic valve.
- **Fainting (syncope):** Decreased circulation of oxygenated blood can cause temporary loss of consciousness.
- **Palpitations:** Increase in the heart rate is the result of compensation of the heart for the reduced blood flow through the aortic valve.
- **Edema:** Decreased systematic blood flow to aortic stenosis causes heart failure, resulting in swelling usually in the legs.

## Common/Interpreting Test Results

A heart murmur is detected on a routine assessment. The following tests are then ordered:

- **ECG:** The ECG (see Chapter 4) measures impulse condition of the heart and will indicate atrial fibrillation.

- **Transthoracic echocardiogram:** A device called a *transducer* sends sound waves through the chest wall. The heart deflects sound waves back to the transducer, which send a corresponding image of the heart on a screen. A trained practitioner can visualize the structure and function of the heart.

- **Transesophageal echocardiogram:** A transducer is passed into the patient's esophagus, which sends sound waves to the heart. The image is similar to transthoracic echocardiogram.

- **Chest X-ray:** A chest X-ray shows the size and shape of the heart. An enlarged heart is a complication of mitral stenosis.

- **Cardiac catheterization:** This is a procedure that involves passing a thin flexible tube called a *catheter* through blood vessels either in the groin or arm or into the heart. Dye is injected through the catheter, making the heart visible on an X-ray.

- **Stress test:** The heart is placed under increased stress in a controlled environment during which cardiac functions are monitored. The stress test reveals symptoms of AS that only appear when the heart is under stress.

- **Magnetic resonance imaging (MRI):** A detailed image of the heart and heart valves is produced by using magnets and radio waves.

- **Magnetic resonance angiography (MRA):** MRA uses MRI technology and dye is injected into the bloodstream to create a detailed image of blood vessels.

- **Computed tomography (CT) scan:** CT scan uses X-rays to create a detailed image of the heart and the aortic valve.

- **CT angiography:** CT angiography uses CT technology and dye is injected into the bloodstream to create a detailed image of blood vessels.

## Treatment

Symptoms are treated with the following medications. In severe cases, surgical procedures are used to repair the aortic valve.

- **Diuretics:** A diuretic (furosemide [Lasix]) reduces fluid retention by excreting excess fluids.

- **Beta-blockers:** These are a class of medications that slow the contractions of the ventricles. The most commonly prescribed is metoprolol (Toprol, Lopressor).
- **Calcium channel blocker:** This medication also slows the contractions of the ventricles. The most commonly prescribed are verapamil (Calan) and diltiazem (Cardizem).
- **Valvuloplasty:** This is a nonsurgical procedure where a balloon-tipped catheter is inserted into a blood vessel in the patient's groin or arm and is moved into the aortic valve. The balloon is then inflated, widening the aortic valve. The balloon is then deflated and removed.
- **Commissurotomy:** This is an open-heart surgery during which the aortic valve is cleared of scar tissue or calcium deposits, increasing blood flow through the aortic valve.
- **Aortic valve replacement:** The aortic valve is surgically removed and replaced by either a mechanical device or tissues from a pig, cow, or deceased human donor. Mechanical aortic valves carry an ongoing risk for blood clots.

## Nursing Diagnoses

- Anxiety
- Decreased cardiac output
- Activity intolerance

## Nursing Interventions

- Place patient in a high Fowler's position to facilitate breathing.
- After surgery, monitor for
  - Pulmonary edema to look for blood flowing back into lungs.
  - Heart failure to assess for a poorly functioning heart.
  - Thrombus because of a prosthetic valve.
  - Arrhythmias because the heart may be irritated after surgery.
  - ABG to check for adequate oxygenation and acid-base balance.
- Weigh the patient daily to assess for fluid overload.
- Explain to the patient
  - Proper recovery from major surgery.

- Schedule rest periods during the day.
- Restrict to low-sodium and low-fat diets.

## Aortic Valve Regurgitation

Aortic valve regurgitation (**incompetence**) occurs when blood flows back from the aorta to the left ventricle because the aortic valve fails to properly seal the left ventricle after the latter contracts, forcing blood into the aorta. As a result, the heart is unable to efficiently pump blood to the body. Some patients have had aortic valve regurgitation for years without any symptoms. Other patients become symptomatic suddenly.

### What Went Wrong?

There are a number of conditions that can cause aortic valve regurgitation. These are

- **Infective endocarditis:** Endocarditis is an infection of the inner lining of the heart called the *endocardium* and can cause tissue damage to the aortic valve.
- **Rheumatic fever:** Rheumatic fever is the result of untreated strep throat that can leave scar tissues on the aortic valve.
- **Congenital heart defects:** A congenital heart defect is a malformation of the heart at birth.

### Prognosis

Prognosis depends on the severity of the valve damage and the acuteness of the symptoms in the patient.

### Hallmark Signs and Symptoms

Patients who become symptomatic report the following symptoms:

- **Fatigue:** Fatigue is caused by decreased circulation of oxygenated blood.
- **Shortness of breath when lying flat (orthopnea) or during activity:** The backward blood flow through the aortic valve increases pressure that backs up blood into the lungs. Lying down causes increased pressure on the lungs.

- **Chest pains:** These are associated with increased activity of the heart related to the backflow of blood into the left ventricle.
- **Fainting (syncope):** Decreased circulation of oxygenated blood can cause temporary loss of consciousness.
- **Edema:** Decreased systematic blood flow to aortic valve, resulting in heart failure that leads to swelling usually in the legs.
- **Arrhythmia:** Arrhythmia is an irregular heartbeat caused by disruption of oxygenated blood flow.
- **Palpitations:** Increase in the heart rate is the result of compensation of the heart for the blood flowing backward through the aortic valve.

## Common/Interpreting Test Results

When the patient is symptomatic, heart murmur (abnormal sound) is initially detected when listening to the patient's heart. If heart murmur is suspected, then the following tests are performed:

- **Chest X-ray:** A chest X-ray shows the size and shape of the heart. An enlarged heart is a complication of mitral stenosis.
- **ECG:** The ECG (see Chapter 4) measures impulse condition of the heart and will indicate atrial fibrillation.
- **Transthoracic echocardiogram:** A device called a *transducer* sends sound waves through the chest wall. The heart deflects sound waves back to the transducer, which send a corresponding image of the heart on a screen. A trained practitioner can visualize the structure and function of the heart.
- **Transesophageal echocardiogram:** A transducer is passed into the patient's esophagus, which sends sound waves to the heart. The image is similar to transthoracic echocardiogram.
- **Cardiac catheterization:** This is a procedure that involves passing a thin flexible tube called a *catheter* through blood vessels either in the groin or arm or into the heart. Dye is injected through the catheter, making the heart visible on an X-ray.
- **Stress test:** The heart is placed under increased stress in a controlled environment during which cardiac functions are monitored. The stress test reveals symptoms of aortic valve stenosis that only appear when the heart is under stress.

- **Cardiac magnetic resonance imaging (CMRI):** A detailed image of the heart and its valves is produced by using magnets and radio waves.

## Treatment

Treatment depends on the severity of symptoms presented by the patient. Patients who experience severe symptoms undergo a surgical procedure. These are as follows:

- **Surgical repair:** Surgical repair of the aortic valve is performed to tighten or replace the ring around the valve (**annuloplasty**) or to reconnect torn cords or remove excess tissue.
- **Aortic valve replacement:** The aortic valve is surgically removed and replaced by either a mechanical device or tissues from a pig, cow, or deceased human donor. Mechanical aortic valves carry an ongoing risk for blood clots.

## Nursing Diagnoses

- Anxiety
- Decreased cardiac output
- Activity intolerance

## Nursing Interventions

- Place patient in a high Fowler's position to facilitate breathing.
- Oxygen.
- Pain management.
- Monitor for
  - Pulmonary edema because of backflow of blood to the lungs.
  - Thrombus because a foreign object (valve) is in place and may cause clotting.
  - Arrhythmias because the heart may be irritable secondary to surgery.
- Weigh the patient daily to be aware of fluid overload.
- Explain to the patient
  - Schedule rest periods during the day.
  - Restrict to low-sodium and low-fat diets.

# Aortic Insufficiency

Aortic insufficiency can be a congenital defect in the aortic valve or secondary to another cardiac disorder. The patient may not realize that aortic insufficiency exists. Symptoms may develop slowly or appear suddenly.

## What Went Wrong?

Leakage of the aortic valve causes blood to flow back into the left ventricle. This results in increased blood volume in the left ventricle, causing it to dilate and become hypertrophic, thus reducing blood flow from the heart. The usual causes are incompetent cusps or leaflets of the valve caused by endocarditis, valve structural problems, connective tissue disorders, rheumatic heart disease, hypertension, arteriosclerosis, and other conditions.

## Prognosis

Prognosis depends on the severity of the valve damage and the acuteness of the symptoms in the patient.

## Hallmark Signs and Symptoms

- Difficulty breathing (dyspnea) because of ineffective pumping.
- Fatigue.
- Orthopnea.
- Palpations because the heart is irritable as a result of improper blood flow.

## Common/Interpreting Test Results

- X-ray shows an enlarged left ventricle.
- Echocardiogram confirms the left ventricle is enlarged and the valve is working inefficiently.

## Treatment

- Treatment is based on the gravity of the symptoms of the patient.
- Aortic valve replacement or repair.

- Administer anticoagulant medication following surgery to prevent thrombus around the aortic valve.
  - Heparin
  - Warfarin (Coumadin)
  - Dalteparin (Fragmin)
  - Enoxaparin (Lovenox)

## Nursing Diagnoses

- Anxiety
- Decreased cardiac output
- Activity intolerance

## Nursing Interventions

- Place patient in a high Fowler's position to facilitate breathing.
- Oxygen.
- Pain management.
- Monitor for
  - Pulmonary edema because of backflow of blood to the lungs.
  - Thrombus because a foreign object (valve) is in place and may cause clotting.
  - Arrhythmias because the heart may be irritable secondary to surgery.
- Weigh the patient daily to be aware of fluid overload.
- Explain to the patient
  - Schedule rest periods during the day.
  - Restrict to low-sodium and low-fat diets.

# Papillary (Chordae) Muscle Rupture

Papillary chordae are tendons that connect the papillary muscles to the tricuspid valve and connect the mitral valve to the ventricle. These are also referred to as heart strings. The chordae can break or the papillary muscle can rupture, resulting in the malfunction of the tricuspid and mitral valves and leading to backflow of blood.

## What Went Wrong?

Papillary muscle can rupture and the chordae can be stretched or torn as a result of the following:

- **Infective endocarditis:** Endocarditis is an infection of the inner lining of the heart called the *endocardium* and can cause tissue damage to the chordae and papillary muscle.

- **Heart attack (acute myocardial infarction):** A heart attack can cause damage to the chordae and papillary muscle.

- **Cardiac tumor:** A growth in the heart within the location of mitral valve and the tricuspid valve can lead to rupture of the papillary muscle and chordae.

## Prognosis

Prognosis depends on several factors, especially which papillary muscle ruptured and the degree of the rupture. Prognosis is generally poor due to the underlying cardiac disorder that might have led to the rupture and complications from the rupture.

## Hallmark Signs and Symptoms

A patient who experiences papillary muscle rupture or torn chordae will report the following symptoms:

- **Chest pains:** These are associated with increased activity of the heart related to the tear and malfunction of the mitral valve and the tricuspid valve.

- **Fainting (syncope):** Decreased circulation of oxygenated blood can cause temporary loss of consciousness.

- **Distension of the jugular vein:** Backflow of blood due to malfunctioning of mitral valve and tricuspid valve causes increased pressure in the jugular veins.

## Common/Interpreting Test Results

When symptoms are presented, the following tests are ordered:

- **Transthoracic echocardiogram:** A device called a *transducer* sends sound waves through the chest wall. The heart deflects sound waves back to the transducer, which send a corresponding image of the heart on a screen. A trained practitioner can visualize the structure and function of the heart.

- **Transesophageal echocardiogram:** A transducer is passed into the patient's esophagus, which sends sound waves to the heart. The image is similar to transthoracic echocardiogram.

## Treatment

If the patient reports mild symptoms, then the treatment is the same as mitral valve and tricuspid valve malfunctions (see Mitral Valve Stenosis, Mitral Valve Regurgitation, Tricuspid Valve Stenosis, and Tricuspid Valve Regurgitation). In severe cases, surgical repair is necessary.

## Nursing Diagnoses

- Anxiety
- Decreased cardiac output
- Activity intolerance

## Nursing Interventions

- Place patient in a high Fowler's position to facilitate breathing.
- After surgery, monitor for
  - Pulmonary edema to look for blood flowing back into lungs.
  - Heart failure to assess for a poorly functioning heart.
  - Thrombus because of a prosthetic valve.
  - Arrhythmias because the heart may be irritated after surgery.
  - ABG to check for adequate oxygenation and acid-base balance.
- Weigh the patient daily to assess for fluid overload.
- Explain to the patient
  - Proper recovery from major surgery.
  - Schedule rest periods during the day.
  - Restrict to low-sodium and low-fat diets.

# CASE STUDY

### CASE 1

A 45-year-old man presents with chest pains on exertion, orthopnea, palpitations, fatigue, and coughing with a tinge of blood in the sputum. Upon examination, you notice swelling of the ankles. The patient asks the following questions. What is the best response?

QUESTION 1. Why did the practitioner order an ECG?
ANSWER: The ECG measures electrical activity of the heart. The practitioner ordered the ECG to rule out a heart attack. Furthermore, your symptoms may indicate a heart valve disorder such as mitral valve stenosis. A heart valve disorder may cause atrial fibrillation, which can be identified by the ECG.

QUESTION 2. Why do I have shortness of breath when lying flat?
ANSWER: Mitral valve stenosis is the narrowing of the mitral valve. When the mitral valve narrows, there is a decrease in blood flow through the mitral valve, causing back pressure throughout the cardiovascular system prior to reaching the mitral valve. As a result blood backs up in to the lungs, causing increased fluid in the lungs. When you sit or stand, fluid falls to the bottom of the lungs. However, the fluid is distributed throughout the lungs when you lie down, making it difficult for you to breathe and resulting in shortness of breath.

QUESTION 3. Why did the practitioner order an X-ray of my heart?
ANSWER: Disruption of blood flow through the mitral valve into the left ventricle causes the heart to work harder to pump blood through the system in order to oxygenate blood in the lungs and distribute oxygenated blood throughout the body. The heart is a muscle. Working harder increases the size of the heart similar to how bodybuilders increase the size of skeletal muscles by working out. The X-ray can determine if the heart is enlarged.

QUESTION 4. Why did the practitioner order an echocardiogram?
ANSWER: An echocardiogram is a test where a device called a *transducer* sends sound waves through the chest wall (transthoracic echocardiogram). The heart deflects sound waves back to the transducer, which sends a corresponding image of the heart to a screen. The practitioner can then visualize the structure and function of the heart since the series of images create a moving image of the heart. The practitioner may also order a transesophageal echocardiogram, which is similar to the transthoracic echocardiogram except the transducer is passed into the patient's esophagus.

# FINAL CHECKUP

1. **A 53-year-old man who is diagnosed with MVP asks you why he should take antibiotics before every dental procedure. What is your best response?**

   A. Antibiotics lower the risk of a blood clot during the procedure.

   B. MVP puts the patient at risk for infective endocarditis. A dental procedure exposes the patient to bacteria and the antibiotic reduces the risk of infection, building the therapeutic level of antibiotics in the blood before the procedure.

   C. MVP puts the patient at risk for infective endocarditis.

   D. MVP puts the patient at risk for infective endocarditis, and the antibiotics reduce the risk by killing bacteria before the procedure.

2. **A 63-year-old woman diagnosed with mitral stenosis is prescribed Lasix. Within minutes of taking the medication, the patient reports urinating. She asks you why she is prescribed Lasix for a heart problem. What is your best response?**

   A. Mitral stenosis disrupts blood flow to the left ventricle causing a buildup of fluid that leads to swelling. Lasix is a diuretic that causes the kidney to increase urine to reduce excess fluid, decreasing swelling.

   B. Mitral stenosis disrupts blood flow to the right ventricle causing a buildup of fluid that leads to swelling. Lasix is a diuretic that causes the kidney to increase urine to reduce excess fluid, decreasing swelling.

   C. Mitral stenosis disrupts blood flow to the left ventricle causing a buildup of fluid that leads to swelling. Lasix is a beta-blocker that causes the kidney to increase urine to reduce excess fluid, decreasing swelling.

   D. Mitral stenosis disrupts blood flow to the left ventricle causing a buildup of fluid that leads to swelling. Lasix is a diuretic that causes the bladder to increase urine to reduce excess fluid, decreasing swelling.

3. **A 45-year-old woman was recently diagnosed with MVR. She is prescribed warfarin. She asks if the practitioner was mistaken to prescribe warfarin because she has no history of blood clots. What is the best response?**

   A. You should ask the practitioner. I am not permitted to answer your question.

   B. MVR places you at risk for atrial fibrillation, which is an irregular contraction of the atria. As a result, there is a chance that blood might pool, leading to blood clots.

   C. MVR places you at risk for atrial fibrillation, which is an irregular contraction of the atria. As a result, there is a chance that blood might pool, leading to blood clots. Warfarin reduces the formation of blood clots.

   D. MVR places you at risk for atrial fibrillation, which is an irregular contraction of the ventricles. As a result, there is a chance that blood might pool, leading to blood clots. Warfarin reduces the formation of blood clots.

4. **A 60-year-old woman diagnosed with tricuspid valve stenosis is told by the practitioner that she should undergo a valvuloplasty. She tells you that she is afraid of undergoing heart surgery. What is your best response?**

    A. Valvuloplasty is a nonsurgical procedure.

    B. Valvuloplasty is a surgical procedure during which a balloon-tipped catheter is inserted into a blood vessel and then moved into the tricuspid valve where the balloon is inflated, opening the tricuspid valve.

    C. Valvuloplasty is a surgical procedure during which a balloon-tipped catheter is inserted into a blood vessel in your arm or groin and then moved into the tricuspid valve where the balloon is inflated, opening the tricuspid valve.

    D. Valvuloplasty is a surgical procedure during which a balloon-tipped catheter is inserted into a blood vessel in your arm or groin and then moved into the tricuspid valve where the catheter scrapes excess tissue around the tricuspid valve.

5. **A 65-year-old male patient who has been diagnosed with pulmonary valve regurgitation reports periods of rapid breathing. He reports that the practitioner told him this is a normal symptom of pulmonary valve regurgitation. The patient asks why this happens. What is your best response?**

    A. You are experiencing respiratory acidosis.

    B. There is a buildup of oxygen in your blood because disruption in blood flow prevents the lung from oxygenating the blood. As a result, your body compensates by breathing rapidly to quickly remove the excess carbon dioxide.

    C. There is a buildup of carbon dioxide in your blood because disruption in blood flow prevents the lung from oxygenating the blood. As a result, your body compensates by breathing rapidly to quickly remove the excess oxygen.

    D. There is a buildup of carbon dioxide in your blood because disruption in blood flow prevents the lung from oxygenating the blood. As a result, your body compensates by breathing rapidly to quickly remove the excess carbon dioxide.

6. **A 42-year-old woman who was recently diagnosed with tricuspid valve regurgitation asks you why her practitioner asked if she had an untreated throat infection. What is your best response?**

    A. An untreated bacterial throat infection can lead to infective endocarditis, which is an underlying cause of tricuspid valve regurgitation.

    B. An untreated bacterial throat infection can lead to complications for a patient who is diagnosed with tricuspid valve regurgitation.

    C. An untreated bacterial throat infection is always the cause of tricuspid valve regurgitation.

    D. The practitioner might have noticed signs of a throat infection during your physical assessment.

7. **A 52-year-old woman diagnosed with tricuspid valve stenosis asks you why the practitioner is prescribing treatment when no treatment was given to her friend who had the same diagnosis. What is your best response?**

   A. Some patients diagnosed with tricuspid valve stenosis don't have any symptoms, and therefore, the practitioner monitors the patient regularly without prescribing treatment.

   B. Your friend probably was diagnosed with mitral valve stenosis.

   C. You friend likely had a different diagnosis.

   D. Some practitioners prefer to monitor the patient regularly without prescribing treatment.

8. **A 64-year-old mam diagnosed with MVR asks why he feels so tired. What is your best response?**

   A. MVR disrupts normal blood flow, resulting in increased circulation of oxygenated blood, which can make you feel tried.

   B. MVR disrupts normal blood flow, resulting in decreased circulation of carbon dioxide in the blood, which can make you feel tried.

   C. MVR disrupts normal blood flow, resulting in decreased circulation of oxygenated blood, which can make you feel tried.

   D. Your fatigue is a side effect of warfarin, which is prescribed for MVR.

9. **A 55-year-old man diagnosed with mitral valve stenosis was told by his practitioner that if his symptoms do not improve he needs to undergo commissurotomy. He asks you to explain commissurotomy. What is your best response?**

   A. Commissurotomy is a nonsurgical procedure during which the mitral valve is cleared of scar tissue, increasing blood flow through the mitral valve.

   B. Commissurotomy is an open-heart surgery during which the mitral valve is cleared of scar tissue or calcium deposits, increasing blood flow through the mitral valve.

   C. Commissurotomy is a nonsurgical procedure during which the mitral valve is cleared of calcium deposits, increasing blood flow through the mitral valve.

   D. Commissurotomy is an open-heart surgery during which the ring around the mitral valve is replaced.

10. **A 21-year-old man diagnosed with pulmonary valve stenosis asks you how he caught the disease. What is the best response?**

    A. You likely caught pulmonary valve stenosis by not going to the practitioner the last time you had a throat infection.

    B. The most common cause of pulmonary valve stenosis is congenital abnormal development of the pulmonary valve.

    C. You can only catch pulmonary valve stenosis from rheumatic fever.

    D. The cause of pulmonary valve stenosis is unknown.

## CORRECT ANSWERS AND RATIONALES

1. B. MVP puts the patient at risk for infective endocarditis. A dental procedure exposes the patient to bacteria and the antibiotic reduces the risk of infection, building the therapeutic level of antibiotics in the blood before the procedure.

2. A. Mitral stenosis disrupts blood flow to the left ventricle causing a buildup of fluid that leads to swelling. Lasix is a diuretic that causes the kidney to increase urine to reduce excess fluid, decreasing swelling.

3. C. MVR places you at risk for atrial fibrillation, which is an irregular contraction of the atria. As a result, there is a chance that blood might pool, leading to blood clots. Warfarin reduces the formation of blood clots.

4. A. Valvuloplasty is a nonsurgical procedure.

5. D. There is a buildup of carbon dioxide in your blood because disruption in blood flow prevents the lung from oxygenating the blood. As a result, your body compensates by breathing rapidly to quickly remove the excess carbon dioxide.

6. A. An untreated bacterial throat infection can lead to infective endocarditis, which is an underlying cause of tricuspid valve regurgitation.

7. A. Some patients diagnosed with tricuspid valve stenosis don't have any symptoms, and therefore, the practitioner monitors the patient regularly without prescribing treatment.

8. C. MVR disrupts normal blood flow, resulting in decreased circulation of oxygenated blood, which can make you feel tried.

9. B. Commissurotomy is an open-heart surgery during which the mitral valve is cleared of scar tissue or calcium deposits, increasing blood flow through the mitral valve.

10. B. The most common cause of pulmonary valve stenosis is congenital abnormal development of the pulmonary valve.

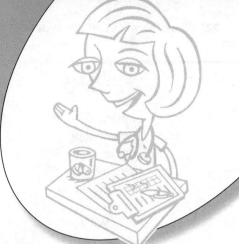

chapter 7

# *Hematology and Hematologic Disorders*

## KEY TERMS

| | |
|---|---|
| Clotting Factors | Monocytes |
| Erythropoiesis | Petechiae |
| Erythropoietin | Plasma |
| Granulocytes | Prothrombin |
| Hemoglobin | Reticulocytes |
| Hemolysis | Stem Cells |
| Koilonychia | Thrombocytopenia |
| Leukopenia | Thrombophlebitis |
| Lymphocytes | Vasoocclusive Crisis |
| Macrophages | |

# Hematology

The hematologic system refers to the *blood* and *blood-forming organs*. The formation of red blood cells (RBCs), white blood cells (WBCs), and platelets begins in the bone marrow (Figure 7–1). **Stem cells** are produced in the bone marrow. Initially, these cells are not differentiated and may become RBCs, WBCs, or platelets. In the next stage of development, the stem cell becomes committed to a particular precursor cell, to become either a myeloid or lymphoid type of cell, and will differentiate into a particular cell type when in the presence of a specific growth factor.

**Erythropoiesis** (the production of RBCs) is stimulated by hypoxia and controlled by erythropoietin. **Erythropoietin** is produced in the kidneys. Iron, vitamin $B_{12}$, and folic acid are necessary for production of RBCs. *Reticulocytes* are immature RBCs that mature within 48 hours of release into the bloodstream. Healthy RBCs survive for about 120 days. WBCs or leukocytes protect the body from infection and are composed of *granulocytes*, *monocytes*, and *lymphocytes*. **Granulocytes** and **monocytes** remove bacteria and other foreign particles by phagocytosis. Platelet aggregation (or clumping) is necessary to prevent blood loss.

Plasma comprises the majority, about 55%, of blood volume, and the cells comprise about 45% (Figure 7–2). The spleen is found in the left upper quadrant (LUQ) of the abdomen. The spleen filters whole blood. It removes old and imperfect WBCs (lymphocytes and **macrophages**) and RBCs. The spleen also

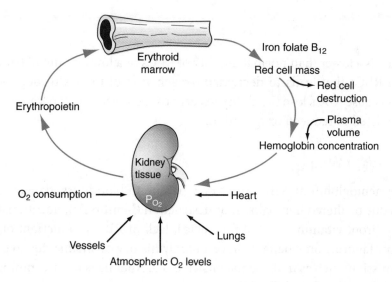

**FIGURE 7–1** · The formation of red blood cells (RBCs), white blood cells (WBCs), and platelets begins in the bone marrow.

breaks down **hemoglobin** and stores of RBCs and platelets. The liver is found in the right upper quadrant of the abdomen and is the main production site for many of the **clotting factors**, including **prothrombin**. Normal liver function is important for vitamin K production in the intestinal tract. Vitamin K is necessary for clotting factors VII, IX, X, and prothrombin.

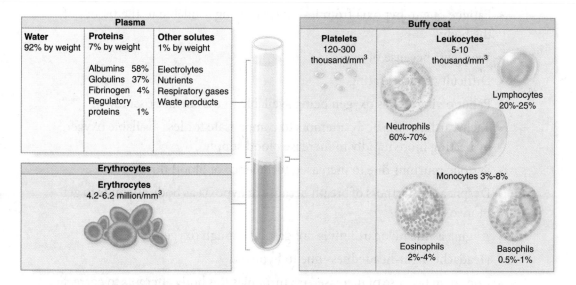

**FIGURE 7–2** · Plasma comprises the majority, about 55%, of blood volume and the cells comprise about 45%.

# Anemia

Anemia is a lower than normal number of RBCs or a low amount of hemoglobin in RBCs that leads to decreased oxygenation of tissues throughout the body because RBCs lose the ability to carry oxygen. Anemia can lead to symptoms related to reduced oxygenation.

## What Went Wrong?

A low hemoglobin or RBC count may be due to blood loss, damage to the RBCs due to altered hemoglobin or destruction (**hemolysis**), nutritional deficiency (iron, vitamin $B_{12}$, and folic acid), lack of RBC production, or bone marrow failure. Some patients have a family history of anemia due to genetic transmission, such as thalassemia or sickle cell. Anemia is fairly common during pregnancy and in chronic disease states.

## Prognosis

Anemia is a symptom of another disorder in the body. The cause of the anemia needs to be determined in order to correct the anemia and its symptoms.

## Hallmark Signs and Symptoms

- Fatigue due to hypoxia from less oxygen being available to the tissues of the body.
- Weakness because of hypoxia.
- Difficulty concentrating.
- Pallor owing to less oxygen being available to the surface tissues.
- Tachycardia as the body attempts to compensate for less available oxygen by beating more rapidly to increase blood supply.
- Systolic murmur due to increased turbulence of blood flow.
- Dyspnea or shortness of breath because of hypoxia as body attempts to get more oxygen.
- Angina as the myocardium is not getting enough oxygen.
- Headache, light-headedness due to hypoxia.
- Bone pain because of increased erythropoiesis as body attempts to correct anemia.

- Jaundice in hemolytic anemia owing to increased levels of bilirubin as RBCs break down.

## Common/Interpreting Test Results

- Hemoglobin level is low.
- Hematocrit level is low.
- RBC count is low.
- Mean corpuscular volume (MCV) shows size of cell—normocytic (normal), microcytic (low), or macrocytic (high).
- Mean corpuscular hemoglobin (MCH) shows color of cell—normochromic (normal) or hypochromic (low).
- Red cell distribution width (RDW) elevated—shows the variation of the cell sizes; there is greater variation in cell size when body is attempting to compensate for anemia.
- Reticulocyte count is elevated when RBC production is increased to compensate for the anemia.

## Treatment

Correction of the underlying cause is necessary. Treatment may include dietary modifications and supplementations, corticosteroids (to suppress the immune system), erythropoietin (to stimulate bone marrow to produce cells), or blood transfusions. See specific anemias to follow.

## Nursing Diagnoses

- Fatigue
- Activity intolerance

## Nursing Interventions

- Check vital signs for changes.
- Monitor complete blood count (CBC)—hemoglobin, RBC, MCV, MCH, RDW.
- Plan nursing care based on patient's tolerance of activity.
- Monitor for angina.

# Aplastic Anemia (Pancytopenia)

Aplastic anemia is a disorder that occurs when bone marrow stops producing a sufficient amount of new RBCs, WBCs, and platelets, thereby increasing the risk of infection and hemorrhage. Aplastic anemia is rare but can develop at any age.

## What Went Wrong?

The red cells remaining in circulation are normal in size and color. This may be due to chemical exposure, high-dose radiation exposure, or exposure to toxins (such as pesticides, arsenic, or benzene). Cancer treatments, such as radiation therapy and chemotherapeutic agents, may suppress bone marrow function, which will result in anemia (low RBC), **thrombocytopenia** (low platelets), and **leukopenia** (low WBC). Disorders such as rheumatoid arthritis (RA), Epstein-Barr virus, hepatitis, cytomegalovirus, HIV infection, and parvovirus may cause anemia. The cause may also be unknown or idiopathic.

## Prognosis

The bone marrow dysfunction may be of slow onset or sudden. The life span of the RBC is longer than the platelets and WBC, so the anemia may show up later than the effects of losing the other cells. Some exposures to toxic agents or medications are severe and potentially fatal in susceptible individuals. Patients with severe aplastic anemia typically need hospital care. In some individuals with severe aplastic anemia, the disease will be fatal.

## Hallmark Signs and Symptoms

- Fatigue due to hypoxemia.
- Weakness owing to tissue hypoxia.
- Shortness of breath as oxygen-carrying capability is diminished.
- Pallor because of lack of oxygen reaching superficial tissues due to anemia.
- Arrhythmias, murmurs, or heart failure as the cardiovascular system has difficulty with decreased oxygen supply.
- Infections due to low WBC production, causing decreased ability to fight infection.
- Fever because of infection.

- Bruising (**ecchymosis**) and tiny subcutaneous (SC) hemorrhages (**petechiae**) due to decrease in platelets, altering clotting ability.
- Bleeding from mucous membranes (gastrointestinal [GI] tract, mouth, nose, and vagina).

## Common/Interpreting Test Results

- Low hemoglobin—decreases oxygen-carrying capabilities.
- Low hematocrit—fewer RBCs within circulation.
- Low RBC count.
- Thrombocytopenia—low platelet count.
- Leukopenia—low WBC.
- Reticulocyte count low—no immature cells available for release into circulation.
- Positive fecal occult blood test.
- Decreased cell counts in bone marrow biopsy as body stops producing RBCs, WBCs, and platelets.
- Bone marrow aspiration to determine components of bone marrow.

## Treatment

- Administer hematopoietic growth factor to correct anemia in patients with low erythropoietin levels.
  - Erythropoietin, epoetin alfa (recombinant human erythropoietin) by SC injection or intravenously.
- Administer human granulocyte colony-stimulating factor (G-CSF) to correct low WBC levels.
  - Filgrastim by SC injection or intravenously
  - Granulocyte-macrophage colony-stimulating factor (GM-CSF) sargramostim by intravenous (IV) infusion
- Packed RBC transfusions when anemia is symptomatic.
- Platelet transfusion for severe bleeding.
- Bone marrow transplant replaces functioning stem cells.
- Administer immunosuppressive drugs, antithymocyte globulin, and corticosteroids.
- Splenectomy when spleen is enlarged and destroying RBCs.

## Nursing Diagnoses

- Risk for infection
- Activity intolerance
- Risk for deficient fluid volume

## Nursing Interventions

- Monitor vital signs for changes.
- Record intake and output of fluids.
- Protect patient from falls.
- Avoid intramuscular (IM) injections due to altered clotting ability.
- Explain to the patient
  - Do not take aspirin due to its effect on platelet aggregation (clotting ability).
  - Plan to take rest periods during activities because of fatigue.
  - Only use an electric razor to decrease risk of bleeding owing to decreased platelet count.
  - Call your physician, nurse practitioner, or physician assistant for signs of bleeding or bruising.

# Iron Deficiency Anemia

Iron deficiency anemia is decreased formation of hemoglobin because there is insufficient iron in the blood to form hemoglobin; as a result the blood loses capacity to carry oxygen. Iron deficiency anemia is an acute disorder that can be resolved with treatment.

## What Went Wrong?

Iron stores are typically depleted first, followed by serum iron levels. Iron deficiency may be due to blood loss, dietary deficiency, or increased demand owing to pregnancy or lactation. As RBCs age, the body breaks them down and the iron is released. This iron is reused for the production of new blood cells. A small amount of iron is lost daily through the GI tract, necessitating dietary replacement. When RBCs are produced without a sufficient amount of iron, the cells are smaller and paler than usual.

## Prognosis

Iron deficiency anemia is a very common type of anemia. Typically patients respond to oral supplementation of iron. Occasionally a patient will have problems absorbing iron from the intestinal tract. These patients will need parenteral supplementation. Once iron stores are replaced, the anemia should correct and hemoglobin levels return to normal. Some patients may need lifelong supplementation, depending on the cause of the deficiency.

## Hallmark Signs and Symptoms

- Weakness because of anemia and tissue hypoxia.
- Pallor due to decreased amount of oxygen getting to surface tissues.
- Fatigue owing to anemia and hypoxemia.
- Koilonychia—thin, concave nails raised at edges, also called spoon nails.
- Tachycardia and tachypnea on exertion due to increased demand for oxygen.

## Common/Interpreting Test Results

- Decrease in serum hemoglobin as fewer RBCs are made.
- Serum ferritin is low.
- MCV initially normal until iron stores are depleted, then low—microcytic anemia as the RBCs produced are smaller than usual due to decreased level of available iron.
- MCH initially normal, then low—hypochromic anemia.
- Serum iron level is low.
- Serum iron-binding capacity is increased.
- Transferrin saturation decreases.
- Peripheral blood smear shows poikilocytosis (RBCs of different shapes).
- Platelet count may increase.

## Treatment

Iron replacement therapy is continued to correct the deficiency and replace the lost stores of iron in the body. The typical time frame for oral therapy is to continue therapy for 3 to 6 months after the anemia has been corrected. If oral treatment is not adequate, parenteral treatment may be necessary. There have been documented incidents of anaphylactic reactions to iron dextran. Patients new to this treatment typically have a smaller test dose initially, before the initiation of treatments.

- Administer iron to replace what has been lost to return stores to normal levels.
- Oral replacement in split doses (three times a day).
  - Ferrous sulfate
  - Ferrous gluconate
  - Ferrous fumarate
- Parenteral iron replacement for those who cannot tolerate or do not respond to oral therapy, have GI illness, or have continued bleeding.
  - Iron dextran given deep intramuscularly or intravenously.
  - Iron sodium gluconate given intravenously.
  - Iron sucrose complex given intravenously.
- Intramuscular (IM) injection of iron using Z-track method.
- Increase dietary intake of iron.

## Nursing Diagnoses

- Imbalanced nutrition, less than what body requires
- Activity intolerance

## Nursing Interventions

- Monitor intake and output.
- Monitor vital signs for tachycardia or tachypnea.
- Monitor for reactions to parenteral iron therapy.
- Explain to the patient
  - Check for bleeding.
  - Increase iron in diet.
- Teach dietary sources of iron.

# Pernicious Anemia

Pernicious anemia is a disorder when the body is unable to absorb vitamin $B_{12}$ that is needed to produce RBCs, resulting in a decreased RBC count. Deficiency of vitamin $B_{12}$ inhibits the ability of RBCs to divide normally. As a result, RBCs become large and have difficulty in exiting bone marrow.

## What Went Wrong?

The anemia typically develops in adulthood and is more common in people of northern European descent. Family history and autoimmune diseases increase the risk for developing the disease. Intrinsic factor is normally secreted by the parietal cells of the gastric mucosa and is necessary to allow intestinal absorption of vitamin $B_{12}$. Destruction of the gastric mucosa due to an autoimmune response results in loss of parietal cells within the stomach. The ability of vitamin $B_{12}$ to bind with intrinsic factor is lost, decreasing the amount that is absorbed. Vitamin $B_{12}$ is commonly found in meat, poultry, shellfish, eggs, and dairy products. Typical onset is between the ages of 40 and 60.

## Prognosis

Ongoing replacement of vitamin $B_{12}$ is necessary to correct the deficit and alleviate symptoms that may have developed. Without treatment, the neurologic effects will continue, ultimately leading to dementia. Patients have an increased risk for gastric polyps, gastric cancer, and gastric carcinoid tumors.

## Hallmark Signs and Symptoms

- Asymptomatic initially.
- Pallor due to anemia.
- Weakness and fatigue owing to anemia.
- Tingling in hands and feet—"stocking-glove paresthesia"—because of bilateral demyelination of dorsal and lateral columns of spinal cord nerves.
- Diminished vibratory and position sense.

- Poor balance due to effect on cerebral function.
- Dementia appears later in the disease.
- Atrophic glossitis—beefy red tongue.
- Nausea may lead to anorexia and weight loss.
- Shortness of breath on exertion as disease progresses.
- Premature graying of hair.

## Common/Interpreting Test Results

- Decreased hemoglobin due to decreased production of RBCs.
- Increased MCV—macrocytic anemia.
- Intrinsic factor antibodies positive.
- Parietal cell antibodies positive.
- Cobalamin level is low.
- Elevated fasting gastrin level.
- Decreased pepsinogen level.
- Decreased amount of hydrochloric acid in the stomach (hypochlorhydria) due to changes within the parietal cells of the gastric mucosa.
- Positive Romberg test owing to ataxia and neurologic changes.
- Diminished sensation when testing for vibration, position sense, or proprioception of extremities.
- Gastric biopsy shows atrophic gastritis.
- False +ve Pap test—vitamin $B_{12}$ alters appearance of epithelial cells.

## Treatment

Lifelong repletion of vitamin $B_{12}$ will correct the anemia and improve the neurologic changes that have occurred. Initially the patient is given weekly injections of $B_{12}$ to combat the deficiency. The injections eventually become monthly for lifelong maintenance. Oral supplementation is not effective in these patients because they cannot adequately absorb vitamin $B_{12}$ due to insufficient intrinsic factor.

- Administer vitamin $B_{12}$ by IM injection.
- Transfusion of packed RBCs if anemia is severe.

## Nursing Diagnoses

- Impaired gas exchange
- Imbalanced nutrition, less than what body requires
- Risk for injury

## Nursing Interventions

- Prevent injuries.
- Explain to the patient
  - Use soft toothbrush due to oral changes.
  - Avoid activities that could lead to injury because of paresthesias or changes in balance.
  - Inspect feet each day for injury due to paresthesia.

# Sickle Cell Anemia

Sickle cell anemia is a sickle cell disorder where RBCs take on a sickle (crescent) shape rather than the traditional disc shape. Sickle cells are stiff and sticky and block blood flow in vessels usually in the limbs and organs, leading to pain and organ damage.

## What Went Wrong?

Sickle cell anemia is an autosomal recessive disorder in which an abnormal gene causes damage to the RBC membrane. The abnormal hemoglobin within the RBC is called *hemoglobin S*. Dehydration or drying of the RBC makes it more vulnerable to sickling (forming a crescent-like shape), as do hypoxemia and acidosis. Hemolytic anemia results as RBCs are destroyed due to the damage to the outer membrane. The sickled cells can also clump together, causing difficulty getting through the smaller vessels.

## Prognosis

Sickle cell anemia may become a chronic multisystem disease. Causes of death in these patients are usually related to organ failure. Patients may also inherit a single gene for sickle cell. These patients may develop sickle cell trait, in which symptoms are only present in the setting of extreme circumstances (vigorous exercise at high altitude, especially with rapid ascent).

## Hallmark Signs and Symptoms

- Acute pain (especially back, chest, and long bones) from vascular occlusion of the small vessels as the sickled cells clump.
- Fever as body responds to acute sickling episode and accompanying provoking event.
- Painful, swollen joints due to vasoocclusive crisis.
- Fatigue because of chronic anemia.
- Stroke (cerebrovascular accident) owing to vasoocclusive process.
- Enlarged liver (hepatomegaly).
- Enlarged heart and systolic murmur.

## Common/Interpreting Test Results

- Low RBC count due to chronic hemolytic anemia; the RBCs have a shorter life span.
- Elevated WBCs.
- Increased reticulocytes.
- Presence of Howell-Jolly bodies and target cells.
- Sickle cells appear in blood smear.
- Indirect bilirubin level elevated.
- Hemoglobin electrophoresis shows majority of hemoglobin S (80%-98%).

## Treatment

During acute episodes, pain control, hydration, and oxygenation are the focus of treatment. The underlying cause that sent the patient into crisis will also need to be treated concurrently.

- Administer analgesics to alleviate the pain associated with the vasoocclusive process.
- Narcotic pain control becomes necessary when pain is severe.
- Warm compresses on joint.

- Blood transfusion of packed RBCs when anemia is indicated.
- Supplemental oxygen if hypoxic.
- Adequate hydration, using IV fluids.
- Treat infections.

## Nursing Diagnoses

- Fatigue
- Acute pain
- Impaired gas exchange

## Nursing Interventions

- Increase fluid intake.
- Monitor IV fluids.
- Monitor pain control.
- Record fluid intake and output to monitor renal function.
- Administer supplemental oxygen to increase available oxygen.
- Explain to the patient
  - Avoid the cold.
  - No cold compresses.
  - Plan for rest periods during the day.

# Deep Vein Thrombosis

Deep vein thrombosis (DVT) is the formation of a clot within the deep veins (Figure 7–3). It is most common over the age of 60 years. There is an increased risk with bed rest, recent surgery, cancer, smoking, fractures (especially involving lower extremities), heart failure, obesity, or estrogen use.

## What Went Wrong?

Initially platelets and white cells clump together, sticking to the inside of the vessel wall. As blood flows over the area, other cells may deposit onto the area, making the thrombus larger. Compression of blood flow, which will increase the venous pressure or sluggishness of the blood flow, can increase the risk of

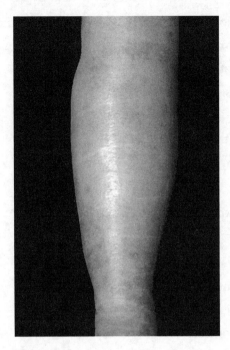

**FIGURE 7-3** • Deep vein thrombosis (DVT) is the formation of a clot within the deep vein.

clot formation. Immobility, obesity, and hormonal changes such as occur in pregnancy can all contribute to increased risk.

## Prognosis

The clot may develop without any outward signs for some time. It may also be due to another disease process or medication that affects clotting abilities. A small piece of the clot may break free to become an embolus and travel elsewhere in the body. This embolus may lodge in a vessel in the lung (a pulmonary embolism), causing acute respiratory symptoms and possibly even death.

## Hallmark Signs and Symptoms

- Some patients will be asymptomatic.
- Unilateral leg (or arm) pain or tenderness (calf, thigh, groin, upper or lower arm) depending on location of thrombosis.

- Unilateral swelling (edema) of leg (or arm) due to vascular occlusion.
- Positive Homan sign (pain on dorsiflexion of foot) seen in minority of patients with DVT.
- Warmth and redness over the site.

## Common/Interpreting Test Results

- Doppler flow studies.
- Venous duplex ultrasound.
- Impedence plethysmography looks at venous outflow; better at diagnosis in thigh than in calf.
- Venography uses contrast dye to visualize the thrombus; not commonly done due to need for dye and other available tests.
- Magnetic resonance imaging, called direct thrombus imaging, is useful to examine the inferior vena cava and pelvic vein locations.
- Prothrombin time (PT), partial thromboplastin time (PTT), international normalized ratio (INR), and CBC with platelet count as baseline.
- D-dimer to test for hypercoagulable state.

## Treatment

Most patients undergo medical treatment and are prescribed rest. Preventive measures are instituted for future occurrences. Patients with repeat occurrences may have an umbrella filter implanted.

- Bed rest with elevation of extremity.
- Warm, moist soaks of the area.
- Monitor PT, PTT, INR.
- Weight-dosed heparin IV.
- Low-molecular-weight heparin.
- Begin warfarin at therapeutic levels for 2 days, then stop heparin, continue for 3 months.
- Thrombolytic therapy to dissolve clot with drugs such as recombinant tissue plasminogen activator (t-PA).
- Umbrella filter is inserted into the inferior vena cava for patients with recurring lower extremity DVT.

- *Thrombectomy* is the surgical removal of the thrombus.
- Antiembolic (elastic) stockings.

## Nursing Diagnoses

- Impaired physical mobility
- Risk for acute pain

## Nursing Interventions

- Monitor vital signs for changes.
- Monitor for signs of pulmonary embolism, shortness of breath, chest pain, tachycardia (rapid heart rate), tachypnea (rapid respirations), and diaphoresis (sweating).
- Avoid massaging the area to lessen the possibility of dislodging the clot.
- Intermittent warm, moist soaks; assess skin between changes.
- Follow weight-dosed heparin protocol.
- Monitor laboratory results: PT, PTT, INR, and CBC with platelets.
- Low-molecular-weight heparin (enoxaparin, dalteparin).
- Take warfarin orally.
- Monitor for signs of bleeding or bruising.
- Explain to the patient
  - Report signs of bleeding or bruising to physician, nurse practitioner, or physician assistant.
  - Avoid injury.
  - Use electric razor and soft toothbrush; avoid flossing between teeth.
  - Observe diet restrictions, and check with health care provider or pharmacist about interactions of any medications, if on warfarin as outpatient.
  - Take warfarin as directed.
  - Continue to have blood tests to monitor anticoagulant therapy.
  - Call 911 or go to emergency room (ER) if there is chest pain, difficulty breathing, and hemoptysis.

# Disseminated Intravascular Coagulation

Disseminated intravascular coagulation (DIC) is a disorder where proteins involved in blood clotting become overactive, resulting in excessive blood coagulation and leading to the depletion of platelets and the body's ability to coagulate, which leads to hemorrhaging.

## What Went Wrong?

DIC occurs as a complication of some other condition. The coagulation sequence is activated, causing many microthrombi to develop throughout the body. The clots that form are the result of coagulation proteins and platelets, resulting in the risk of bleeding or severe hemorrhage. It is often due to obstetric complications, post-trauma, sepsis, cancer, or shock.

## Prognosis

The prognosis varies depending on the underlying disease process and the ability to reverse the coagulopathy.

## Hallmark Signs and Symptoms

- Unexpected bleeding (**epistaxis**, mucous membranes)—oozing from puncture sites (venipuncture, IVs, surgical wounds).
- Petechiae as clotting factors are lost.
- Purpura as clotting factors are lost.
- Severe hemorrhage as clotting factors are lost.
- Uncontrolled postpartum bleeding.
- Tissue hypoxia from microemboli (small blood clots in the bloodstream).
- Hemolytic anemia, as cells are destroyed trying to pass through partially blocked vessels.
- Thrombosis may lead to organ failure.

## Common/Interpreting Test Results

- PT prolonged (may be normal in early disease or chronic disease).
- PTT normal or prolonged.
- Thrombin time may be elevated due to consumption of fibrinogen.

- Platelet count low—thrombocytopenia.
- Fibrin degradation products elevated (may be normal in early disease).
- D-dimer may be elevated (best single test).

## Treatment

Treatment needs to decrease coagulation ability (to prevent further clot development) and replace clotting components (to prevent further bleeding). Other interventions may be necessary depending on the locations of clot development and any compromise of body system function due to clot formation.

- Transfusion.
- Packed RBCs to replace what has been lost due to bleeding.
- Fresh frozen plasma replaces coagulation factor deficiency.
- Platelets replace needed cells.
- Cryoprecipitate replaces fibrinogen.
- Administer anticoagulant drugs to decrease coagulation; not done in all patients.
  - Heparin
- Bed rest.

## Nursing Diagnoses

- Ineffective tissue perfusion
- Risk for deficient fluid volume

## Nursing Interventions

- Monitor for bleeding from obvious sites (wounds, suture lines, venipuncture, etc.) and occult sites (GI, urine).
- Avoid cleaning clots from exposed areas—may start bleeding from the site and not have sufficient clotting factors to stop.
- Explain to the patient
  - Avoid situations that might cause bleeding—use electric razor and soft toothbrush and avoid flossing between teeth.

# Hemophilia

Hemophilia is a disorder where the patient is missing a coagulation factor that is essential for normal blood clotting and, as a result, the blood does not clot when the patient bleeds (Figure 7–4). Hemophilia is a chronic disorder that can lead to bleeding at the slightest trauma.

## What Went Wrong?

Hemophilia is an X-linked recessive inherited disorder, passed on so that it presents symptoms in males and rarely in females. Hemophilia A is the result of missing clotting factor VIII. Hemophilia B is the result of missing clotting factor IX and is also known as *Christmas disease*.

## Prognosis

The most common sites of bleeding are into the joints or muscles or from the GI tract. Mild forms of the disease will only cause bleeding after surgery or trauma, whereas severe forms of the disease will cause bleeding without any prior cause.

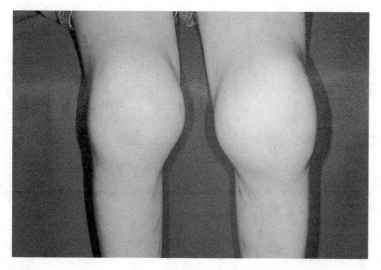

**FIGURE 7–4** · Enlarge joints indicate bleeding into the joints and is a sign of hemophilia.

## Hallmark Signs and Symptoms

- Tender joints due to bleeding.
- Swelling of knees, ankles, hips, and elbows because of bleeding.
- Blood in stool (tarry stool) owing to GI blood loss.
- Blood in the urine (hematuria).

## Common/Interpreting Test Results

- PTT prolonged.
- PT normal.
- Bleeding time is normal.
- Fibrinogen level is normal.
- Decrease in clotting factor VIII found in blood serum in hemophilia A.
- Decrease in clotting factor IX found in blood serum in hemophilia B.

## Treatment

- Avoid aspirin.
- For hemophilia A, administer factor VIII concentrates.
- Cryoprecipitate.
- DDAVP for patients with mild deficiency.
- For hemophilia B, administer factor IX concentrates.

## Nursing Diagnoses

- Acute pain
- Impaired gas exchange

## Nursing Interventions

- Avoid IM injections.
- No aspirin.
- To stop bleeding
  - Elevate site.
  - Apply direct pressure to the site.

- Explain to the patient
  - Wear a medical alert identification.
  - Contact physician for any injury.
  - Avoid situations where injury might occur.

# Idiopathic Thrombocytopenic Purpura

Idiopathic thrombocytopenic purpura (ITP) is an autoimmune disorder in which antibodies to the patient's own platelets are developed. ITP is a chronic condition in adults and children that is developed after a viral infection.

## What Went Wrong?

Antibodies attach to the platelets and macrophages within the spleen. The body destroys the platelets within the spleen. Normal clotting is affected. ITP in adults is typically more common in women and may become chronic in adults who are in early to mid-adulthood.

## Prognosis

Problems for the patient are most likely the result of bleeding due to inadequate platelets. Prednisone can control the majority of cases of ITP. Remission is common.

## Hallmark Signs and Symptoms

- Bleeding in mucous membranes or skin due to low platelet count.
- Epistaxis.
- Oral bleeding.
- Menorrhagia (heavy menstrual bleeding).
- Purpura.
- Petechiae.

## Common/Interpreting Test Results

- Thrombocytopenia—low platelet count.
- Mild anemia—usually secondary to bleeding.
- PT is normal.
- PTT is normal.

- Bleeding time is prolonged.
- Antibodies are detected.
- Bone marrow aspiration shows increased megakaryocytes (immature platelets).

## Treatment

The use of prednisone in patients with ITP is to decrease the body's action on the antibody-tagged platelets. Initially, the use of prednisone will also help enhance vascular stability. High-dose therapy needs to be tapered down. Most patients will be on long-term maintenance doses of prednisone. Splenectomy provides complete or partial remission.

- Prednisone—bleeding will stop even before platelet count begins to rise.
- High-dose IV immunoglobulin (gamma globulin).
  - Danazol
- Immunosuppressive therapy.
  - Vincristine, azathioprine, cyclosporine, cyclophosphamide
  - Rituximab
- Stem cell transplantation.
- Splenectomy (not commonly done).

## Nursing Diagnoses

- Risk for infection
- Disturbed body image
- Risk for ineffective individual coping

## Nursing Interventions

- Monitor vital signs for changes.
- Monitor for signs of bleeding or bruising.
- Decrease chance of bleeding.
- Use soft toothbrushes, no flossing, and use only electric razors.
- Protect from potential infection, sick visitors, etc.
- Encourage patient to discuss feelings about illness.
- Avoid aspirin or nonsteroidal anti-inflammatory drugs.

# Leukemia

Replacement of bone marrow by abnormal cells results in unregulated proliferation of immature WBCs entering the circulatory system. The WBCs do not function properly, grow faster than normal, and don't stop growing. The abnormal cells crowd out the normal cells. Leukemic cells enter the liver, spleen, or lymph nodes, causing these areas to enlarge.

## What Went Wrong?

Leukemia is classified according to the type of cell it is derived from, lymphocytic or myelocytic, and is either acute or chronic. Lymphocytic leukemia involves immature lymphocytes originating in the bone marrow and typically infiltrates the spleen, lymph nodes, or central nervous system. Myelogenous or myelocytic leukemia involves the myeloid stem cells in the bone marrow and interferes with the maturation of all blood cell types (granulocytes, erythrocytes, thrombocytes). People who have been exposed to high levels of radiation, who have had exposure to benzene, or who have a history of aggressive chemotherapy for a different type of cancer are at risk for leukemia. There may be a genetic predisposition to develop acute leukemia. Patients with Down syndrome, Fanconi anemia, or a family history of leukemia also have a higher-than-average incidence of this disease.

## Prognosis

Patients with acute leukemia typically have a more aggressive disease process, which may have a shorter course from the time of diagnosis. Patients have increased incidence of anemia, bleeding, and infections. Patients with chronic leukemia are more likely to have a less aggressive disease process that runs over a longer course. The chronic patients typically have an insidious onset and a better prognosis. Adults typically develop acute myeloid leukemia (AML) or chronic lymphocytic leukemia (CLL).

## Hallmark Signs and Symptoms

- Acute patients
  - Fatigue and weakness due to anemia.
  - Night sweats.
  - Frequent infections.

- Fever due to increased susceptibility to infection.
- Bleeding, petechiae, ecchymosis (bruising), epistaxis (nosebleed), gingival (gum) bleeding—owing to decreased platelet count.
- Bone pain because of bone infiltration and marrow expansion.
- Lymph nodes (lymphadenopathy) enlarged as leukemic cells invade nodes.
- Liver (hepatomegaly) and spleen (splenomegaly) enlarged as leukemic cells invade. Enlarged spleen may cause swollen, tender abdomen (typically left upper quadrant).
- Headache, nausea, anorexia, vomiting, and weight loss.
- Papilledema, cranial nerve palsies, seizure if there is central nervous system involvement.
- Chronic patients
  - Fatigue due to anemia.
  - Weight loss because of chronic disease process and poor or loss of appetite.
  - Enlarged lymph nodes (lymphadenopathy) due to infiltration of lymph nodes.
  - Enlarged spleen (splenomegaly) owing to involvement of the spleen.

## Common/Interpreting Test Results

- Low RBC count, low hemoglobin—anemia.
- Low platelet count—thrombocytopenia.
- Elevated WBC count—leukocytosis.
- Abnormal amount of immature WBCs shown in bone marrow biopsy.

## Treatment

- Acute myelogenous leukemia
  - Chemotherapy.
  - Administer an anthracycline (idarubicin or daunorubicin) plus cytarabine.
  - Combination: Daunorubicin, vincristine, prednisone, asparaginase.
  - Radiation therapy.
  - Administer platelet transfusions.

- Administer filgrastim for neutropenia.
- Administer antibiotics for infections.
- Bone marrow or stem cell transplant.
- Administer immunosuppressives to avoid transplant rejection.
- Chronic myelogenous leukemia
  - Administer signal transduction inhibitor.
    - Imatinib
    - Interferon-alpha
    - Busulfan
    - Hydroxyurea
- Chronic lymphocytic leukemia
  - Administer alkylating agents.
    - Cyclophosphamide
    - Chlorambucil
  - Administer antineoplastics.
    - Vincristine
    - Prednisone
    - Doxorubicin
  - Monoclonal antibody-targeted therapy.
    - Alemtuzumab
    - Combination of fludarabine and rituximab
  - Transfusion if hemolytic anemia or bleeding.
  - Packed RBCs.
  - Whole blood.
  - Platelets.
  - Bone marrow transplant and immunosuppression.
  - High-protein diet.

## Nursing Diagnoses

- Risk for infection
- Chronic pain
- Imbalanced nutrition, less than what body requires

## Nursing Interventions

- Monitor for bleeding—platelet count may be decreased.
- Monitor for infection—patients have increased susceptibility to infection.
- Monitor pain control.
- Small, frequent meals.
- Teach patients about infection control.
- Avoid others with infection.
- Report signs of infection, sore throat, fever, etc.
- Explain to the patient
  - Use an electric razor.
  - Use soft toothbrush.
  - Watch for bleeding or bruising.
  - Maintain a healthy diet.
  - Balance rest and exercise, and avoid overexertion.

# Multiple Myeloma

Multiple myeloma is a malignancy of the plasma cells that causes an excessive amount of plasma cells in the bone marrow. Plasma cells grow out of control within the marrow. Platelets and blood cells have difficulty forming within the crowded marrow.

## What Went Wrong?

Masses within the bone marrow cause destructive lesions in the bone. Normal bone marrow function is reduced as the abnormal plasma cells continue to grow. Immune function is diminished because plasma cells make antibodies, and the patient develops anemia. The disease typically affects older adults. There is an increased risk for patients with a history of radiation therapy.

## Prognosis

Patients are susceptible to infection and often have significant pain from bone involvement of the disease. The survival time from diagnosis averages about 3 years.

## Hallmark Signs and Symptoms

- Severe bone pain due to involvement in back or ribs.
- Anemia owing to invasion of the bone marrow.
- Fatigue because of anemia.
- Bleeding due to decreased platelet count.
- Fever.
- Shortness of breath owing to anemia.
- Skeletal fractures because of loss of normal bone structure (osteoporosis).
- Numbness and weakness of extremities if spine is affected.
- Increased risk of infection because of bone marrow failure to produce WBCs.
- Spinal cord compression as mass enlarges.
- Renal failure due to protein effect in renal tubules.

## Common/Interpreting Test Results

- Presence of the Bence Jones protein in urine.
- Serum protein electrophoresis shows a monoclonal protein spike.
- CBC shows anemia.
- Rouleaux formation on peripheral smear, a group of RBCs clump together in a stack (like a stack of coins).
- Abnormal plasma cells in bone marrow biopsy.
- X-rays of bone show lytic lesions.
- Elevated level of calcium in blood (hypercalcemia).
- Protein in urine (proteinuria).
- Elevated erythrocyte sedimentation rate.
- Decreased bone density.

## Treatment

Treatment regimens are based on patient response and current research findings. Combination therapy is common in treatment of multiple myeloma.

- Pain management.

- Combination chemotherapy.
  - Alkylating agent (melphalan) and prednisone
  - Thalidomide and dexamethasone
  - Nonalkylating combination (vincristine, doxorubicin, and dexamethasone)
  - Proteasome inhibitor (bortezomib) and thalidomide derivative (lenalidomide)
  - Dexamethasone, cyclophosphamide, Doxil, thalidomide, lenalidomide
  - Bortezomib alone or in combination
- Diet high in protein, carbohydrates, vitamins, and minerals.
- Small frequent meals.
- Transfusion of packed RBCs if anemia is severe.
- Bone marrow transplantation.
- Autologous (patient's own cells—increased survival in younger patients) or allogeneic (donor cells—more risk).
- Radiation therapy for bone pain or bone tumors.
- Bisphosphonates to decrease bone pain and prevent fractures.

## Nursing Diagnoses

- Pain
- Impaired mobility
- Risk for injury

## Nursing Interventions

- Protect the patient from falling.
- Monitor input and output due to renal function changes.
- Perform muscle-strengthening exercises.
- Increase fluids to enhance kidney clearance.
- Explain to the patient
  - Not to lift anything.
  - Be alert for fractures.

# Polycythemia Vera

Polycythemia vera is a disorder of the bone marrow (myeloproliferative disorder), resulting in an overproduction of blood cells and thickening of blood. This disorder is chronic and progressive. Researchers believe the *JAK2* gene mutation plays a role in this disorder.

## What Went Wrong?

Polycythemia vera predominantly causes increased RBCs, but WBCs and platelets may also be increased. The hallmarks of polycythemia vera include excessive production of RBCs, WBCs, and platelets. The excess of cells present in the blood causes problems with the flow of blood through vessels, especially the smaller ones. There will be an increase in peripheral vascular resistance, causing increased pressure, and vascular stasis in the smaller vessels, potentially causing thrombosis or tissue hypoxia. Organ damage may result because of these changes.

## Prognosis

After diagnosis of polycythemia vera, the average survival time is 10 to 15 years with appropriate treatment and less than 2 years without treatment. Some patients may go on to develop acute leukemia. Complications usually arise from thrombosis or tissue hypoxia. Polycythemia vera is associated with a gene mutation (*JAK2V617F*). It is more common in men and those over the age of 40 years.

## Hallmark Signs and Symptoms

- Facial skin and mucous membranes are dark and flushed (plethora).
- Hypertension due to increased peripheral vascular resistance and thickening of the blood.
- Difficulty breathing when lying flat (orthopnea).
- Itching worse after warm shower because of histamine release from increased basophils within dilated vessels.
- Headache and difficulty concentrating.
- Vision blurred, tinnitus (ringing in ears), and hearing changes.
- Thrombosis owing to vascular stasis.

- Spleen enlargement (splenomegaly).
- Sensation of fullness in the LUQ of the abdomen due to enlarged spleen.
- Tissue hypoxia and possible infarction of heart, spleen, kidneys, and brain as a result of thrombosis.

## Common/Interpreting Test Results

- Increased RBC count.
- Increased hemoglobin.
- Increased hematocrit level.
- Increased WBC count.
- Increased basophils.
- Increased eosinophils.
- Increased platelet count.
- Increased uric acid level.
- Increased potassium.
- Increased vitamin $B_{12}$ level.
- Bone marrow panhyperplasia; iron stores absent.
- Genetic testing may show *JAK2V617F* mutation.

## Treatment

Treatment is aimed at maintaining blood flow to the smaller vessels and diminishing the amount of excess blood cells being made by the bone marrow.

- Periodic scheduled phlebotomy—the removal of 500 mL of blood—to reduce the hematocrit level to below 45 in males or 42 in females may be done weekly.
- Adequate hydration.
- Administer anticoagulants such as aspirin.
- Administer myelosuppressive medication to reduce the number of RBCs being made.
  - Hydroxyurea
  - Anagrelide
  - Radioactive phosphorus 32

- Administer medication to lower uric acid level if necessary.
  - Allopurinol
  - Alkylating agents
  - Melphalan
  - Busulfan
- Radiation therapy.
- Antihistamine for pruritus.
- Aspirin to reduce risk of clotting.
- Ultraviolet B light therapy may decrease itching.

## Nursing Diagnoses

- Ineffective tissue perfusion
- Disturbed sensory perception
- Risk for injury

## Nursing Interventions

- Monitor vital signs.
- Monitor for bleeding.
- Monitor for signs of infections.
- Keep the patient mobilized to decrease chance of clot formation.
- Increase fluid intake.
- Explain to the patient
  - Maintain activity.
  - Use electric razor, use soft toothbrush, and avoid flossing to decrease chances of bleeding.
  - Avoid activities that could cause injury.

# CASE STUDY

## CASE 1

A 43-year-old mother of five children reports feeling tired for the past several months. She reports getting sufficient sleep, and she usually drinks several cups of black coffee a day; however, she is still fatigued. She reports feeling weak but can still function. She has headaches frequently and at time feels dizzy but denies fainting. She reports no pain or shortness of breath. She has pallor and is slightly tachycardic. The practitioner performed a CBC that came back with a low RBC count and low hemoglobin level. The patient is diagnosed with anemia and asks you the following questions. What is the best response?

**QUESTION 1.** The patient tells you that she feels that she is going to die from anemia. She asks you, "how long do I have to live a productive life?"
**ANSWER:** After looking at the patient's laboratory report, you notice that she has a low iron level. You then tell the patient that she has acute iron deficiency anemia. Iron deficiency anemia is very common and is not fatal. Taking oral iron supplements typically resolves the issue.

**QUESTION 2.** What happens if the oral supplements don't work?
**ANSWER:** If oral treatment is not adequate, the practitioner may admit the patient to the hospital or require the patient to be treated at an outpatient infusion center where the patient will receive iron supplements intravenously.

**QUESTION 3.** The patient tells you that her sister-in-law had anemia too. The patient then asks, "how frequently do I get $B_{12}$ injections?"
**ANSWER:** Your sister-in-law probably was diagnosed with pernicious anemia. Pernicious anemia is a disorder when the body is unable to absorb vitamin $B_{12}$ that is needed to produce RBCs, resulting in a decreased RBC count. Deficiency of vitamin $B_{12}$ inhibits the ability of RBCs to divide normally. As a result, RBCs become large and have difficulty in exiting bone marrow. Injections of vitamin $B_{12}$ are a typical treatment for pernicious anemia. However, you have iron deficiency anemia and will not require vitamin $B_{12}$ injections.

**QUESTION 4.** The patient asks, "how long must I take the iron supplement?"
**ANSWER:** Iron replacement therapy is continued to correct the deficiency and replace the lost stores of iron in the body. The typical time frame for oral therapy is to continue therapy for 3 to 6 months after the anemia has been corrected.

# FINAL CHECKUP

1. **A 12-year-old boy diagnosed with sickle cell anemia is undergoing inpatient treatment for an episode. He asks why you are administering morphine. What is your best response?**

   A. Morphine will prevent the cells from becoming stiff and sticky.

   B. Morphine prevents cells from clumping together.

   C. Morphine will ease the pain experienced in severe episodes of sickle cell anemia.

   D. Morphine dilates smaller vessels allowing cells to pass easily.

2. **A patient who was brought to the hospital for hemorrhaging was diagnosed with DIC. She asks what is happening to her body. What is your best response?**

   A. Proteins involved in blood clotting become overactive, resulting in excessive blood coagulation and leading to the depletion of platelets.

   B. There is a depletion of platelets, preventing your body from coagulating blood and leading to hemorrhaging.

   C. You are at risk for microthrombi.

   D. This is not a serious condition. Your body is missing an element that you can obtain from the pharmacy.

3. **A 78-year-old woman was recently diagnosed with leukemia. She asks you to describe the disorder. What is the best response?**

   A. There is an unregulated proliferation of immature RBCs that do not function properly.

   B. Leukemia is a form of cancer.

   C. Abnormal and immature WBCs enter the circulatory system and do not function properly, increasing the risk of other disorders.

   D. This is a blood condition that makes you susceptible to infection.

4. **A 32-year-old woman who travels by air many hours every week reports swelling of the lower right leg. You assess the lower right leg to find it is warm to the touch. What is your best response?**

   A. Lay down and bend your right foot toward your face.

   B. Lay down and bend your left foot toward your face.

   C. Call 911.

   D. Tell her not to move and call 911.

5. **A 45-year-old patient received a diagnosis of ITP after several episodes of bleeding. She asks if she is dying. What is your best response?**

   A. ITP is an autoimmune disorder in which antibodies to the patient's own platelets are developed.

   B. ITP is a chronic condition in adults and children that is developed after a viral infection.

C. Avoid situations where injury might occur.

D. Medication can control the majority of cases of ITP. Remission is common.

6. **A patient tells you that the practitioner said he has polycythemia vera and briefed him on the condition. The practitioner asks you to educate the patient about the importance of compliance with treatment. What is your best response?**

A. You should always follow treatment prescribed by a practitioner.

B. If you follow the treatment prescribed by the practitioner, the average survival time is between 10 and 15 years. Without treatment, survival time is less than 2 years.

C. Following the prescribed treatment will eliminate your blurry vision and ringing in your ears.

D. Your enlarged spleen will return to normal if you follow the treatment prescribed by the practitioner.

7. **A 52-year-old man recently diagnosed with DVT tells you he was told that he needs to inject himself in the stomach daily. He asks why this is so. What is your best response?**

A. You are injecting low-molecular-weight heparin, which will dissolve the blood clot.

B. The injections are SC injections. You should rotate the injection site with each injection.

C. You are injecting low-molecular-weight heparin, which will reduce formation of new blood clots.

D. You are injecting low-molecular-weight heparin, which will prevent formation of new blood clots.

8. **A 77-year-old woman was told she has aplastic anemia. She is confused and asks you if this disorder was acquired from drinking from plastic cups. What is your best response?**

A. Aplastic means that a part of the body is failing to develop. Aplastic anemia occurs when bone marrow stops producing a sufficient amount of new RBCs.

B. Drinking from plastic cups does not cause aplastic anemia.

C. You can continue to use plastic cups. Plastic cups have no effect on your condition.

D. Aplastic means that a part of the body is failing to develop. Aplastic anemia occurs when bone marrow stops producing a sufficient amount of new WBCs.

9. **A 56-year-old man who is newly diagnosed with leukemia tells you that he has no more good RBCs. What is your best response?**

A. You have a mix of abnormal WBCs, immature WBCs, and mature WBCs (good WBCs). However, there are more abnormal and immature WBCs than there are normal WBCs.

B. You have a mix of abnormal RBCs, immature RBCs, and mature RBCs (good RBCs). However, there are more abnormal and immature RBCs than there are normal RBCs.

C.  A bone marrow transplant will fix this problem.

D.  Let's focus on finding a bone marrow match for you.

10.  **A 41-year-old man diagnosed with multiple myeloma asks why the practitioner told him that his immune system is weakened because multiple myeloma doesn't affect WBCs. What is your best response?**

A.  Multiple myeloma is a malignancy of WBCs. WBCs create antibodies that fight invading microorganisms such as bacteria. There are decreased antibodies in your blood.

B.  Multiple myeloma is a malignancy of RBCs. RBCs create antibodies that fight invading microorganisms such as bacteria. There are decreased antibodies in your blood.

C.  Multiple myeloma is a malignancy of plasma cells. Plasma cells create antibodies that fight invading microorganisms such as bacteria. There are decreased antibodies in your blood.

D.  Plasma makes antibodies.

# CORRECT ANSWERS AND RATIONALES

1.  C.  Morphine will ease the pain experienced in severe episodes of sickle cell anemia.
2.  B.  There is a depletion of platelets, preventing your body from coagulating blood and leading to hemorrhaging.
3.  C.  Abnormal and immature WBCs enter the circulatory system and do not function properly, increasing the risk of other disorders.
4.  A.  Lay down and bend your right foot toward your face.
5.  D.  Medication can control the majority of cases of ITP. Remission is common.
6.  B.  If you follow the treatment prescribed by the practitioner, the average survival time is between 10 and 15 years. Without treatment, survival time is less than 2 years.
7.  C.  You are injecting low-molecular-weight heparin, which will reduce formation of new blood clots.
8.  A.  Aplastic means that a part of the body is failing to develop. Aplastic anemia occurs when bone marrow stops producing a sufficient amount of new RBCs.
9.  A.  You have a mix of abnormal WBCs, immature WBCs, and mature WBCs (good WBCs). However, there are more abnormal and immature WBCs than there are normal WBCs.
10.  C.  Multiple myeloma is a malignancy of plasma cells. Plasma cells create antibodies that fight invading microorganisms such as bacteria. There are decreased antibodies in your blood.

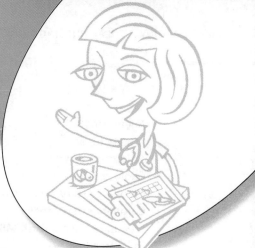

# chapter 8

# Vascular Disorders

## LEARNING OBJECTIVES

1. Vascular Disease
2. Aortic Aneurysm
3. Angina (Angina Pectoris)
4. Coronary Artery Disease
5. Hypertension
6. Hypovolemic Shock
7. Myocardial Infarction
8. Peripheral Arterial Disease
9. Raynaud Disease
10. Thrombophlebitis

## KEY TERMS

| | |
|---|---|
| Aneurysm | Nitrates |
| Atherectomy | Partial Thromboplastin Time (PTT) |
| Atherosclerosis | Percutaneous Transluminal Coronary |
| Cholesterol |    Angioplasty |
| Coronary Artery Bypass Graft (CABG) | PQRST Pain Assessment |
| Coronary Artery Stent | Pro-Brain Natriuretic Peptide (proBNP) |
| Creatine Kinase-MB (CK-MB) | Prothrombin Time (PT) |
| Duke Treadmill Score | Stable Angina |
| Embolectomy | Troponins |
| Femoropopliteal Bypass Graft | Unstable Angina |
| Laser Angioplasty | Vasospastic Angina |

# What Is Vascular Disease?

Vascular disease is a disruption of blood flow through blood vessels, which prevents adequate blood from reaching tissues and organs; as a result, tissues and organs do not get nutrition and oxygen, leading to tissue necrosis and organ failure. Vascular disease can involve arteries and veins. Nearly half the population will experience vascular disease as result of age, obesity, and type II diabetes.

A buildup of fat and cholesterol on the walls of blood vessels, referred to as *plaque*, decreases blood flow through the vessels in patients who have atherosclerosis. Eventually plaque could block blood flow, referred to as a *blockage*. A blocked blood vessel is an ischemic attack that results in the patient becoming symptomatic. Some ischemic attacks last for a fraction of a second. These are referred to as *transient ischemic attacks* (TIAs) and usually have no prolonged effect on the patient.

Other ischemic attacks can have long-term effects. Ischemic attack of coronary arteries causes chest pains (angina) that can lead to a heart attack. Ischemic attack of the carotid arteries that supply blood to the brain can lead to a stroke. Ischemic attack of arteries supplying the legs can result in cramps during activities (claudication) and leg pain, and can lead to ulcers, gangrene, and amputation. Ischemic attack of renal arteries can lead to hypertension, congestive heart failure, and kidney failure.

In addition to disorders that decrease circulation, there are other vascular diseases that affect circulation, which are discussed in this chapter.

# Aortic Aneurysm

An **aneurysm** is a weakening in the wall or a portion of the aorta, resulting in a balloon-like bulge as blood flows through the aorta. The blood flow within this bulging area of the aorta becomes very turbulent. Over time this turbulence can cause the dilated area to increase in size, creating an aneurysm (Figure 8–1). The aneurysm can rupture, causing a disruption in blood flow to everything below the affected area, and may even result in death.

## What Went Wrong?

An aneurysm is commonly due to **atherosclerosis** where fatty substances, **cholesterol**, calcium, and the clotting material fibrin, referred to as *plaque*, build up in the inner lining of an artery, resulting in thickening and hardening of the arteries. It may also be caused by degeneration of the smooth muscle layer (middle) of the aorta, trauma, congenital defect, or infection. The aneurysm may be found incidentally on radiographic studies done for other reasons, or the patient may have developed symptoms, indicating that something was wrong, such as severe back or abdominal pain or a pulsating mass. Severe hypotension and syncope (fainting caused by insufficient blood supply to the brain) may indicate rupture.

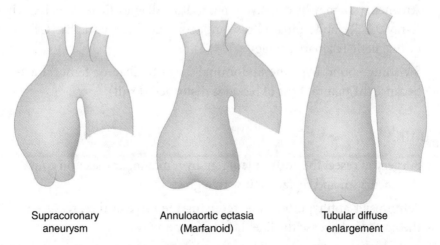

Supracoronary
aneurysm

Annuloaortic ectasia
(Marfanoid)

Tubular diffuse
enlargement

**FIGURE 8–1** · Three common patterns of ascending aortic aneurysm: supracoronary, annuloaortic ectasia, and tubular.

## Prognosis

Outcome will vary depending on size and location of an aneurysm. Some patients have aneurysms for months before a diagnosis is made, because they are asymptomatic. Treatment decisions will depend on the size and location of the aneurysm. Some patients with an aneurysm will be managed with watchful waiting with periodic imaging to monitor the size of the aneurysm, while other patients may need emergent surgery.

## Hallmark Signs and Symptoms

- Asymptomatic
- Abdominal pain
- Back pain that may radiate to posterior legs
- Abdominal pulsation
- Diminished femoral pulses
- Anxiety
- Restlessness
- Decreased pulse pressure
- Increased thready pulse

## Common/Interpreting Test Results

- An aneurysm may be displayed in a routine diagnostic test, such as chest X-ray (CXR), abdominal ultrasound, computed tomography (CT) scan, or magnetic resonance imaging (MRI).
- Swishing sound over the abdominal aorta or iliac or femoral arteries because the natural flow of blood is disturbed (bruit).

## Treatment

- Surgery to resect the aortic aneurysm by removing the section containing the aneurysm and replacing it with a graft.
- Administer antihypertensives, reducing the force of the pressure within the aorta to decrease the likelihood of rupture.
- Administer analgesics to treat patients who may be having pain from pressure on nearby structures (nerves, etc.) or tearing of the vessel.

- Administer oxycodone or morphine sulfate as needed to decrease oxygen demand.

## Nursing Diagnoses

- Ineffective peripheral tissue perfusion
- Risk for deficient fluid volume
- Acute pain
- Anxiety

## Nursing Interventions

- Monitor vital signs by looking for changes in blood pressure (BP) or elevated pulse and respiratory rates. During aortic dissection, the BP may initially increase due to severity of pain. It may then become difficult or impossible to obtain both the BP and pulse in one or both arms because of disruption of blood flow to the arm(s). The patient may go into shock quickly if the aneurysm ruptures.
- Monitor cardiovascular system by checking heart sounds, peripheral pulses (upper and lower extremities), and for abdominal bruits (swishing sounds heard over the blood vessel when flow is disturbed).
- Measure intake and output.
- Hypovolemia is suspected if there is a low urine output and high specific gravity of urine.
- Palpate abdomen for distention or pulsatile mass.
- Abdominal distention, which is an enlarged abdomen, may signify imminent rupture of the aneurysm.
- Check for
  - Signs of severe decrease in blood or fluid volume (hypovolemic shock).
  - The BP decreases as less blood circulates. Pulse rate increases as the heart tries to pump the blood faster to meet the oxygen demands of the body. Respiratory rate increases to meet oxygen needs while peripheral pulse sites are harder to find as BP lowers. The farther the pulse is from the heart, the more difficult it will be to find; it will be harder to locate the dorsalis pedis and posterior tibialis pulses earlier than the radial pulses.
  - Pale, clammy skin will be present as circulation decreases.

- Severe back pain due to rupture or dissection.
- Anxiety due to uncertainty of what is happening.
- Restlessness due to anxiety, discomfort, and decreased oxygenation.
- Decreased pulse pressure due to less circulating volume, increased heart rate, and less filling time between heartbeats.
- Increased thready pulse.
- Limit patient's activity to a prescribed exercise and rest regimen.
- Explain to the patient
  - Decreased peripheral circulation.
  - Numbness.
  - Tingling.
  - Decrease in temperature of extremities.
  - Change in skin color in extremities.
  - Absence of peripheral pulses.
  - Reduce patient anxiety.
  - Maintain a quiet place.
  - Have the patient express his or her feelings.

## Angina (Angina Pectoris)

Angina is the narrowing of blood vessels to the coronary artery, resulting in inadequate blood flow through blood vessels of the heart muscle, causing chest pain. An episode of angina is typically precipitated by physical activity, excitement, or emotional stress. There are three categories of angina.

- **Stable angina**—pain is relieved by rest or nitrates and symptoms are consistent.
- **Unstable angina**—pain occurs at rest; is of new onset; is of increasing intensity, force, or duration; isn't relieved by rest; and is slow to subside in response to nitroglycerin.
- **Prinzmetal or vasospastic angina**—usually occurs at rest or with minimal formal exercise or exertion; often occurs at night.

### What Went Wrong?

Angina is caused by arteriosclerosis. Atherosclerotic heart disease occurs when there is a buildup of plaque within the coronary arteries. Angina is often the first symptom of heart disease. When the demand for oxygen by the heart muscle exceeds the available supply, chest pain occurs.

## Prognosis

Patients can often be managed with lifestyle modifications and medications to control symptoms of angina. The most important factor is patient education. Patients need to understand the importance of their symptoms and when to seek medical attention. The pain must be evaluated initially and whenever a change in pattern or lack of response to treatment occurs. Additionally, a **Duke Treadmill score** is often used to determine an individual's prognosis.

## Hallmark Signs and Symptoms

- Chest pain lasting 3 to 5 minutes—not all patients get substernal pain; it may be described as pressure, heaviness, squeezing, or tightness. Use the patient's words.
- Can occur at rest or after exertion, excitement, or exposure to cold—due to increased oxygen demands or vasospasm.
- Usually relieved by rest—a chance to reestablish oxygen needs.
- Pain may radiate to other parts of the body such as the jaw, back, or arms—angina pain is not always felt in the chest. Ask if the patient has had similar pain in the past.
- Sweating (diaphoresis)—increased work of body to meet basic physiologic needs; anxiety.
- Tachycardia—heart pumping faster trying to meet oxygen needs as anxiety increases.
- Difficulty breathing, shortness of breath (dyspnea)—increased heart rate increases respiratory rate and increases oxygenation.
- Anxiety—not getting enough oxygen to heart muscle, the patient becomes nervous.

## Common/Interpreting Test Results

- Electrocardiogram (ECG) during episode.
- T wave inverted with initial ischemia, which is reduced blood flow due to an obstructed vessel, usually first sign.

- ST segment changes occur with injury to the myocardium (heart muscle).
- Abnormal Q waves due to infarction of myocardium.
- Laboratory tests: **Troponins, creatine kinase-MB (CK-MB)**, which is an enzyme released by damaged cardiac tissue 2 to 6 hours following an infarction, electrolytes.
- CXR to determine signs of heart failure.
- Holter monitoring: A portable electrocardiograph that the patient wears for 24 to 48 hours, giving that many hours of continuous cardiac monitoring.
- Coronary angiography to determine plaque buildup in coronary arteries.
- Cardiac positron emission tomography (PET) to determine plaque buildup in coronary arteries.
- Stress testing to determine symptoms/ECG changes when at exercise or under pharmacologic stress.
- Echocardiogram or stress echo to determine any abnormality of wall's motion due to ischemia.
- Consult cardiologist.
- Nonemergent laboratory tests: Complete blood count (CBC) (used to determine the general health status of the patient), chemistry (provides information about the status of electrolytes, kidneys, acid-base balance, blood sugar, and calcium levels), prothrombin time /international normalized ratio (PT/INR), activated partial thromboplastin time (PTT) (helps detect and diagnose bleeding disorders and determine the effectiveness of anticoagulants), and **pro-brain natriuretic peptide (proBNP)** (measures the presence and severity of heart failure).
- Cholesterol panel to evaluate risk.
- Increased risk for coronary artery disease (CAD) with increased total cholesterol, increased low-density lipoproteins (LDLs), increased triglycerides, and decreased high-density lipoproteins (HDLs).

## Treatment

The goal of treatment is to deliver sufficient oxygen to the heart muscle to meet its need. When suspecting chest pain, always give oxygen as the first line of defense. Medications are used initially to treat symptoms and increase blood flow to the heart muscle. Medications are used for symptom control and cholesterol management in the long term. Cardiovascular interventions are used to maintain adequate blood flow through the coronary arteries.

- 2 to 4 L of oxygen.
- Administer beta-adrenergic blocking agents—this class has a cardioprotective effect, decreasing cardiac workload, and likelihood of arrhythmia.
  - Propranolol (Inderal), nadolol (Corgard), atenolol (Tenormin), metoprolol (Lopressor)
- Administer nitrates—aids in getting oxygenated blood to heart muscle.
  - Nitroglycerin—sublingual tablets or spray; timed-release tablets.
  - Topical nitroglycerin—paste or timed-release patch.
- Aspirin for antiplatelet effect.
- Analgesic—typically morphine intravenously during acute pain. The medicine is very fast-acting when given this way and will decrease myocardial oxygen demand as well as decrease pain.
- **Percutaneous transluminal coronary angioplasty**—this is a nonsurgical procedure in which a long tube with a small balloon is passed through blood vessels into the narrowed artery. The balloon is inflated, causing the artery to expand.
- **Coronary artery stent**—this is a small, stainless steel mesh tube placed within the coronary artery to keep it open.
- **Coronary artery bypass graft (CABG)**—this is a surgical procedure in which a vein from a leg or an artery from an arm or the chest is removed and grafted to coronary arteries, bypassing the blockage and restoring free flow of blood to heart muscles.
- Restrict to low-cholesterol, low-sodium, and low-fat diet.

## Nursing Diagnoses

- Anxiety
- Decreased cardiac output
- Acute pain

## Nursing Interventions

- Monitor vital signs—look for change in BP, pulse, respiration; irregular pulse; pulse deficit; when a discrepancy is found between an atrial rate and a radial rate when measured simultaneously; pulse oximetry.

- Notify physician if systolic blood pressure (SBP) is less than 90 mm Hg.
- **Nitrates** dilate arteries to the heart and increase blood flow. You may have an order to hold nitrates if SBP is less than 90 mm Hg to reduce risk of patient passing out from lack of blood flow to brain.
- Notify physician if heart rate is less than 60 beats/min. Beta-adrenergic blocking agents slow conduction through the atrioventricular (AV) node and reduce the heart rate and contractility. You may have an order to hold beta-blockers if heart rate goes below 60; you should continuously monitor the patient's pulse rate.
- Assess chest pain each time the patient reports it.
- Remember **PQRST pain assessment** as follows:
  - Determine the
    - *P*lace.
    - *Q*uality (describe the pain—stabbing, squeezing, etc.).
    - *R*adiation (does the pain travel anywhere else?).
    - *S*everity (on a scale of 0 to 10).
    - *T*iming (when it started and how long it lasts and what preceded the pain).
- Monitor cardiac status using a 12-lead ECG while the patient is experiencing an angina attack. Each time the patient has pain, a new 12-lead ECG is done to assess for changes, even if one was already done that day.
- Record fluid intake and output. Assess for renal function.
- Place patient in a semi-Fowler's position (semisitting with knees flexed).
- Explain to the patient
  - Rest when pain begins to decrease oxygen demands.
  - Take nitroglycerin when any pain begins—it helps dilate coronary arteries and get more oxygen to heart muscle.
  - Avoid stress and activities that bring on an angina attack.
  - Call 911 if the pain continues for more than 10 minutes or if the patient is taking the third nitroglycerine dose (one sublingual dose every 5 minutes, if BP allows, for maximum of three doses).
  - Stop smoking! Smoking is associated with heart disease.
  - Adhere to the prescribed diet and exercise plan. Lower cholesterol and fat intake to decrease further plaque buildup, and decrease excess salt

intake to help BP control. Slowly increase exercise to build up activity tolerance. Possibly exercise with cardiac rehabilitation.

- How to recognize the symptoms of a myocardial infarction: Pay attention to chest pains as well as changes in patterns of pain and response to treatment. Be aware of changes in respiratory patterns, increase in shortness of breath, swelling, and general feelings of malaise.

# Coronary Artery Disease

Coronary artery disease (CAD) is the narrowing of coronary arteries that supply heart muscle with blood. Plaque builds up within the artery, resulting in decreased blood flow to the heart. Cardiac tissue is deprived of oxygen and nutrients, ultimately damaging the heart muscle (Figure 8–2).

## What Went Wrong?

Cholesterol, calcium, and other elements carried by the blood are deposited on the wall of the coronary artery, resulting in the narrowing of the artery and the

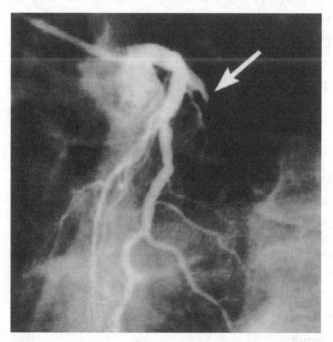

**FIGURE 8–2** · The white arrow points to severe stenosis in this coronary arteriogram, which is a sign of coronary artery disease.

reduction of blood flow through the vessel. This impedes blood supply to the heart muscle. These deposits start out as fatty streaks and eventually develop into plaque that inhibits blood flow through the artery. Elevated cholesterol levels and fat intake can contribute to this plaque buildup, as can hypertension, diabetes, and smoking.

## Prognosis

Lifestyle changes and medications can significantly impact the risks of the individual. Dietary modification, activity, and medications can help alter the disease process. Patients who continue with previous bad habits will continue with disease progression. Risk factors include age, male gender, and family history.

## Hallmark Signs and Symptoms

- Asymptomatic.
- Chest pain (angina) because of decreased blood flow to heart muscle and/or increase in myocardial oxygen demand resulting from stress.
- Pain may radiate to the arms, back, and jaw.
- Chest pain occurs after exertion, excitement, or when the patient is exposed to cold temperatures because there is an increase in blood flow throughout the body, raising the heart rate.
- Chest pain lasts between 3 and 5 minutes.
- Chest pain can occur when the patient is resting.

## Common/Interpreting Test Results

- Blood chemistry.
- Increased total cholesterol.
- Decreased HDL—helps with reverse transport of cholesterol.
- Increased LDL.
- ECG during chest pain.
- T-wave inversion—sign of ischemia.
- ST segment depressed—sign of injury to muscle.
- The waves are depressed because of tissue injury.
- Stress testing.

# Treatment

Treatment consists of risk factor modification, lifestyle changes, medications, and revascularization.

- Lose weight.
- Diet change: Lower sodium, lower cholesterol and fat, decrease calorie intake, increase dietary fiber.
- Administer low doses of aspirin.
- Administer beta-adrenergic blocking agents to reduce workload of heart.
  - Propranolol (Inderal), nadolol (Corgard), metoprolol (Lopressor)
- Administer calcium channel blockers to reduce heart rate, BP, and muscle contractility; helps with coronary vasodilation; slows AV node conduction.
- Administer nitrate if patient has symptomatic chest pains to reduce discomfort and enhance blood flow to myocardium.
- Administer platelet inhibitors.
  - Dipyridamole (Persantine)
  - Clopidogrel (Plavix)
  - Ticlopidine (Ticlid)
  - Prasugrel (Effient)
- Administer HMG CoA reductase inhibitors (statins)—lowers cholesterol.
  - Lovastatin (Mevacor)
  - Simvastatin (Zocor)
  - Atorvastatin (Lipitor)
  - Fluvastatin (Lescol)
  - Pravastatin (Pravachol)
  - Rosuvastatin (Crestor)
- Administer fibric acid derivatives to reduce synthesis and increase breakdown of very-low-density lipoprotein (VLDL) particles.
  - Gemfibrozil (Lopid)
- Bile acid binding resins bind bile acid in the intestine.
  - Colestipol (Colestid)

- Nicotinic acid reduces production of VLDL.
  - Niacin (vitamin B$_3$)

## Nursing Diagnoses

- Acute pain
- Activity intolerance
- Impaired gas exchange

## Nursing Interventions

- Monitor vital signs—signs of hypertension, irregular heart rate.
- Monitor ECG—look for end-organ damage, signs of heart disease.
- Monitor labs—periodic lipid panel, liver function for patients on statins.
- Monitor for myalgias (muscle aches).
- Explain to the patient
  - Smoking cessation.
  - Reduce alcohol consumption.
  - Change to a lower-fat, lower-cholesterol diet and increase dietary fiber intake.
  - Increase daily activity.
  - Weight reduction.
  - Stress management.
  - Hospital-based cardiac rehabilitation programs.

## Hypertension

Hypertension (HTN) is increased pressure within the blood vessels. Normal BP is 140 mm Hg **systolic** and 90 mm Hg **diastolic**.
  BP is classified as

- **Normal:** Less than 120 mm Hg systolic/less than 80 mm Hg diastolic
- **Prehypertension:** 120 to 139 mm Hg systolic/80 to 89 mm Hg diastolic
- **Stage 1 HTN:** 140 to 159 mm Hg systolic/90 to 99 mm Hg diastolic

- **Stage 2 HTN:** More than or equal to 160 mm Hg systolic/more than or equal to 100 mm Hg diastolic
- **In diabetic patients:** HTN is defined as 130/80 mm Hg or higher.

## What Went Wrong?

Primary (essential) HTN develops gradually over years without an identifiable cause. Secondary HTN appears suddenly and is caused by an underlying condition. These include kidney disease; thyroid disease; use of amphetamines, cocaine, alcohol, or tobacco; ingesting too much sodium or too little potassium; stress; or sleep apnea.

## Prognosis

The vast majority of patients have primary HTN, or high BP, that is not caused by other disease. Patients are typically asymptomatic and need to understand the importance of treatment to avoid long-term complications. End-organ damage can affect the heart, kidneys, brain, or eyes. Adequate control of BP is possible with medications and lifestyle modification, but these need to be maintained for the long term, often for the rest of the patient's life. Many patients will ultimately need to be on multiple medications to achieve adequate BP control.

## Hallmark Signs and Symptoms

- Asymptomatic
- Headache
- Dizziness

## Common/Interpreting Test Results

- BP readings higher than 140/90 mm Hg on at least three occasions.
- Ventricular hypertrophy depicted on ECG or CXR.
- Blood test to look for associated cardiovascular risks.
- High cholesterol—often associated with HTN.
- Check electrolytes for imbalance—sodium, potassium, chloride, and $CO_2$.
- Monitor BUN and creatinine (Cr) for renal function, a sign of impaired organ damage.
- Chemistry to check for diabetes mellitus.

## Treatment

Treatment is aimed at decreasing the risk of cerebral vascular accident (CVA), CAD, heart failure, renal disease, and other long-term sequelae of HTN.

- Lifestyle changes
  - Reduce caloric intake and exercise to reduce weight.
  - Low-sodium diet.
  - No smoking.
  - Reduce alcohol intake.
  - Reduce caffeine intake.
- Medication
  - Administer diuretics to reduce circulating blood volume.
    - Furosemide (Lasix), spironolactone (Aldactone), hydrochlorothiazide (HCTZ), bumetanide (Bumex)
  - Beta-adrenergic blocking agents to lower heart rate and cardiac output.
    - Propranolol (Inderal), atenolol (Tenormin), metoprolol (Lopressor)
  - Calcium channel blockers to cause peripheral vasodilation, less tachycardia.
    - Verapamil (Calan), diltiazem (Cardizem), nicardipine (Cardene)
  - Administer angiotensin-converting enzyme (ACE) inhibitors to inhibit the renin-angiotensin-aldosterone system. In diabetes, ACE inhibitors also delay the progression of renal disease.
    - Enalapril (Vasotec), lisinopril (Zestril), benazepril (Lotensin), captopril (Capoten), fosinopril (Monopril), quinapril (Accupril), perindopril (Aceon)

## Nursing Diagnoses

- Imbalanced nutrition: more than the body requires
- Knowledge deficit
- Excess fluid volume

## Nursing Interventions

- Monitor BP with multiple readings—lying, sitting, and standing, bilateral both arms.
- Reduce stress by providing a quiet environment.

- Explain to the patient
  - No smoking—smoking contributes to cardiovascular disease, raising BP.
  - Change to a low-sodium and low-cholesterol diet—salt adds to elevated BP in some patients by contributing to fluid retention; lowering cholesterol intake lowers risk for associated hyperlipidemia.
  - Reduce alcohol intake—reduces risk for end-organ damage from alcohol intake.
  - Reduce weight—decreased risk for obesity, better BP control with better weight control.
  - Exercise.
  - Call physician when BP is elevated.
  - Side effects of medications.

# Hypovolemic Shock

Rapid fluid loss causes inadequate circulation, resulting in inadequate perfusion of organs. A sufficient amount of blood is not available within the cardiovascular system, resulting in tissues and organs being deprived of sufficient amounts of oxygen and nutrients.

## What Went Wrong?

Hypovolemic shock can be caused by external hemorrhage, fluids moving in the body from vessels into tissue (third spacing), or dehydration. External hemorrhage is loss of blood, plasma, fluids, and electrolytes due to trauma, gastrointestinal (GI) bleed, vomiting, or diarrhea. Third spacing can result from ascites or pancreatitis.

## Prognosis

Prognosis depends on the etiology of the low volume; there may occasionally be more than one reason.

## Hallmark Signs and Symptoms

- Hypotension because blood volume in the body is decreased.
- Urine output less than 25 mL/h because less blood is perfusing the kidneys, causing decreased urinary output.

- Heart rate more than 100 (tachycardia), because the heart attempts to compensate for the decreased volume.
- Cold skin, because of peripheral vasoconstriction due to decreased volume.
- Restlessness, agitation; may be seen due to poor perfusion of the brain.

## Common/Interpreting Test Results

- Blood tests.
- CBC anemia.
- Chemistry to look at volume as depicted by the Cr and BUN.
- Coagulation studies.
- Type and cross-match for blood transfusion.
- Arterial blood gas (ABG).
- Decreased pH—if not perfusing well, acidosis will occur.
- Metabolic acidosis—by-products of metabolism will accumulate.
- Increased partial pressure of arterial carbon dioxide and decreased partial pressure of arterial oxygen due to poor perfusion.

## Treatment

Treatment depends on severity of symptoms. As always, maintaining open airway, breathing, circulation, and fluid resuscitation are of vital importance. After stabilization, the focus is on determining and treating the cause of the shock.

- Control bleeding—CBC, stool guaiac test (to find hidden [occult] blood in stool), assess for bleeding.
- Replace fluid—proper fluid replacement depends on the etiology of the shock; intravenous (IV) fluid and/or blood products are the choices.

## Nursing Diagnoses

- Deficient fluid volume
- Ineffective tissue perfusion
- Decreased cardiac output

## Nursing Interventions

- IV using 14-gauge (G) catheter (16 or 18 gauge also adequate if not able to obtain 14 gauge; use largest possible).
- Lactated Ringer solution (which contains electrolytes) or normal saline (0.9%).
- Blood replacement—type-specific or type O negative, which is the universal donor type.
- Monitor BP every 15 minutes.
- If systolic pressure is lower than 80 mm Hg, then oxygen flow rate may be increased.
- Monitor vital signs every 15 minutes.
- Measure urine output each hour with indwelling urinary catheter.
- Increase fluid rate if urine output is less than 30 mL/h. Be alert for signs of fluid overload. These include, but are not limited to, crackles in the lungs and dyspnea.
- Assess for cool, pale, clammy skin, indicating hypovolemic shock.
- Explain to the patient
  - Causes of hypovolemia and how to avoid a recurrence.
  - The purpose of the treatment.

# Myocardial Infarction

Myocardial infarction (MI) is commonly known as a heart attack. Blood supply to the myocardium is interrupted for a prolonged time due to the blockage of coronary arteries. This results in insufficient oxygen reaching cardiac muscle, causing cardiac muscles to die (**necrosis**).

## What Went Wrong?

The area of infarction is often caused by a buildup of plaque over time (atherosclerosis). It may also be caused by a clot that develops in association with the atherosclerosis within the vessel. Patients are typically (not always) symptomatic, but some patients will not be aware of the event; they will have what is called a *silent MI*.

## Prognosis

The outcome depends on the coronary artery that is affected. The earlier the person enters the health care system, the better the prognosis is, because emergency measures will be available for otherwise fatal arrhythmias. There is a better outcome for patients who receive adequate medical attention and make appropriate lifestyle changes post-MI. Cardiac rehabilitation can help patients make these changes safely.

## Hallmark Signs and Symptoms

- Chest pain that is unrelieved by rest or nitroglycerin, unlike angina.
- Pain that radiates to arms, jaw, back, and/or neck.
- Shortness of breath, especially in the elderly or women.
- Nausea or vomiting possible.
- May be asymptomatic, known as a *silent MI*, which is more common in diabetic patients.
- Heart rate more than 100 (tachycardia) because of sympathetic stimulation, pain, or low cardiac output.
- Variable BP.
- Anxiety.
- Restlessness.
- Feeling of impending doom.
- Pale, cool, clammy skin; sweating (diaphoresis).
- Sudden death due to arrhythmia usually occurs within first hour.

## Common/Interpreting Test Results

- ECG.
- T-wave inversion—sign of ischemia.
- ST segment elevated or depressed—sign of injury.
- Significant Q waves—sign of infarction.
- Decreased pulse pressure because of diminished cardiac output.
- Increased white blood count (WBC) due to inflammatory response to injury.
- Blood chemistry.

- Elevated CK-MB—usually done serially, the numbers will rise along a predetermined curve to signify myocardial damage and resolution.
- Elevated troponin I and troponin T proteins elevated within an hour of myocardial damage.
- Less than 25 mL/h of urine output due to lack of renal blood flow.

## Treatment

Treatment is focused on reversing and preventing further damage to the myocardium. Early intervention is needed to have the best possible outcome. Thrombolytic therapy is instrumental in reducing mortality. A 3-hour time window is ideal for maximizing benefit. Medications are used to enhance blood flow to the heart muscle while reducing the workload of the heart. Supplemental oxygen is used to help meet myocardial oxygen demand. Data from coronary angioplasty and percutaneous coronary intervention (stenting) of an occluded artery have been impressive. Following the acute management, the patient will have to make lifestyle changes—altering diet and exercise, stopping smoking, and so on.

- Administer oxygen, aspirin.
- Administer antiarrhythmic because arrhythmias are common, as are conduction disturbances.
  - Amiodarone
  - Lidocaine
  - Procainamide (Pronestyl)
- Electrical cardioversion for unstable ventricular tachycardia. In cardioversion, an initial shock is administered to the heart to reestablish sinus rhythm.
- Administer antihypertensive to keep BP low.
  - Hydralazine (Apresoline)
- Percutaneous revascularization.
- Administer thrombolytic therapy within 3 to 12 hours of onset because it can reestablish blood flow in an occluded artery, reduce mortality, and halt the size of the infarction.
  - Alteplase (Activase)
  - Streptokinase (Streptase)
  - Anistreplase (Eminase)
  - Reteplase (Retavase)

- Heparin following thrombolytic therapy.
- Administer calcium channel blockers as they appear to prevent reinfarction and ischemia, only in non-Q wave infarctions.
  - Verapamil (Calan)
  - Diltiazem (Cardizem)
- Administer beta-adrenergic blocking agents because they reduce the duration of ischemic pain and the incidence of ventricular fibrillation and decrease mortality.
  - Propranolol (Inderal)
  - Nadolol (Corgard)
  - Metoprolol (Lopressor)
- Administer analgesics to relieve pain, reduce pulmonary congestion, and decrease myocardial oxygen consumption.
  - Morphine
- Administer nitrates to reduce ischemic pain by dilation of blood vessels; helps lower BP.
  - Nitroglycerin
- Place patient on bed rest in coronary care unit.
- No bathroom privileges. Provide bedside commode.
- Low-fat, low-calorie, low-cholesterol diet.

## Nursing Diagnoses

- Ineffective tissue perfusion
- Decreased cardiac output

## Nursing Interventions

- Monitor for
  - Cardiovascular—look for changes or instability in pulse, heart sounds, murmur.
  - Respiration—look for changes, fluid in lung fields, shortness of breath.
  - ECG during attack—12-lead during any episode of pain.
  - ECG continuous monitoring for arrhythmias.

- Vital signs—check for changes in BP, pulse quality, peripheral pulses.
- Pulse oximetry monitoring.
- Explain to the patient
  - Change to a low-fat, low-cholesterol, and low-sodium diet.
  - The difference between angina pain and MI pain.
  - To take nitroglycerin when the patient feels angina pain.
  - To call 911 if the pain doesn't subside after 5 minutes of medication.
  - Smoking cessation.
  - Limit activities.
  - Need for cardiac rehabilitation.
  - Stress reduction.
  - Lifestyle changes such as increase in exercise and diet changes.

# Peripheral Arterial Disease

Large peripheral arteries become narrowed and restricted (**stenosis**), leading to the temporary (acute) or permanent (chronic) reduction of blood flow to tissues (**ischemia**). Severe peripheral arterial occlusive disease can lead to skin ulceration and gangrene.

## What Went Wrong?

Peripheral arterial disease is most commonly due to atherosclerosis (plaque on the inner walls of arteries), but may also be caused by a blood clot (**embolism**), or from an inflammatory process. Peripheral arterial occlusive disease is more common in patients with diabetes or hypertension, in older adults, in those with hyperlipidemia, and in those who smoke, as these conditions can predispose to diminished circulation. Vascular disease that happens in one area of the body, for example, the coronary arteries, is not an isolated process. The plaque buildup caused by long-term elevated cholesterol levels will happen throughout the body. The most common area of involvement is the lower extremities.

## Prognosis

Patients typically have progressive disease. It is a chronic problem, getting worse with age. Symptoms may not be present until there is a 50% or greater

**occlusion** (blockage) of the vessel. Suspect disease in patients who have risk for other cardiovascular diseases. Medications can help improve blood flow to the area, and increased activity will improve exercise tolerance and quality of life. Vascular intervention may be necessary as the disease progresses.

## Hallmark Signs and Symptoms

- Femoral, popliteal arteries.
- Sudden pain in the affected area because of spontaneous muscle contractions due to the reduced oxygenation of tissue.
- Intermittent claudication—pain, numbness, and/or weakness with walking due to increased oxygen demand of the muscle during activity.
- Weak or absent pulse in affected area because blood flow is reduced or blocked.
- Decreased temperature distal to the blockage because of restricted blood flow.
- Pallor or patchy coloring (mottling) of affected area because of reduced tissue oxygenation.
- Dependent rubor (increased redness when legs are lowered).
- Hair loss on extremities.

## Common/Interpreting Test Results

- Doppler ultrasonography of affected area.
- Arteriography—dye is injected into the affected artery enabling an outline of the artery and blockage to be seen in an X-ray.
- Ankle-brachial index (ABI) helps determine the amount of arterial insufficiency.

## Treatment

The goal of treatment is to maintain adequate blood flow to the area and avoid tissue damage. Patients are encouraged to maintain activity and reduce risk for disease, such as smoking, as well as to control BP and monitor diabetes.

- Exercise.
- Smoking cessation.
- Decrease in lipids, depending on what the lab work shows.

- Surgical treatment
  - **Femoropopliteal bypass graft:** A vessel from another part of the body is removed and grafted to the affected artery, permitting blood to bypass the blockage.
  - **Percutaneous transluminal angioplasty:** A catheter containing a balloon is inserted into the affected artery. The balloon is inflated, stretching the artery; this causes a healing response that breaks up plaque on the artery wall.
  - **Atherectomy:** A catheter containing a grinding tool is inserted into the affected artery and is used to grind plaque from the artery wall.
  - **Embolectomy:** Surgical removal of a blood clot from the affected artery.
  - **Thromboendarterectomy:** Surgical removal of atherosclerotic tissue from the affected artery.
  - **Laser angioplasty:** A laser-tipped catheter is inserted into the affected artery to remove the blockage.
  - **Stent:** A metal mesh tube is inserted into the affected artery to keep the artery open.
  - **Amputation:** Surgical removal of the affected limb that contains gangrene caused by low blood flow or complete blockage of blood to the affected limb.
- Administer antiplatelet medications to enhance blood flow to the lower extremities. This helps get blood through the vessels and alleviates symptoms.
  - Pentoxifylline (Trental)
  - Cilostazol (Pletal)
  - Aspirin
  - Clopidogrel (Plavix)
  - Dipyridamole (Persantine)
  - Ticlopidine (Ticlid)

## Nursing Diagnoses

- Fear
- Ineffective tissue perfusion
- Risk for injury

## Nursing Interventions

- Monitor most distal pulse to assure circulation exists.
- Compare bilateral pulses.
- Monitor temperature and color of affected area indicating tissue perfusion.
- Support hose.
- Check capillary refill.
- Don't elevate leg or apply heat if occlusion affects the femoral or popliteal arteries.
- Elevation of the lower extremities makes it harder for the blood flow to get to the tissues.
- Avoid prolonged sitting, which increases the risk of compression to vessels (impeding blood flow to lower extremities) and increases risk of clot formation in lower extremities.
- Explain to the patient
  - How to check pulses in the affected area if there is an absence of a pulse.
  - Call the physician if the patient experiences numbness, paralysis, or pain.
  - Don't wear tight clothes; avoid tight knee-high hose, which constricts at the popliteal space; avoid tight waistbands; wide shoes.
  - Change his/her lifestyle to reduce the risk of peripheral arterial occlusive disease.
  - The importance of regular examinations.
  - Foot check daily for open wounds, redness.
  - Regular visits to podiatrist.
  - Regular consults to vascular MD.

# Raynaud Disease

Blood flow to the extremities decreases as peripheral arteries narrow from vasospasm when exposed to cold or emotional stress. This results in the fingers, toes, nose, and ears blanching to a pale shade and/or turning blue and red as blood flow decreases (Figure 8–3). It usually occurs bilaterally, often sparing the thumbs, and begins to resolve with warming of affected areas.

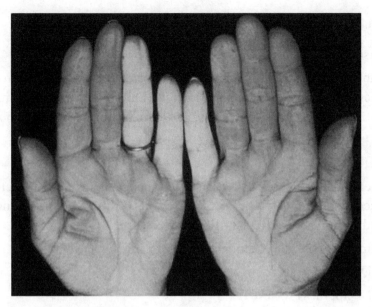

**FIGURE 8–3 ·** Raynaud disease's ischemic phase is shown with marked pallor of the ring finger and the little finger of the left and right hands.

## What Went Wrong?

Raynaud disease is a benign condition usually controlled by avoidance of underlying factors, that is, cold and stress. Secondary Raynaud disease can be seen with other disorders, mostly inflammatory and/or connective tissue diseases. This is more common in older men, usually involves the hands, and can have other complications.

## Prognosis

Prognosis for primary Raynaud disease is good. Symptoms may be controlled by avoidance or by medications. In secondary Raynaud disease, long-term ischemic complications may develop, such as loss of fat pads of fingers, gangrene due to diminished sensation, and propensity to develop frostbite.

## Hallmark Signs and Symptoms

- Discoloration of extremities progressing from pale, to blue, and then red because of decreased blood flow.
- Tingling and numbness in the extremities because of poor perfusion.

## Common/Interpreting Test Results

- Vasospasm is detected in an arteriograph.
- Laboratory tests to look for underlying disease process—CBC may show anemia; erythrocyte sedimentation rate (ESR), rheumatoid arthritis (RA), antinuclear antibodies (ANA) (these autoimmune tests will be positive).

## Treatment

Treatment is outpatient and consists of avoidance of aggravating factors and may need medication for primary disease and treatment of underlying disorders and ischemia for secondary Raynaud disease.

- Administer calcium channel blockers to ameliorate symptoms.
  - Diltiazem (Cardizem)
  - Nifedipine (Procardia)
- Administer vasodilators to aid in blood flow.
- Avoid cold and stress because this may causes vasospasms.
- Avoid smoking because it causes vasoconstriction.
- Surgical removal of a part of a sympathetic nerve (sympathectomy) because it can eliminate symptoms.

## Nursing Diagnoses

- Risk for injury
- Risk for peripheral neurovascular dysfunction
- Ineffective tissue perfusion

## Nursing Interventions

- Teach patient to wear mittens rather than gloves when exposed to the cold because it allows for air flow around fingers to hold body heat.
- Explain to the patient
  - Stop smoking.
  - Avoid cold.
  - Inspect skin regularly for cracks and treat immediately to prevent infections.
  - Use moisturizers.

# Thrombophlebitis

Thrombophlebitis is the inflammation of a vein as a result of the formation of one or more blood clots (thrombus). It is usually seen in the lower extremities, calves, or pelvis (Figure 8–4).

## What Went Wrong?

Thrombophlebitis may be the result of injury to the area, may be precipitated by certain medications or poor blood flow, or may be the result of a coagulation disorder.

## Prognosis

Prognosis is usually good unless embolization or moving of the clot occurs. It may move to the lung or brain, which can be life-threatening.

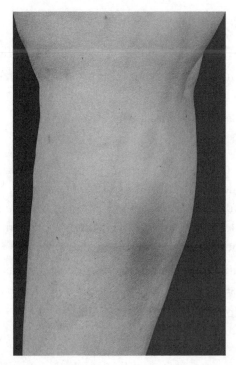

**FIGURE 8–4** · Thrombophlebitis in the mid-calf.

## Hallmark Signs and Symptoms

- May be asymptomatic
- Edema, tenderness, and warmth in the affected area as part of an inflammatory response.
- Palpable tender cord.
- Positive Homan sign (pain on dorsiflexion of the ipsilateral foot) is an unreliable sign.
- Cramping because blood flow to the area is impaired due to the presence of the clot.
- If the clot dislodges from the vein and travels to the lung, other symptoms will develop.
- Difficulty breathing (dyspnea) when the clot has traveled to the lungs.
- Rapid breathing, more than 20 breaths/min (tachypnea), because of a clot in the lungs.
- Chest pain in the area of clot.
- Crackle sounds in lungs in the area of clot.

## Common/Interpreting Test Results

- Ultrasound to determine if blood is flowing to the affected area.
- Photoplethysmography to depict any defects in venous filling in the affected area.
- Laboratory tests to look for clotting disorders.

## Treatment

Patients with large deep vein thrombosis (DVT), with comorbidities (a disease coexisting with, and often impacting on, another disease present), and/or of advanced age should be treated in the hospital. Treatment consists of anticoagulation to prevent further occurrences.

- Administer anti-inflammatory medication to decrease the inflammation within the vessel.
  - Aspirin, indomethacin

- Administer anticoagulant medication to prevent the clot from becoming larger.
  - Heparin, warfarin (Coumadin), dalteparin (Fragmin), enoxaparin (Lovenox)
- Limit activity initially to diminish risk of moving clot—bed rest with bathroom privileges.

## Nursing Diagnoses

- Ineffective tissue perfusion
- Acute pain
- Impaired skin integrity

## Nursing Interventions

- Monitor breathing because changes in respiratory status can signal that a clot has dislodged and moved to the lung.
- Monitor laboratory tests because the patient is receiving anticoagulants.
- Monitor for therapeutic effect.
- Apply warm moist compresses over affected area because this enhances blood flow to area.
- Explain to the patient
  - Report signs of bleeding—anticoagulant may be too much.
  - Report signs of clotting—pain in affected area, shortness of breath—patient may have underlying clotting disorder.
  - Move about frequently when allowed—discourages chances of developing another clot.
  - Don't cross legs—avoid constriction of lower extremity vessels.
  - Don't use oral contraceptives—increases risk of clot formation.
  - Support hose.
  - Elevate affected area.

# CASE STUDY

## CASE 1

The practitioner asks you to meet a 54-year-old woman who has just been diagnosed with angina. The practitioner tells the patient about the diagnosis and asks you to answer the patient's other questions. Here are questions asked by the patient. What is the best response?

QUESTION 1. How come I get chest pains?

ANSWER: Angina is caused by arteriosclerosis. Atherosclerotic heart disease occurs when there is a buildup of plaque within the coronary arteries. Angina is often the first symptom that heart disease exists. When the demand for oxygen by the heart muscle exceeds the available supply, chest pain occurs.

QUESTION 2. Am I going to die?

ANSWER: Patients can often be managed with lifestyle modifications and medications to control symptoms of angina. It is important to understand the symptoms and when to seek medical attention. You must contact your practitioner if medication does not relieve the pain or whenever a change in pattern occurs.

QUESTION 3. What should I do when I get chest pain again?

ANSWER: Take nitroglycerin when any pain begins—it helps dilate coronary arteries and get more oxygen to heart muscle. Rest when pain begins to decrease the demand for oxygen. Call 911 if the pain continues for more than 10 minutes or when you take the third nitroglycerine dose.

QUESTION 4. Is there any way to prevent chest pain?

ANSWER: Avoid stress and activities that bring on an angina attack. Stop smoking! Adhere to the prescribed diet and exercise plan. Lower cholesterol and fat intake to decrease further plaque buildup, and decrease excess salt intake to help BP control. Slowly increase exercise to build up activity tolerance. Pay attention to chest pains as well as changes in patterns of pain and response to treatment. Be aware of changes in respiratory patterns, increase in shortness of breath, swelling, and general feelings of malaise.

# FINAL CHECKUP

1. **A 46-year-old man was diagnosed with an aneurysm during follow-up to his annual physical examination. He said that he feels fine and questions the diagnosis. What is your best response?**

   A. It is best to speak with the practitioner about your concerns.

   B. Some patients have aneurysms for months before a diagnosis is made because they don't have any symptoms.

   C. You are lucky they caught it in time because you can die from an aneurysm.

   D. Aneurysms are common. You shouldn't be concerned unless you experience symptoms.

2. **A 53-year-old woman reports chest pains at night when she is resting. She asks what might be the problem. What is your best response?**

   A. You might have vasospastic angina. Let's speak with your practitioner.

   B. You might have vasospastic angina.

   C. Speak with your practitioner.

   D. I'm not permitted to answer your question.

3. **A 58-year-old woman tells you that she is considering undergoing percutaneous transluminal coronary angioplasty. She asks you to describe that procedure. What is the best response?**

   A. This is a nonsurgical procedure that uses X-rays to expand narrowed arteries.

   B. This is a nonsurgical procedure in which a long tube is passed through the urethra into the narrowed artery. The balloon is inflated, causing the artery to expand.

   C. This is a surgical procedure in which a long tube with a small balloon is passed through blood vessels into the narrowed artery. The balloon is inflated, causing the artery to expand.

   D. This is a nonsurgical procedure in which a long tube with a small balloon is passed through blood vessels into the narrowed artery. The balloon is inflated, causing the artery to expand.

4. **A 64-year-old man is told that he must undergo emergency CABG. He asks you to explain the procedure. What is your best response?**

   A. This is a nonsurgical procedure in which a long tube with a small balloon is passed through blood vessels into the narrowed artery. The balloon is inflated, causing the artery to expand.

   B. This is a surgical procedure in which a vein from a leg or an artery from an arm or the chest is removed and grafted to coronary arteries, bypassing the blockage and restoring free flow of blood to heart muscles.

C. This is a small, stainless steel mesh tube that is placed within the coronary artery to keep it open.

D. This is a nonsurgical procedure in which a vein from a leg or an artery from an arm or the chest is removed and grafted to coronary arteries, bypassing the blockage and restoring free flow of blood to heart muscles.

5. **A 55-year-old patient who has been diagnosed with primary HTN disorder asks you what underlying disorder caused his HTN. What is your best response?**

   A. Primary HTN develops gradually over years without an identifiable cause.

   B. Diabetes.

   C. Kidney disease.

   D. Too much salt.

6. **An 18-year-old woman was in a motor vehicle accident and was taken to the emergency department with multiple internal injuries. Which of the following conditions do you need to rule out?**

   A. Raynaud disease

   B. Coronary artery disease

   C. Hypovolemic shock

   D. Atherosclerosis

7. **A 52-year-old woman was diagnosed with thrombophlebitis. She asks how serious this disorder is. What is the best response?**

   A. You must avoid all movement until the thrombophlebitis is resolved.

   B. Prognosis is usually poor because a clot will move to the lung or brain, which can be life-threatening.

   C. Prognosis is usually good unless embolization or moving of the clot occurs. It may move to the lung or brain, which can be life-threatening.

   D. This is not serious as long as you take your medication.

8. **A 54-year-old man was told by the practitioner that he must undergo laser angioplasty. He doesn't understand the procedure. What is your best response?**

   A. A laser-tipped catheter is used to correct your eyesight so you no longer require corrective glasses.

   B. A laser-tipped catheter is inserted into the affected artery and a balloon is inflated to remove the blockage.

   C. A laser-tipped catheter is inserted into the affected artery to install a stent.

   D. A laser-tipped catheter is inserted into the affected artery to remove the blockage.

9. **A 69-year-old man tells you that the practitioner suggested an embolectomy. He asks you to explain this procedure. What is your best response?**

   A. A catheter containing a grinding tool is inserted into the affected artery and is used to grind plaque from the artery wall.

   B. A metal mesh tube is inserted into the affected artery to keep the artery open.

   C. Embolectomy is the surgical removal of a blood clot from the affected artery.

   D. A vessel from another part of the body is removed and grafted to the affected artery, permitting blood to bypass the blockage.

10. **A 41-year-old man tells you that the practitioner suspects he has a blockage in an artery. He asks you how the practitioner will confirm that the blockage exists. What is your best response?**

    A. The practitioner may use Doppler ultrasonography to examine the affected area. If this test indicates there might be a blockage, the practitioner will likely order an arteriography where dye is inserted into your arteries and an X-ray of your artery is taken.

    B. The practitioner will use the ankle-brachial index to confirm the blockage.

    C. The practitioner will perform exploratory surgery under a local anesthetic.

    D. The practitioner will perform exploratory surgery under a general anesthetic.

## CORRECT ANSWERS AND RATIONALES

1. B. Some patients have aneurysms for months before a diagnosis is made because they don't have any symptoms.
2. A. You might have vasospastic angina. Let's speak with your practitioner.
3. D. This is a nonsurgical procedure in which a long tube with a small balloon is passed through blood vessels into the narrowed artery. The balloon is inflated, causing the artery to expand.
4. B. This is a surgical procedure in which a vein from a leg or an artery from an arm or the chest is removed and grafted to coronary arteries, bypassing the blockage and restoring free flow of blood to heart muscles.
5. A. Primary HTN develops gradually over years without an identifiable cause.
6. C. Hypovolemic shock.
7. C. Prognosis is usually good unless embolization or moving of the clot occurs. It may move to the lung or brain, which can be life-threatening.
8. D. A laser-tipped catheter is inserted into the affected artery to remove the blockage.
9. C. Embolectomy is the surgical removal of a blood clot from the affected artery.
10. A. The practitioner may use Doppler ultrasonography to examine the affected area. If this test indicates there might be a blockage, the practitioner will likely order an arteriography where dye is inserted into your arteries and an X-ray is of your artery is taken.

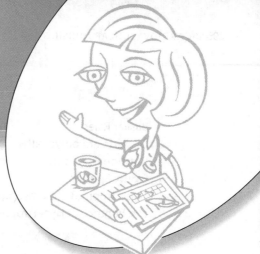

chapter 9

# Cardiac Disorders

## LEARNING OBJECTIVES

1. Cardiac Tamponade
2. Cardiogenic Shock
3. Cardiomyopathy
4. Heart Failure (Congestive Heart Failure)
5. Pulmonary Edema
6. Rheumatic Heart Disease

---

## KEY TERMS

Basilar Rales

Dilated Cardiomyopathy

Exertional Dyspnea

Frothy Sputum

Hypertrophic Cardiomyopathy

Left Ventricular Hypertrophy

Pericardiocentesis

Pericardium

Positive Hepatojugular Reflux

Pulsus Paradoxus

Restrictive Cardiomyopathy

Swan Ganz Catheter

---

# What Are Cardiac Disorders?

A *cardiac disorder* is a term used to describe many different conditions that cause the heart to function abnormally. A cardiac disorder disrupts the heart's ability to pump blood throughout the body. As a result, the patient may experience shortness of breath, light-headedness, and irregular heartbeat and chest pains.

There are a number of underlying causes of a cardiac disorder. These include trauma, infection, postoperative effects, myocardial infarction (MI), and heart disease. These underlying causes may lead to fluid retention in the lungs, around the heart, and in the legs. Some cardiac disorders are idiopathic and have no obvious underlying cause.

Most cardiac disorders are manageable through procedures or ongoing treatment with medication. Prognosis varies depending on the cardiac disorder and compliance with treatment.

# Cardiac Tamponade

Cardiac tamponade occurs when a large amount of liquid accumulates in the sac around the heart (pericardium), creating pressure on the heart that reduces the filling of ventricles with blood. This results in a low volume of blood being pumped with each contraction. The accumulating pressure within the pericardium may be due to fluid, pus, or blood. The end result is decreased stroke volume and cardiac output.

## What Went Wrong?

The cause of cardiac tamponade may be trauma, postoperative, post-MI, uremia, or cancer. The fluid may develop rapidly or over time, depending on cause. Cardiac tamponade is a life-threatening condition. The seriousness is related to the amount of pressure within the heart and the resulting decrease in ventricular filling.

## Prognosis

Cardiac tamponade is a medical emergency requiring immediate intervention, such as drainage of the fluids. Stabilization occurs quickly once the fluid is removed and pressure is alleviated. If fluid recurs, surgery may be necessary. The prognosis depends on the etiology of the cardiac tamponade.

## Hallmark Signs and Symptoms

- Neck vein distention—accumulation of fluid within the pericardium causes pressure on the heart, which prevents the venous return from the jugular veins. This causes distention, which is more pronounced on inspiration.
- Restlessness due to decreased oxygen to the brain.
- Muffled (dull) heart sounds on auscultation because it's harder to hear through fluid.
- **Pulsus paradoxus**—decrease of 10 mm Hg or more in systolic blood pressure (SBP) during inspiration—change in pressure within the chest during inspiration, resulting in decreased ventricular filling, decreased output, and fall in SBP.
- Sweating (diaphoresis).
- Difficulty breathing (dyspnea).
- Tachycardia.
- Hypotension.
- Fatigue.

## Common/Interpreting Test Results

- **Echocardiogram:** Ultrasound imaging of the heart to assess the heart's position, structure, and motion. Ventricles and atria are compressed. Fluid found within pericardial sac.
- Cardiac catheterization.
- Chest X-ray (CXR): This shows an enlarged heart if large effusion present.
- Electrocardiogram (ECG) used to rule out other cardiac problems.

## Treatment

Treatment is directed at reducing the pressure on the heart from the accumulating fluids in the pericardial sac. The following may be necessary to support and stabilize the patient.

- **Pericardiocentesis:** A needle is inserted into the pericardium and fluid is aspirated or drained.
- **Adrenergic agent:** This increases heart rate and blood pressure (BP).

## Nursing Diagnoses

- Anxiety
- Ineffective tissue perfusion
- Decreased cardiac output

## Nursing Interventions

- Monitor vital signs.
- Ensure adequate oxygenation.

# Cardiogenic Shock

The heart is unable to pump blood, resulting in a cardiac emergency. Blood pools in the left ventricle, which causes a backup of blood into the lungs, resulting in pulmonary edema.

Contractions increase to compensate for the decreased cardiac output, causing an increase in demand for oxygen by the heart. However, the lungs are not oxygenating the blood sufficiently due to decreased blood flow, and therefore heart muscles are starved for oxygen.

## What Went Wrong?

A drop in BP and blood flow is caused by the heart's inability to pump blood as a result of cardiac tamponade, myocardial ischemia, myocarditis, cardiomyopathy (a disease of the heart that deteriorates the heart muscle), or cardiac trauma.

## Prognosis

Treatment needs to find a balance between improving cardiac output and reducing oxygen needs and cardiac workload of the myocardium. This balance must be achieved while maintaining perfusion of the heart muscle. Prognosis depends on finding and treating the underlying cause. Cardiogenic shock requires immediate treatment, often before the cause is known.

## Hallmark Signs and Symptoms

- Hypotension, because blood flow decreases below normal.
- Tachycardia, because the heart is trying to pump faster to maintain adequate blood flow to the body, or occasionally bradycardia, where the heart rate is less than 60 beats/min due to myocardial damage.
- Arrhythmias—when the heart muscle does not have enough oxygen, it becomes irritable, making arrhythmias more likely.
- Clammy skin, because oxygenation to tissues is reduced.
- Drop in skin temperature because of reduced circulation as a result of hypotension.
- Urine output less than 30 mL/h (oliguria) because the kidneys are not being perfused.
- Crackles heard in the lungs secondary to pulmonary edema, indicating fluid is building up in lungs.
- Confusion due to poor perfusion.
- Distended jugular veins—sign of fluid overload, inability of heart to manage fluid flowing into heart.
- Narrow pulse pressure.
- Cyanosis of lips, peripheral extremities due to poor perfusion.

## Common/Interpreting Test Results

- Chemistry—check electrolytes, kidney function to ascertain kidney perfusion; calcium level is increased or decreased secondary to muscle contractility.
- Echocardiogram—to look for ventricular rupture, pericarditis, or valve dysfunction.
- ECG
  - Q wave enlarged due to heart failure.
  - Elevation of ST waves is a sign of ischemia.

## Treatment

Treatment is based on medical support for the heart until etiology (cause) can be determined. In cardiogenic stroke, the stroke volume and the heart rate must be increased to keep the organs perfused. The effects of the following medications should accomplish this.

- Administer vasodilator—dilates blood vessels (arterial and venous) to decrease the venous return to the heart and reduces the peripheral arterial resistance.
- Administer adrenergic agent—to increase the heart rate and BP.
  - Epinephrine
- Administer inotropes—strengthens the heartbeat, improves contractions, produces peripheral vasoconstriction.
  - Dopamine (Intropin)
  - Dobutamine
  - Inamrinone (Amrinone)
  - Milrinone (Primacor)
- Administer vasopressor—decreases blood flow to all organs except the heart and brain.
  - Norepinephrine
- Provide supplemental oxygen—may need to be through intubation.

## Nursing Diagnoses

- Ineffective tissue perfusion
- Decreased cardiac output

## Nursing Interventions

- Monitor vital signs—look for changes in BP, pulse (P), and respiration (R).
- Monitor heart sounds.
- Monitor **Swan Ganz catheter.** This is a catheter placed into the pulmonary artery to check for pressures in the heart, vessels, and lungs.
- Test capillary refill.
- Monitor arterial blood gas (ABG) to determine the pH level, acidosis or alkalosis, bicarbonate level.

- Monitor respiratory status—due to poor perfusion, these patients are in respiratory distress; mechanical ventilation may be needed.
- Place the patient on bed rest.
- Monitor intake and output of fluids—look for adequate renal perfusion.
- Without sufficient cardiac function, the patient will not have enough blood flow to the kidneys to get adequate filtration.
- Explain to the patient
  - Be aware of particular symptoms and call the doctor.
  - Take rest periods.
  - Call the physician if there are signs of fluid overload—weight increase, shortness of breath, fatigue, dependent edema.
  - Record weight each day and call the physician, nurse practitioner, or physician assistant if there is an increase of 3 lb (1.4 kg).
  - Change to a low-sodium, low-fat diet.

# Cardiomyopathy

The middle layer of the heart wall that contains cardiac muscle (myocardium) weakens and stretches, causing the heart to lose its pumping strength and become enlarged. Cardiac contractions are weak, resulting in decreased cardiac output; however, cardiac functions remain normal.

## What Went Wrong?

Most are idiopathic and not related to the major causes of heart disease. The three types of cardiomyopathy are as follows:

- **Dilated cardiomyopathy (common):** The heart muscle thins and enlarges, leading to congestive heart failure (CHF). Progressive hypertrophy and dilatation result in problems with pumping action of ventricles.
- **Hypertrophic cardiomyopathy (HCM):** The ventricular heart muscle thickens, resulting in outflow obstruction or restriction. There is some blood flow present.
- **Restrictive cardiomyopathy (rare):** The heart muscle becomes stiff and restricts blood from filling ventricles, usually as a result of amyloidosis, radiation, or myocardial fibrosis after open-heart surgery.

## Prognosis

Prognosis is variable. Sudden cardiac death is a possible outcome in dilated cardiomyopathy or HCM; arrhythmia is often a precursor to sudden death.

## Hallmark Signs and Symptoms

- **Asymptomatic:** Many patients with HCM are asymptomatic. The first sign is often cardiac arrest. Those with signs do not present until their mid-twenties.

- **Dyspnea:** The most frequent symptom is shortness of breath due to increased pressure in the lungs. The heart may not sufficiently relax, resulting in higher pressure and a backup of blood into the lungs.

- **Angina:** Patients experience chest pain related to increased oxygen demand of the extra heart muscle and due to thick, narrowing coronary blood vessels within the heart's wall.

- **Syncope:** Fainting is caused by heart arrhythmias related to the inability of the cardiac muscle to conduct electrical impulses.

- **Sudden death:** Young adults are at risk of sudden death during physical exercise, resulting from ventricular fibrillation—a cardiac arrhythmia.

- Abnormal heart sounds.

- **Murmur:** The sound of turbulence and results from abnormal blood flow.

- $S_3$, which is a third heart sound commonly heard in heart failure. $S_3$ is a soft sound made by the vibration of the ventricular wall when the ventricle fills too rapidly. $S_3$ is heard after the $S_2$ heart sound and is best found over the apex of the left ventricle, which is the fourth intercostal space along the mid-clavicular line.

- $S_4$, which is the heart sound heard before the $S_1$ heart sound is the result of the heart being too stiff. This is a vibration of the valves and the ventricular walls when the atria contract and the ventricles fill.

## Common/Interpreting Test Results

- CXR shows enlarged heart, pulmonary congestion.

- Echocardiography shows **left ventricular hypertrophy** (LVH) and dysfunction in dilated cardiomyopathy and HCM; small ventricular size and function in restrictive cardiomyopathy.

- ECG: ST changes, conduction abnormalities:
  - LVH shows as a broad QRS wave, usually in leads 4, 5, and 6 because of high voltage.
- **Cardiac catheterization:** To measure chamber pressures, cardiac output, ventricular function, but is often unable to add to information that has already been received from the echocardiogram.
- Exercise testing may show poor cardiac function not evident in a resting state.

## Treatment

Treatment is based on the specific cause. Avoiding the offending drug/treatment is imperative. Manage the underlying disease and provide cardiac support; however, few therapies can halt the process of cardiomyopathy.

- Change to a low-sodium diet.
- Beta-adrenergic blocking agents cause the heart to beat slowly, allowing more time for ventricular filling and improving contractile function.
  - Propranolol (Inderal), nadolol (Corgard), metoprolol (Lopressor) (for HCM)
- Angiotensin-converting enzyme (ACE) inhibitors—to decrease left ventricular filling pressures.
- Calcium channel blockers reduce cardiac workload by increasing contractility.
  - Verapamil (Calan) (for HCM)
- Diuretics reduce fluid retention.
  - Furosemide (Lasix), bumetanide (Bumex), metolazone (Zaroxolyn) (for dilated cardiomyopathy)
  - Spironolactone (aldosterone antagonist)
- Administer inotropic agent to enable the heart to have greater contractile force.
  - Dobutamine
  - Milrinone (Primacor)
  - Digoxin (Digitalis) (for dilated cardiomyopathy)
- Administer oral anticoagulant to reduce the coagulation of blood.
  - Warfarin (Coumadin) (for dilated and HCM)

- Implantable cardioverter-defibrillator for high risk.
- Myectomy—incision into septum and removal of tissue.

## Nursing Diagnoses

- Activity intolerance
- Impaired gas exchange
- Decreased cardiac output

## Nursing Interventions

- Place patient in a semi-Fowler's position for comfort, which eases respiratory effort.
- Record intake and output of fluids.
- Monitor vital signs to assess for increased respiratory rate, arrhythmias.
- Monitor ECG to look for changes from previous tracing.
- Explain to the patient
  - Fluids restriction may be necessary if the patient has heart failure and dilated cardiomyopathy.
  - Record daily weight and call physician if weight increases by 3 lb (1.4 kg).
  - No smoking or drinking alcohol.
  - No straining during bowel movements.
  - Increase exercise.

## Heart Failure (Congestive Heart Failure)

In CHF, the heart is unable to pump sufficient blood to maintain adequate circulation. This results in a backup of blood, and the extra pressure may cause accumulation of fluid into the lungs.

## What Went Wrong?

The heart muscle is too weak to adequately push blood forward or the heart is not able to sufficiently relax and receive enough blood, returning back to the heart. Heart failure is primarily due to problems with ventricular pumping action of the cardiac muscle, which may be caused by diseases such as MIs (heart attacks), endocarditis (infection in the heart), hypertension (high BP), or valvular insufficiency.

When disease affects primarily the left side of the heart, the blood will back up into the lungs. When disease affects primarily the right side of the heart, the systemic circulation may be overloaded. When the heart failure becomes significant, the whole circulatory system may be compromised.

## Prognosis

Medications can help the heart to pump more efficiently. Some medications are used for disease management; others are used for symptom control. Monitoring dietary intake of sodium and fluids can also help with symptom control. Heart failure is the main complication of heart disease, produced by an abnormality of pumping function. The heart is unable to carry blood effectively to meet metabolic needs. The resulting problems include acute left ventricular dysfunction usually due to arrhythmias and MI, and chronic failure due to fluid overload, usually in valvular heart disease.

Heart failure is a compromise of any of the following:

- Contractility of the muscle
- Heart rate
- Ventricular preload
- Ventricular afterload

While most hearts can tolerate some changes in the above items, some diseased, older hearts may not be able to do so, resulting in heart failure. Treatment results of early disease are usually good. Long-term prognosis can be variable, depending on the severity of the disease and associated conditions.

## Hallmark Signs and Symptoms

- Extra heart sounds (Chapter 2).
- $S_3$: Soft sound caused by vibration of the ventricular wall because of rapid filling; heard after $S_2$ heart sound; heard over the apex of the left ventricle, fourth intercostal space along the mid-clavicular line. Best heard when patient lies on left side. Usually indicates heart failure.
- $S_4$: Vibration of valves and the ventricular walls during the second phase of ventricular filling when the atria contract; heard before $S_1$, in the same location as $S_3$, usually due to a "stiff heart."

- **Murmur:** Sounds of turbulence caused by blood flow through the valves; heard anywhere around the heart.
- CHF.
- Fatigue.
- Syncope.
- Chest pain.

Early symptoms

- **Basilar rales** from fluid overload.
- Nocturia.
- **Exertional dyspnea.**
- Fatigue.
- **Positive hepatojugular reflux** from liver congestion—the distension of the neck veins precipitated by the maneuver of firm pressure over the liver.
- S$_3$ heart sound.

Moderate stage symptoms

- Cough
- Orthopnea
- Discomfort in right upper abdomen due to hepatomegaly
- Cardiac rales
- Edema
- Cardiomegaly

Late symptoms

- Anasarca—generalized edema from ineffective pump function.
- Frothy or pink sputum from capillary permeability.

## Common/Interpreting Test Results

- B-type natriuretic peptide (BNP)—elevated levels in CHF; produced when the ventricles are stretched.
- ECG may show signs of ischemia (T-wave inversion), tachycardia, or extrasystole (extra beats).
- CBC may show anemia—hemoglobin (Hgb) less than 12 in female, less than 14 in male; hematocrit (HCT); less than three times the Hgb.

- Chemistry may show renal problems, electrolyte disturbance.
- CXR.
- Left-sided heart failure.
  - Pulmonary congestion because of accumulation of fluid in the lungs.
  - Enlarged left ventricle (LVH) because of the increased stress on the heart to pump blood.
- Right-sided heart failure.
  - Pulmonary congestion because of accumulation of fluid in the lungs.
  - Accumulation of fluid in the pleural cavity (pleural effusion).
  - Enlarged heart (cardiomegaly) because of the increased stress on the heart to pump blood.

## Treatment

Treatment is aimed at the underlying disease, that is, ischemia, valve defects, and arrhythmias.

Excreting volume with diuretics, supplemental oxygen, use of medications to reduce workload of heart muscle, peripheral vascular resistance (afterload), and venous return to the heart (preload) may all be used. Dietary indiscretions may be a contributing factor, that is, consuming too much salt or too many calories.

- Administer diuretics for symptom control, resulting in patient comfort by reducing blood volume.
  - Furosemide (Lasix), bumetanide (Bumex), metolazone (Zaroxolyn), hydrochlorothiazide (HCTZ), spironolactone (Aldactone)—be aware of electrolyte imbalance—these medications may alter the potassium level.
- Administer ACE inhibitors to decrease afterload.
  - Captopril (Capoten), enalapril (Vasotec), lisinopril (Zestril)
- Administer beta-adrenergic blocking agents that help raise ejection fraction and decrease ventricular size.
- Administer inotrope to strengthen myocardial contractility.
  - Digoxin (Digitalis)
- Administer vasodilator to reduce preload, relieve dyspnea.
  - Nitroprusside (Nitropress), nitroglycerin ointment
- Administer anticoagulants in patients with severe heart failure, as they have a propensity to develop thrombus and emboli; those with concurrent atrial fibrillation will also need anticoagulation.

- Reduce fluids as fluid overload is a causative factor in CHF.
- High Fowler's position to ease breathing and enhance diaphragmatic excursion.
- Supplemental oxygen to meet increased demand of myocardium.
- Low-sodium diet to prevent additional fluid retention.
- Daily weights to promote close monitoring of fluid status.

## Nursing Diagnoses

- Impaired gas exchange
- Decreased cardiac output
- Excess fluid volume

## Nursing Interventions

- Monitor vital signs and look for changes.
- Record fluid intake and output—weigh daily to assess for fluid overload.
- Position patient in semi-Fowler's position to ease breathing.
- Administer oxygen as ordered because it helps decrease workload of heart.
- Explain to the patient
    - Eat foods low in sodium to avoid fluid retention. (For these patients, there is no such thing as "low-salt" cold cuts.)
    - Raise legs when sitting to lessen dependent edema.
    - Call the physician, nurse practitioner, or physician assistant if experiencing fluid retention, such as a weight gain of several pounds in 1 or 2 days.

## Pulmonary Edema

Fluid builds up in the lungs due to ineffective pumping of blood by the heart; as a result, there is hypoxia leading to tissue necrosis. Typically the left ventricle is overworked and is unable to pump blood received from the lungs. Pressure in the left atrium increases, backing up pressure in the veins in the lungs. Fluid is then pushed through the capillary into the alveoli.

## What Went Wrong?

Pulmonary edema occurs as a result of left-sided heart failure, acute MI, worsening of heart failure, or volume overload. The patient experiences hypoxia, which is insufficient oxygen supply to tissues, caused by decreased oxygenation of the blood. Several noncardiac issues may lead to pulmonary edema. These include acute respiratory distress syndrome (ARDS), neurogenic pulmonary edema, adverse drug reaction, pulmonary embolism, smoke inhalation, viral infections, and aspiration of toxins.

## Prognosis

Poor heart function results in fluid overload, which results in further diminished cardiac function, causing marked dyspnea.

## Hallmark Signs and Symptoms

- Difficulty breathing even when sitting upright (because of the fluid in the lungs).
- Rapid breathing: Greater than 20 breaths/min (tachypnea), because the body is trying to get more oxygen.
- **Frothy sputum** with a tinge of blood due to capillary permeability.
- Cyanosis.
- Cool, clammy skin because the body is diverting blood flow from the periphery.
- Restlessness and fear due to lack of oxygenation.
- Distended jugular veins due to increased pressure within chest.
- Crackles, wheezing heard in the lungs as the air moves through the fluid.

## Common/Interpreting Test Results

- Oxygen saturation less than 90%.
- CXR: Alveolar fluid, large heart.
- Echocardiogram to determine ejection fraction percentages in the heart.
- ABGs will show lower levels of oxygen.

## Treatment

Treatment may continue at home unless a worsening change in condition merits hospitalization. Immediate treatment of heart failure, while searching for underlying correctable conditions, is necessary.

- Administer supplemental oxygen, which increases arterial $PO_2$. Mechanical ventilation may be necessary.
- Administer morphine, which lowers left-atrial pressure, decreases myocardial oxygen demand, lowers anxiety, and relieves pain.
- Administer diuretics to remove excess fluid.
  - Furosemide (Lasix), bumetanide (Bumex), metolazone (Zaroxolyn)
- Administer cardiac glycosides to increase contractions of the heart.
  - Digoxin (Digitalis)
- Administer cardiac inotropics to strengthen the heart.
  - Dobutamine
  - Inamrinone
  - Milrinone (Primacor)
- Administer nitrates to decrease BP and left ventricular filling pressures.
  - Isosorbide dinitrate (Isordil)

## Nursing Diagnoses

- Impaired gas exchange
- Anxiety
- Excess fluid volume

## Nursing Interventions

- Place the patient in full Fowler's position to enhance air exchange and diaphragmatic movement, sitting with legs dangling over sides of bed.
- Monitor cardiovascular function for changes in heart sounds, extra sounds, and murmurs.
- Monitor respirations for changes in lung sounds, chest expansion.
- Check oxygen saturation (pulse oximetry).
- Record fluid intake and output.
- Weigh the patient daily. Call physician if patient gains 2 lb daily.

- Call physician if BUN and creatinine increase.
- Record characteristics of sputum.
- Explain to the patient
    - Call the physician, nurse practitioner, or physician assistant if the patient detects fluid overload, weight gain, shortness of breath, fatigue, or chest pains.
    - Call 911 if in respiratory distress.
    - Decrease sodium in diet.
    - Sleep with head elevated, that is, using three pillows or placing blocks under head of bed frame.

# Rheumatic Heart Disease

Rheumatic heart disease (RHD) is a disease that causes damage to the mitral valve and aortic valve that interferes with blood flowing out of the chambers on the left side of the heart. RHD can also lead to myocarditis and pericarditis.

## What Went Wrong?

RHD is the result of the patient having rheumatic fever as a child or young adult. Rheumatic fever is the result of strep throat or scarlet fever (less common) that is ineffectively treated with antibiotics.

## Prognosis

Prognosis of RHD depends on the amount of damage done to the valves. When progressive valve disease occurs in the mitral valve, it is imperative to recognize the early onset of atrial fibrillation to ensure early initiation of anticoagulation to prevent emboli.

## Hallmark Signs and Symptoms

- A new murmur of insufficiency $S_3$.
- Joint pain because of the inflammation.
- Increased temperature higher than 100.3°F because it may signify infection.
- Carditis—chest pain, heart failure, friction rub.

## Common/Interpreting Test Results

- Increase in cardiac enzymes to look for other causes of chest pain.
- Positive C-reactive protein and erythrocyte sedimentation rate (ESR), which are elevated in inflammation.
- Increase in white blood cell count because it may be of infectious origin.
- Echocardiogram to assess for damage to valves.

## Treatment

Treatment of RHD is based on the severity of the valve damage. Valve replacement may be necessary. If a fibrillation (contracting of the heart) is present, ensure adequate anticoagulation with an international normalized ratio (INR) between 2 and 3. Rheumatic fever prophylaxis may be required; antibiotics are recommended for prevention of recurrent episodes.

- Administer nonsteroidal anti-inflammatory drugs to decrease inflammation and pain.
  - Aspirin
  - Indomethacin (Indocin)
- Administer antibiotics if an infectious process is confirmed.
  - Erythromycin
  - Penicillin
- Repair or replacement of heart valves due to irreparable damage.
- Antibiotic prophylaxis for unsterile procedures—usually penicillin; if allergic to penicillin, clindamycin is usually the drug of choice.
- Anticoagulation if atrial fibrillation.

## Nursing Diagnoses

- Decrease cardiac output
- Activity intolerance
- Risk for infection

## Nursing Interventions

- Monitor for difficulty breathing (dyspnea) and hacking, nonproductive cough, because these are signs of heart failure.

- Determine if patient is allergic to penicillin.
- Monitor for infection because rheumatic fever may recur.
- Red, sore throat with pain when swallowing.
- Swollen cervical lymph glands.
- Headache.
- Temperature higher than 100°F.
- Explain to patient
  - Anticoagulation use, interference with foods and medications, need for frequent laboratory monitoring.
  - Avoid contact with anyone who has a respiratory tract infection.
  - Maintain good dental hygiene.
  - Call the physician, nurse practitioner, or physician assistant if detect signs of heart failure: shortness of breath, weight gain, nonproductive cough.
  - Return to normal activities slowly.

## CASE STUDY

### CASE 1

A 56-year-old man has a preliminary diagnosis of cardiomyopathy. The practitioner continues to order additional tests to confirm the diagnosis. The patient has several questions about the diagnosis, forthcoming tests, and his prognosis. The practitioner asks you to educate the patient. What are the best responses to the following questions raised by the patient?

QUESTION 1. The practitioner made the preliminary diagnosis after my echocardiograph. What could be seen in the echocardiograph?
ANSWER: The practitioner likely noticed that the ventricles on the left side of your heart are enlarged, which is called *left ventricular hypertrophy* and a sign of cardiomyopathy. The left ventricles pump oxygenated blood throughout your body. The practitioner likely saw signs of left ventricular hypertrophy on the X-ray and ECG.

QUESTION 2. Why did the practitioner place me on a diet that restricts my fluids?
ANSWER: There is a possibility that you may experience CHF since it is a common concurrent disorder with some cardiomyopathy. Restricting fluid intake and checking your weight daily reduces the risk of developing excessive fluids. Once the practitioner completes testing, he/she will tell you if you need to maintain fluid restriction.

QUESTION 3. Why did the practitioner place me on a low-salt diet?
ANSWER: Salt causes fluid retention. There is a saying that where salt goes so does water. The practitioner wants to lower your fluid retention. Therefore, lowering salt in your diet prevents unnecessary retention of fluid in your body.

QUESTION 4. The practitioner didn't tell me which type of cardiomyopathy I may have. What are the different types?
ANSWER: The most common is dilated cardiomyopathy. This is where the heart muscle thins and enlarges, leading to CHF. Progressive hypertrophy and dilation result in problems with pumping action of ventricles. A less common form is HCM where the ventricular heart muscle thickens, resulting in outflow obstruction or restriction. There is some blood flow present. A rare form is restrictive cardiomyopathy. This is where the heart muscle becomes stiff and restricts blood from filling ventricles, usually as a result of amyloidosis, radiation, or myocardial fibrosis after open-heart surgery.

## FINAL CHECKUP

1. A 32-year-old man presents to the emergency department with neck vein distention and is restless, sweating, and has difficulty breathing. You realize that the systolic pressure dropped greater than 10 mm Hg during inspiration. He tells you that he feels fatigued. What do you suspect is happening?

   A. Pulsus paradoxus
   B. Cardiac tamponade
   C. Acute myocardial infarction
   D. Acute heart failure

2. A 53-year-old woman is brought in by ambulance to the emergency department following a motor vehicle accident. Her BP is 70/50 with a pulse of 110 beats/min. What do you expect is happening?

   A. Cardiac tamponade
   B. Cardiogenic shock

C. Pulmonary edema

D. CHF

3. **A 48-year-old woman was told by the practitioner that she should be monitored by a Swan Ganz catheter. She is unsure of the procedure. Which is your best response?**

A. Swan Ganz catheter is a catheter placed into the lungs to check for pressures in the heart, vessels, and lungs.

B. Swan Ganz catheter is a catheter placed into the lungs to check for pressures in the lungs.

C. Swan Ganz catheter is a catheter placed into the heart to check for pressures in the heart.

D. Swan Ganz catheter is a catheter placed into the pulmonary artery to check for pressures in the heart, vessels, and lungs.

4. **An 80-year-old woman diagnosed with HCM asks to you explain the disorder. What is your best response?**

A. HCM occurs when the ventricular heart muscle thickens, resulting in outflow obstruction or restriction. There is some blood flow present.

B. HCM occurs when the heart muscle becomes stiff and restricts blood from filling ventricles.

C. HCM occurs when the heart muscle thins and enlarges.

D. HCM occurs when the heart muscle thins and narrows.

5. **A 45-year-old patient was told by the practitioner that he has a positive hepato-jugular reflux. He asks you to explain this condition. What is your best response?**

A. Positive hepatojugular reflux is distension of the gallbladder precipitated by the maneuver of firm pressure over the liver by the practitioner.

B. Positive hepatojugular reflux is distension of the hepatic veins precipitated by the maneuver of firm pressure over the liver by the practitioner.

C. Positive hepatojugular reflux is distension of the neck veins precipitated by the maneuver of firm pressure over the liver by the practitioner.

D. Positive hepatojugular reflux is distension of the liver precipitated by the maneuver of firm pressure over the liver by the practitioner.

6. **A 42-year-old woman is diagnosed with pulmonary edema. She asks you to describe this condition. What is your best response?**

A. Fluid builds up in the legs due to ineffective pumping of blood by the heart.

B. Fluid builds up around the heart due to ineffective pumping of blood by the heart.

C. Fluid builds up in the lungs due to effective pumping of blood by the heart.

D. Fluid builds up in the lungs due to ineffective pumping of blood by the heart.

7. A 34-year-old man is concerned that he has RHD. What should you do?

   A. Ask the patient if he ever had rheumatic fever or scarlet fever as a child.
   B. Ask the patient if he ever had strep throat.
   C. Ask the patient if he ever had strep throat as a child.
   D. Ask the patient if he ever had strep throat recently.

8. A 54-year-old man recently diagnosed with CHF asks you if he is going to die. What is your best response?

   A. Long-term prognosis can be variable, depending on the severity of the disease and associated conditions.
   B. Treatment results of early disease are usually good.
   C. Treatment results of early disease are usually good. Long-term prognosis can be variable, depending on the severity of the disease and associated conditions.
   D. Treatment results of early disease are usually good. Long-term prognosis can be variable, depending on the severity of the disease and associated conditions. Your practitioner is the best person to speak about your prognosis.

9. A 55-year-old man was told by his practitioner to weigh himself daily and to call the practitioner immediately if there is a weight gain of 3 lb. He asks you why he must weigh himself daily since he has already changed his diet. What is your best response?

   A. Weight gain is an early sign that you are retaining fluid.
   B. Weight gain is an early sign that you are retaining fluid. Retaining fluid may indicate a problem with your heart that needs to be addressed immediately.
   C. Weight gain may indicate that you are not adhering to your new diet.
   D. Weight gain may indicate that your new diet needs to be changed.

10. A 41-year-old man asks why the practitioner told him not to strain during a bowel movement. What is your best response?

    A. Straining during a bowel movement increases pressure in the chest and slows return of blood to the heart.
    B. Straining during a bowel movement means that you are constipated.
    C. Straining during a bowel movement means that you are constipated. You should take a stool softener daily.
    D. Straining during a bowel movement means that you are constipated. You shouldn't take a stool softener daily.

## CORRECT ANSWERS AND RATIONALES

1. B.  Cardiac tamponade.
2. B.  Cardiogenic shock.
3. D.  Swan Ganz catheter is a catheter placed into the pulmonary artery to check for pressures in the heart, vessels, and lungs.
4. A.  HCM occurs when the ventricular heart muscle thickens, resulting in outflow obstruction or restriction. There is some blood flow present.
5. C.  Positive hepatojugular reflux is distension of the neck veins precipitated by the maneuver of firm pressure over the liver by the practitioner.
6. D.  Fluid builds up in the lungs due to ineffective pumping of blood by the heart.
7. A.  Ask the patient if he ever had rheumatic fever or scarlet fever as a child.
8. D.  Treatment results of early disease are usually good. Long-term prognosis can be variable, depending on the severity of the disease and associated conditions. Your practitioner is the best person to speak about your prognosis.
9. B.  Weight gain is an early sign that you are retaining fluid. Retaining fluid may indicate a problem with your heart that needs to be addressed immediately.
10. A.  Straining during a bowel movement increases pressure in the chest and slows return of blood to the heart.

# Cardiovascular Emergencies

14. Atrial Fibrillation

15. Atrial Flutter (Aflutter)

16. Asystole

17. Ventricular Fibrillation

18. Ventricular Tachycardia

19. Cardiac Arrest

20. Bradycardia

21. Fibrinolytic Therapy

22. Acute Stroke

23. Acute Coronary Syndrome

24. Cardiac Contusion

## KEY TERMS

Antiarrhythmic Medication
Anticoagulant Medication
Antihypertensive Medication
Antiplatelet Medication
Arterial Blood Gas
Blood Chemistry
Brain Natriuretic Peptide (BNP)
Cardiac Emergency
Cardiac Enzymes
Cardiac Glycoside Medication
Cardiac Marker
Cardioversion
Chest Pain
Coronary Artery Bypass Graft (CABG)
Diuretic Medication

Emergency Assessment
Hematologic Studies
Percutaneous Transluminal Coronary
    Angioplasty (PTCA)
Phosphodiesterase (PDE) Inhibitor
    Medication
PQRST
Pulse Oximetry
Renin Assay Test
Respiratory Distress
Stabilize the Patient
Thrombolytic Medications
Transcutaneous Pacemaker
Vasodilator Medication

# What Is a Cardiovascular Emergency?

A *cardiovascular emergency* is a condition that has the potential of disrupting circulation throughout the patient's body resulting in decreased blood flow to organs and causing malfunction of other systems in the body. This can be from hypertension (HTN), thrombosis, embolus, or anything that disrupts the oxygen and nutrients from reaching tissues and organs.

A *cardiac emergency* is a condition that disrupts the function of the heart. The patient is asymptomatic or experiences discomfort, chest pain, back pain, jaw pain, increased urination at night, swelling of ankles and feet, heart pounding, heart skipping a beat, and shortness of breath. However, there are times when a patient is in **respiratory distress** or respiratory arrest. This is not a cardiac emergency because the patient's heart is working, although respiratory arrest can lead to a cardiac emergency if rescue breathing does not occur.

HTN is an emergency if the systolic pressure is above or equal to 160 mm Hg or diastolic pressure is above or equal to 100 mm Hg. The patient experiences headache, drowsiness, confusion, vision disorders, nausea, and vomiting. Hypotension is an emergency if the systolic pressure is below 90 mm Hg or the diastolic is below 60 mm Hg. The patient experiences light-headedness, dizziness, fainting, loss of consciousness, and fatigue.

*Thrombosis* is a blood clot that reduces blood flow or prevents blood flow to a part of the patient's body. The patient experiences pain in the area, coughing, swelling below the blood clot, and decreased circulation below the blood clot.

*Embolus* is a dislodged blood clot that flows freely through the circulatory system until it enters a small blood vessel causing a disruption of blood flow to that area of the body. The patient is asymptomatic until the embolus no longer moves freely, at which point the patient experiences symptoms of thrombosis.

## Goal of Treating Cardiovascular Emergencies

The goal of the emergency department (ED) staff is to stabilize the patient—not to treat the underlying cause of the problem unless the underlying cause can be addressed within the scope of the ED staff. For example, angina is chest pain due to ischemia, resulting in lack of oxygen supply to cardiac muscle. The ED staff might alleviate angina by administering nitroglycerin, however, the underlying ischemia is likely to be addressed by follow-up care.

Objectives are to

- Maintain airway, respiratory functions, and circulation.

- Diagnose the acute problem. For example, the acute problem might be hypertensive crisis, not the underlying cause of the hypertensive crisis.

- Stabilize the patient by relieving pain and treat the acute problem. For example, administer medication to decrease HTN immediately.

- Refer the patient to follow-up care to treat the underlying cause of the problem.

# Cardiovascular Emergency Assessment

Limit the **emergency assessment** to identifying the problem area and then direct your assessment to the problem area. Stop the assessment if you need to intervene to **stabilize the patient**. Ask the patient to describe the problem. Ask questions that help you quickly identify the problem. Questions should be short and to the point, enabling the patient to answer yes or no. Remember that the patient is typically distressed and anxious because he/she is experiencing an unusual problem that has not been identified.

Take vital signs during triage and monitor vital signs throughout the patient's stay in the ED to assess changes in the patient's condition. Remember that anxiety and pain cause increase in vital signs. The ED staff's therapeutic demeanor can decrease patient's anxiety, reducing the anxiety effect on vital signs and therefore enabling the staff to develop baseline vital signs for the patient.

Ask the following questions:

- Are you in pain? Pain might be a sign of decreased circulation to the heart muscle.
  - Where is the pain?
  - On a scale of 0 to 10, how bad is the pain?
  - Is the pain burning, tight, or squeezing?
  - Does the pain radiate?
  - When did you notice the pain?
  - What were you doing before you noticed the pain?
  - What aggravates the pain?
  - What relieves the pain?
- Are you dizzy? Dizziness is a sign of decreased oxygenation related to decreased circulation.
- Do you urinate frequently at night? Frequent night urination is possibly a sign of right-side heart failure.
- Do you have nausea?
- Are you short of breath? Shortness of breath is a sign of decreased oxygenation related to decreased circulation.
- Do you feel your heart fluttering? Heart fluttering is a sign of irregular heart rhythm.
- Do you feel your heart pounding? Heart pounding might be a sign of hypoxia.

- Do you feel that your heart skips a beat? Skipping a beat is a sign of irregular heart rhythm.
- Do you ever have difficulty awakening? Hypoxia related to decreased circulation is a potential problem.
- Do your ankles or feet swell? Bilateral swelling is a sign of right-side heart failure.

## Inspection

- Look for signs of cyanosis in extremities such as nail beds, tip of the nose, and earlobes, which is a sign of deoxygenation of the blood possibly caused by inadequate circulation.
- Look for clubbing of fingers, which is a possible sign of chronic deoxygenation of the blood.
- Look at mucous membranes in dark-skinned patient for pallor, which is a possible sign of inadequate circulation.
- Look at hair distribution on arms and legs. If hair is missing, then there may be decreased arterial circulation to the area.
- Look for swelling of legs, ankles, and feet. Bilateral swelling is a possible sign of right-side heart failure, venous insufficiency, or varicosities.
- Look for flushed skin, which is a possible sign of increased circulation related to fever.
- Look at the chest wall for indentations called *retractions* that can be related to heart failure or congenital heart defect.
- Look for abnormal thoracic cavity, which may inhibit cardiac movement.

## Palpation

- Squeeze the nail bed to assess capillary refill time. More than 3 seconds may indicate decreased circulation.
- Feel the skin temperature. Cold or cool skin temperature may indicate decreased circulation. Hot or warm skin temperature may indicate increased circulation.
- Feel the precordium of the chest to assess the apical pulse.
  - Fine vibrations might indicate turbulent blood flow related to an aneurysm or heart valve malfunction.
  - Strong longer pulse might indicate increased cardiac output.
  - Diffused pulse might indicate left ventricular hypertrophy.

- Feel each of the carotid arteries separately to compare results. Both pulses should be symmetric and equal, otherwise there may be decreased circulation through one of the carotid arteries.
- Feel pulse sites throughout the body. Compare bilateral pulses.
  - Weak pulse might indicate decreased cardiac output or increased peripheral vascular resistance.
  - Bounding pulse might indicate HTN and high cardiac output.

### Percussion

- Percuss the patient's lung fields. A dull sound might indicate pleural effusion possibly caused by biventricular failure in the heart. This allows fluid to build up between the lung and the chest wall.

### Auscultation

- Listen for fine vibrations throughout the cardiac region of the chest, which might indicate an aneurysm or ventricular hypertrophy.
- Listen for abnormal heart sounds.
  - $S_3$ heart sound might indicate myocardial infarction (MI), left- or right-side heart failure, intracardiac blood shunting, pulmonary congestion, hyperthyroidism, or anemia.
  - $S_4$ heart sound might indicate aortic stenosis, angina, coronary artery disease, cardiomyopathy, or HTN.
- Listen to the patient's lungs for pulmonary congestion. Pulmonary congestion is a sign of left-sided heart failure.
- Listen to the patient's abdominal region for bruits over the abdominal aorta, indicating abdominal aorta aneurysm.

## Chest Pain Assessment

A patient presenting with **chest pain** must be assessed immediately to rule out a cardiac event. The initial assessment is made by asking the patient three questions. These are as follows:

- What does the pain feel like?
- Where is the pain?
- What makes the pain worse?

Here is a quick way to assess the answers to these questions in order to identify the potential cause and immediate treatment to stabilize the patient. Keep in mind that objective testing such as cardiac enzymes and ECG are necessary to reach a diagnosis.

- Sudden, sharp, continuous pain located below the sternum and radiates to the neck or left arm, worse with lying on back or breathing deeply, might indicate pericarditis and require the patient to sit and lean forward to reduce the pain and require anti-inflammatory medications to be administered.

- Sudden, stabbing pain over the back, worse on inspiration, might indicate pulmonary emboli requiring analgesics.

- Sudden, severe pain, located at the side of the chest with difficulty breathing and deviated trachea, worse with normal breathing, might indicate pneumothorax requiring analgesics and reinflation of the affected lung.

- Sudden, severe tearing pain located in the upper abdomen or behind the sternum might indicate dissecting aortic aneurysm requiring analgesics and immediate surgery.

- Squeezing, aching, burning pain below the sternum radiating to the arms, neck, back, and jaw, worse on exertion, stress, eating, and lying, might be caused by angina pectoris, requiring rest and administration of nitroglycerin. The pain may continue if the patient experiences unstable angina pectoris.

- Pressure, aching, burning pain across the chest and radiating to the arms, neck, back, and jaw, worse on exertion, and increased anxiety might be caused by acute MI and require administration of nitroglycerin and opioid analgesic.

The pneumonic **PQRST** is another useful method for pain assessment.

- **Provokes**
  - What causes the pain?
  - What makes the pain better?
  - What makes the pain worse?
- **Quality**
  - What does the pain feel like?
  - Is the pain sharp?
  - Is the pain dull?
  - Is the pain stabbing?
  - Is the pain burning?
  - Is the pain crushing?

- **Radiates**
  - Does the pain radiate?
  - Does the pain remain in one place?
  - Where does the pain radiate?
- **Severity**
  - On a scale from 0 to 10, how severe is the pain where 0 is no pain and 10 is the worst pain?
- **Time**
  - What time did the pain start?
  - How long did the pain last?

# Cardiovascular Emergency Tests

The physical assessment of a patient who enters the ED is performed quickly and methodically. The goal of the physical assessment is to determine if the patient is in a life-threatening situation or find signs and symptoms that lead to a suspected acute disorder or chronic episode of a disorder that causes the patient to be unstable. Suspicions are confirmed by conducting one or more objective tests and analyzing test results.

When a cardiac emergency is suspected, the health care provider will likely order an electrocardiograph (ECG), pulse oximetry, arterial blood gas (ABG), blood chemistry, and hematologic studies. Additional cardiac tests may be ordered once the patient is stabilized in the ED.

## Electrocardiograph

The ECG (see Chapter 3) shows a graphic representation of the electrical activity of the heart in a three-dimensional perspective. An electrical signal is generated each time the heart contracts. Small pads containing electrodes are placed on the surface of the skin to detect the electrical signal. Six electrodes are placed on the chest and six electrodes are placed on the arms and legs. Each electrode is connected with wires to an ECG machine that draws up to 12 different graphical representations of the electrical signal.

## Pulse Oximetry

**Pulse oximetry** assesses the arterial oxygen saturation of the patient's blood by passing an infrared beam of light through the patient's nail bed or skin. The amount of infrared light absorbed by the patient's blood provides an estimate of arterial oxygen saturation. This is referred to as an *abbreviated arterial oxygen saturation value.*

The pulse oximetry value should be between 95% and 100% if the patient is breathing room air and does not have chronic pulmonary disease such as chronic obstructive pulmonary disease (COPD). A patient who has a chronic pulmonary disease may have a lower pulse oximetry value, which might be normal for the patient. A patient who is sedated or sleeping may also have a low pulse oximetry, which is not alarming because the cause of the low value is known.

A patient who has supplemental oxygen should have a pulse oximetry value between 95% and 100%. A lower value may indicate a cardiac or respiratory problem. It may also indicate that a mechanical problem prevents the patient from receiving the supplemental oxygen such as a blockage in the nasal cannula tube.

A value less than 95% on room air or on supplemental oxygen indicates there is instability in the cardiorespiratory systems. If the underlying cause is not obvious, such as the patient is hyperventilating, then the health care provider is likely to order an ABG.

## Arterial Blood Gas

The **ABG** is a blood test where an arterial blood sample is taken from the patient and assessed for oxygen, carbon dioxide, bicarbonate, and pH levels in the blood. It is important that any supplemental oxygen or ventilation assistance administered to the patient shortly before or when the sample is taken is noted on the sample documentation. This enables the laboratory to adjust the results accordingly.

Since the sample is taken from an artery, you must apply pressure to the puncture site for 5 minutes and apply a pressure dressing for 30 minutes once the bleeding stops. The site then needs to be monitored for 1 minute following removal of manual pressure to ensure there is no residual bleeding. Check for hematoma formation and then reassess the pulse.

## Blood Chemistry

**Blood chemistry** is a laboratory test of venous blood and examines levels of enzymes and other elements in blood to develop a profile of the patient's health. This test is usually performed routinely for ED patients because results provide the health care provider with objective information about how well the patient's systems are functioning.

Blood chemistry results typically include the following:

- Electrolyte balance (sodium, potassium, bicarbonate, magnesium, calcium, phosphorus)
- Kidney function (blood urea nitrogen [BUN], creatinine)
- Liver function (aspartate aminotransferase/alanine transaminase [AST/ ALT])
- Diabetes (serum glucose)
- Cholesterol level (cholesterol, low-density lipoproteins [LDL], high-density lipoprotein [HDL], triglycerides)

Enzymes are normally inside the cell. As cells rupture during normal events, enzymes leave the cell and enter the bloodstream. The laboratory determines the normal level of a particular enzyme in the blood. A level greater than the normal level indicates more than the normal amount of cells were injured indicating something unusual is happening with the patient.

Enzyme levels might increase gradually and then return to normal levels. This might occur with a MI when blood supply to a part of cardiac tissue is interrupted leading to the death of some cardiac tissue. Enzyme levels remain normal for several hours and then become abnormal. It takes several hours before enzyme levels return to normal as no more cardiac tissues is injured.

It is important to look for obvious reasons why enzyme levels or other values are abnormal before assuming that the patient is unstable related to the test results. For example, a patient who exercised before coming to the ED will have elevated muscle cell enzymes because exercising injures muscles. Likewise, a patient who ate a normal breakfast before visiting the ED will have high blood glucose levels.

## Hematologic Studies

**Hematologic studies** outline the patient's blood and include the following:

- Red blood cell (RBC) count
- White blood cell (WBC) count indicating inflammation
- Erythrocyte sedimentation rate (ESR)
- Bleeding (prothrombin time [PT], international normalized ratio [INR], partial thromboplastin time [PTT], platelet count)
- Hemoglobin and hematocrit (Hgb, Hct)

# Cardiac Enzymes and Markers

When a patient is suspected of having a MI, the health care provider will order **cardiac enzymes** and **cardiac marker** tests to determine if cardiac muscle enzymes appear in the patient's blood.

- Cardiac muscle contains enzymes.
- In a MI, cardiac muscle is damaged causing the release of cardiac enzymes into the bloodstream.
- It can take between 2 and 24 hours for cardiac muscle enzymes to reach a detectable level in blood.
- The cardiac enzymes and cardiac marker tests are used to confirm a previous acute MI.

# Brain Natriuretic Peptide Test

The heart produces the hormone **brain natriuretic peptide (BNP)**.

- Low level of BNP is normally found in blood.
- BNP level increases when the heart works harder for long periods such as in heart failure.
- The BNP test measures the level of BNP in the blood.
- The health care provider may order the N-terminal pro brain natriuretic peptide (NT-proBNP) test, which measures the NT-proBNP hormone and provides similar diagnostic results as the BNP test.

# Cardiac Enzyme Studies

The cells of heart muscles and other tissues contain the enzyme creatinine phosphokinase (CK or CPK) and the protein troponin (TnT, TnI).

- CPK and troponin enter the blood when heart muscle and other tissues are damaged.
- If levels of CPK and troponin are abnormal, the health care provider orders an ECG to differentiate between heart muscle damage and other tissue damage.
- Troponin and CPK-MB are mostly found in cardiac muscle.
- Blood samples are taken every 8 hours for 2 days following a suspected heart attack.
- It takes 3 to 12 hours for troponin levels to rise after a heart attack.

- The health care provider may order a myoglobin test along with the cardiac enzymes test to help diagnose a heart attack.
- High troponin values may indicate
  - Cardiac muscle injury. Troponin level increases in 3 to 12 hours and reaches the highest level 12 to 24 hours after the cardiac muscle injury. Troponin level returns to normal in 10 to 14 days following the cardiac muscle injury.
- High total CPK values may indicate
  - Cardiac muscle injury or tissue injury. Total CPK increases in 4 to 12 hours and reaches the highest level 10 to 24 hours after the cardiac muscle injury. Total CPK level returns to normal in 3 days following the cardiac muscle injury.
- High CPK-MB values may indicate
  - Cardiac muscle injury. CPK-MB increases in 1 to 6 hours and reaches the highest level 18 hours after the cardiac muscle injury. CPK-MB level returns to normal in 3 days following the cardiac muscle injury. If levels are high after 3 days, then additional cardiac muscle is being damaged and the heart attack is continuing.

## Renin Assay Test for Hypertension

BP is regulated by the renin-angiotensin system (RAS).

- Low BP causes the secretion of the renin enzyme by the kidneys, which increases angiotensin I. Angiotensin I constricts blood vessels resulting in increased BP.
- Angiotensin II induces vasoconstriction leading the kidneys to retain water and sodium and resulting in increased intravascular fluid volume, decreased urine output, and an increase in BP.
- The **renin assay test** measures the level of rennin in blood.
- The health care provider may also order the aldosterone test.
- The renin stimulation test may be ordered if the renin level is low.
- High renin assay test results may indicate the following:
  - Malignant high BP
  - Kidney disease
  - Blocked artery
  - Cirrhosis

- Addison disease
- Hemorrhage

# Cardiovascular Emergency Procedures

There are several cardiac procedures that are used to restore blood flow to the heart and reestablish cardiac rhythm. These are as follows:

- **Percutaneous transluminal coronary angioplasty (PTCA):** This is a nonsurgical procedure used to open a blocked coronary artery by inserting a balloon-tipped catheter into the femoral artery and moving the catheter into the blocked coronary artery using a fluoroscope to help guide the catheter into position. Once in position, the balloon is inflated to push plaque that causes the blockage against the coronary artery wall, allowing blood to flow again.

- **Coronary artery bypass graft (CABG):** This is a surgical procedure performed when a patient experiences myocardial ischemia. Before this procedure is performed, the patient typically undergoes catheterization to determine the severity of the myocardial ischemia. In severe ischemia, the blockage is bypassed by grafting a segment of the saphenous vein from the leg.

- **Cardioversion:** This is a nonsurgical procedure used to treat atrial fibrillation, atrial flutter, supraventricular tachycardia (SVT), and ventricular tachycardia (VT). A low energy level shock is administered that is synchronized with the patient's heart cycle, causing interruption of the reentry circuit and enabling control to resume by the sinoatrial (SA) node.

- **Transcutaneous pacemaker:** This is a nonsurgical procedure that uses an external electrical generator to send impulses through electrodes placed on the patient's chest to the patient's heart to provide external impulses to the heart in an emergency. The transcutaneous pacemaker remains active until a transvenous pacemaker is implemented.

# Cardiovascular Emergency Medications

There are several classifications of medications that are commonly used to stabilize a patient who is experiencing cardiac instability. It is important that the ED nursing staff be familiar with each medication.

## Adrenergic

Adrenergic medication causes an effect similar to the sympathetic nervous system that stimulates the fight or flight response. There are two classifications of adrenergic medication. These are catecholamines and noncatecholamines.

Adrenergic medications can stimulate one or more receptors depending on the medication. These receptors are

- Alpha-adrenergic receptors
- Beta-adrenergic receptors
- Dopamine receptors

### Catecholamines

Catecholamines stimulate the nervous system and increase the depolarization of the SA node, resulting in increased heart rate, increased BP related to constriction of peripheral blood vessels, and bronchial dilation. Catecholamines are referred to as *inotropes* because these medications increase the force of cardiac contractions causing the heart to work harder and use more oxygen than when at rest. Table 10–1 lists commonly used catecholamines.

### Noncatecholamines

Noncatecholamines also stimulate the nervous system but focus on a local or systemic effect rather than a general effect of catecholamines. Noncatecholamines can affect selected beta-adrenergic receptors, and some stimulate alpha-adrenergic receptors. Table 10–2 lists commonly used noncatecholamines.

| TABLE 10–1  Commonly Used Catecholamines | |
|---|---|
| Catecholamine | Use |
| Dobutamine (Dobutrex) | Increases heart rate and cardiac output. |
| Dopamine | Increases cardiac contraction and output. |
| Epinephrine | Restores cardiac rhythm in cardiac arrest. |
| | Reverses anaphylaxis reaction to an antigen. |
| | Relaxes bronchial muscles in bronchospasm. |
| Norepinephrine (Levophed) | Increases BP in acute hypotension caused by peripheral vasodilation. |

| TABLE 10–2 Commonly Used Noncatecholamines | |
|---|---|
| Noncatecholamine | Use |
| Albuterol (Proventil) | Relaxes bronchial muscles in bronchospasm. |
| Metaproterenol (Alupent) | Relaxes bronchial muscles in bronchospasm. |
| Isoetharine | Relaxes bronchial muscles in bronchospasm. |
| Methoxamine (Vasoxyl) | Increase BP in hypotension. |
| Ephedrine | Increase BP in acute hypotension and orthostatic hypotension. |
| Phenylephrine (Neo-Synephrine) | Increase BP in hypotensive emergencies. |

## Adrenergic Blockers

Adrenergic blocker is a class of medication that disrupts the function of the sympathetic nervous system by blocking impulses at the adrenergic receptor site. There are two classifications of the adrenergic blockers.

Alpha-adrenergic blockers block the alpha-adrenergic receptor sites. There are two types of alpha-adrenergic receptor sites referred to as *alpha$_1$* and *alpha$_2$*. Alpha-adrenergic blockers affect both types. The result is dilation of blood vessels, relaxing smooth muscles of blood vessels, decreased BP, and increased blood flow to organs.

Alpha-adrenergic blockers are phentolamine and prazosin (Minipress) used for HTN, peripheral vascular disorders, and pheochromocytoma (an adrenal gland tumor causing too much epinephrine and norepinephrine to be released).

Beta-adrenergic blockers block the beta-receptor sties. There are two kinds of beta-receptor sites referred to as *beta$_1$* and *beta$_2$*. Beta$_1$-receptor sites are in the heart. Beta$_2$-receptor sites are in the bronchi, blood vessels, and uterus.

Beta-adrenergic blockers decrease BP, decrease cardiac contractions by slowing conduction of impulses between the atria and ventricles, and therefore decrease the oxygen requirement for the heart and decrease cardiac output. Peripheral vascular resistance increases.

Beta-adrenergic blockers are further classified as nonselective and selective. Nonselective beta-adrenergic blockers affect both beta$_1$ and beta$_2$ receptors. Selective beta-adrenergic blockers affect beta$_1$-receptors.

Both nonselective and selective beta-adrenergic blockers are used for

- Angina
- Anxiety
- Migraine headaches
- HTN
- Essential tremor
- Pheochromocytoma
- Thyroid crisis (thyrotoxicosis)
- MI complications

Nonselective beta-adrenergic   Nonselective beta-adrenergic blockers decrease cardiac stimulation and cause constriction of bronchioles in the lungs, resulting in bronchospasm in patients who have chronic obstructive lung disorders. Nonselective beta-adrenergic blockers are

- Carvedilol (Coreg)
- Labetalol (Normodyne)
- Penbutolol (Levatol)
- Nadolol (Corgard)
- Pindolol (Visken)
- Propranolol (Inderal)
- Sotalol (Betapace)
- Timolol (Blocadren)

Selective beta-adrenergic   Selective beta-adrenergic blockers are called *cardioselective beta-adrenergic blockers* because they reduce cardiac stimulation. These are

- Acebutolol (Sectral)
- Atenolol (Tenormin)
- Betaxolol (Kerlone)
- Bisoprolol (Zebeta)
- Esmolol (Brevibloc)
- Metoprolol (Lopressor)

# Antianginal

Antianginal medication is used to decrease oxygen demand by the heart and/or increases oxygen to the heart and is used to treat angina (angina pectoris). Angina occurs when the heart requires more oxygen than is supplied, resulting in cardiac ischemia that presents as chest pain.

There are three classes of antianginal medications.

## Nitrates

Nitrates are used for acute angina because nitrates relax smooth muscle around veins causing a decrease in return blood to the ventricles during preload, which is when ventricles are full and before the ventricles contract. Since there is less blood in the ventricles, the ventricles are reduced in size and tension and therefore require less oxygen.

Nitrates cause coronary arteries to dilate and increase the flow of oxygenated blood to cardiac muscle and decrease the ischemia, resulting in decreased chest pain.

Nitrates also dilate peripheral arterioles, reducing peripheral vascular resistance and resulting in decrease of the cardiac afterload that occurs after the left ventricle contracts pumping blood throughout the peripheral vascular system.

Commonly prescribed nitrates are

- Isosorbide dinitrate (Isordil)
- Isosorbide mononitrate (Imdur)
- Nitroglycerin (Nitro-Bid)

### Beta-Adrenergic Blockers

Beta-adrenergic blockers are used to prevent angina in addition to treating HTN (see Adrenergic) by decreasing the heart rate and reducing the force of contractions leading to decreased cardiac oxygen demand.

### Calcium Channel Blockers

Calcium channel blockers are used to prevent angina when other treatments have failed and the patient continues to experience angina. Calcium is used within muscle cells to contract muscles. Calcium channel blockers dilate coronary and peripheral arteries by preventing calcium ions from entering cardiac muscle and smooth muscle of veins and arteries, resulting in decreased resistance against the heart. Calcium is used by muscle cells for muscle contraction. The workload of the heart decreases, and therefore, there is a reduced need for oxygen by the heart. Calcium channel blockers also prevent peripheral arteriole constriction, reducing the afterload oxygen demand. Calcium channel blockers slow conduction of the impulse from the SA node to the atrioventricular (AV) node, resulting in a decrease in heart rate and a lower need for oxygen by the heart.

Commonly prescribed calcium channel blockers are

- Amlodipine (Norvasc)
- Diltiazem (Cardizem)
- Nicardipine (Cardene)
- Nifedipine (Procardia)
- Verapamil (Calan)

## Antiarrhythmic

**Antiarrhythmic medication** is used to resolve disturbances of cardiac rhythm called *arrhythmias* by restoring normal heart rhythm. However, there is a risk that antiarrhythmic medication can cause arrhythmia.

There are four classes of antiarrhythmic medications.

### Class I Antiarrhythmic

Class I antiarrhythmic medication has three divisions, each of which is a sodium channel blocker.

Class IA antiarrhythmic medication interferes with impulses from the autonomic nervous system with pacemaker cells in the heart. They also block impulses from the parasympathetic nervous system of the SA and AV nodes resulting in increased impulse speed between the SA and AV nodes. Normally the impulses from the parasympathetic nervous system slow impulses to the

SA and AV nodes. There is a risk that patients with atrial fibrillation might experience a critical increase in ventricular contractions. In this case, class IA antiarrhythmic medication will not resolve the patient's arrhythmia. Class IA antiarrhythmic medication is used for atrial fibrillation, atrial flutter, paroxysmal atrial tachycardia, and VT.

Commonly prescribed class IA antiarrhythmic medications are

- Disopyramide (Norpace)
- Procainamide (Procanbid)
- Quinidine sulfate
- Quinidine gluconate

Class IB antiarrhythmic medication blocks influx of sodium ions when the heart contracts (depolarizes) resulting in a decrease in the time between contractions (refractory period). Class IB antiarrhythmic medications are used for VT and ventricular fibrillation (VF).

Commonly prescribed class IB antiarrhythmic medications are

- Lidocaine (Xylocaine)
- Mexiletine (Mexitil)

Class IC antiarrhythmic medication slows cardiac impulses resulting in decreased contraction (depolarization) rate. Class IC antiarrhythmic medications are used for VT, VF, and supraventricular arrhythmias.

Commonly prescribed class IC antiarrhythmic medications are

- Flecainide (Tambocor)
- Moricizine (Ethmozine)
- Propafenone (Rythmol)

### Class II Antiarrhythmic

Class II antiarrhythmic medication slows the automatic firing of impulses by the SA node, thereby also slowing impulses of the AV node by blocking the beta-adrenergic receptors in the heart. As a result, class II antiarrhythmic medication decreases the strength of cardiac contractions and therefore reduces the oxygen requirement of the heart.

Commonly prescribed class II antiarrhythmic medications are

- Acebutolol (Sectral)
- Esmolol (Brevibloc)
- Propranolol (Inderal)

### Class III Antiarrhythmic

Class III antiarrhythmic medication converts a unidirectional block to a bidirectional block, resulting in suppressing the arrhythmia in patients with life-threatening arrhythmias and ventricular arrhythmias.

The commonly prescribed class III antiarrhythmic medication is

- Amiodarone (Cordarone)

## Class IV Antiarrhythmic

Class IV antiarrhythmic medication blocks calcium during the second phase of the action potential resulting in slowing conduction and slowing the refractory period of the AV node. This results in resolving supraventricular arrhythmias.

Commonly prescribed class IV antiarrhythmic medications are

- Diltiazem (Cardizem)
- Verapamil (Calan)

One medication does not belong to any of the classes and therefore is considered under the miscellaneous category of cardiac antiarrhythmic medication. This is *adenosine (Adenocard)*. This medication decreases the SA node's ability to send impulses resulting in decreased AV node impulse to the atria and ventricles and leading to a decreased heart rate. This is used in paroxysmal SVT.

# Anticoagulant Medication

**Anticoagulant medication** is used to decrease the formation of blood clots by interfering with platelet aggregation. There are three categories of anticoagulant medications. All anticoagulant medication presents a risk for bleeding, and therefore the effectiveness of these medications must be monitored regularly.

## Heparin

Heparin is used to treat deep vein thrombosis (DVT), embolism prophylaxis, and disseminated intravascular coagulation (DIC) and to reduce the formation of blood clots following a MI. Heparin does not dissolve existing blood clots. Heparin prevents new blood clots from forming by inhibiting the body's ability to create fibrin and thrombin. The side effects of heparin are bleeding and decreased platelets (thrombocytopenia). Heparin is typically administered intravenously. If the patient is maintained on anticoagulant medication, then he/she receives oral anticoagulants in conjunction with heparin. Once oral anticoagulation approaches a therapeutic level, the patient is typically placed on low-molecular-weight (LMW) heparin (Lovenox, Fragmin) subcutaneous injections until the oral anticoagulant is effective. The PTT test is used to measure heparin effectiveness. The INR and PT tests are used to measure the effectiveness of oral anticoagulants.

Commonly prescribed heparin medications are

- Heparin
- Dalteparin (Fragmin)
- Enoxaparin (Lovenox)

### Oral Anticoagulant Medication

Oral anticoagulant medication is used to prevent DVT, atrial arrhythmias, and complications from malfunctioning heart valves. Oral anticoagulant medications do not have an immediate effect on preventing the formation of blood clots. Oral anticoagulant medications disrupt the ability of the liver to create vitamin K-related clotting factor. The effectiveness of oral anticoagulant medications occurs once free floating clotting factors in the blood dissipate.

The commonly prescribed oral anticoagulant medications are

- Warfarin (Coumadin)
- Rivaroxaban (Xarelto)
- Rivaroxaban (Xarelto)
- Dabigatran (Pradaxa)

## Antiplatelet Medication

**Antiplatelet medications** reduce platelet aggregation and are used for patients who are at risk for complications from prostatic heart valve surgery and who experience acute coronary syndrome or a MI.

Commonly prescribed antiplatelet medications are

- Aspirin (low dose)
- Dipyridamole (Persantine)
- Sulfinpyrazone (Anturane)
- Ticlopidine (Ticlid)
- Clopidogrel (Plavix)

## Thrombolytic Medication

**Thrombolytic medications** dissolve blood clots by transforming plasminogen to plasmin, dissolving plasma protein thrombi and fibrinogen. Thrombolytic medications are used to treat blood clots related to acute ischemic stroke, catheter occlusion, pulmonary embolus, acute MI, and arterial thrombosis.

Commonly prescribed thrombolytic medications are

- Alteplase (Activase)
- Reteplase (Retavase)
- Streptokinase (Streptase)

## Antihypertensive Medication

**Antihypertensive medication** is used to decrease BP when beta-adrenergic blockers (see Adrenergic) and diuretics (see Diuretic Medication) are ineffective. There are three categories of antihypertensive medication. These are sympatholytics, vasodilators, and angiotensin-converting enzyme (ACE) inhibitors.

### Sympatholytic Medication

Sympatholytic medication is used to decrease impulses from the sympathetic nervous system resulting in dilation of peripheral blood vessels and decreasing cardiac output, leading to decreased BP. Sympatholytic medications are classified by their action.

Commonly prescribed central-acting sympathetic nervous system inhibitor (sympatholytic) medications are

- Clonidine (Catapres)
- Guanabenz (Wytensin)
- Guanfacine (Tenex)
- Methyldopa (Aldomet)

Commonly prescribed alpha-blocker sympatholytic medications are

- Doxazosin (Cardura)
- Phentolamine (Minipress)
- Terazosin (Hytrin)

A commonly prescribed mixed alpha- and beta-adrenergic blocker sympatholytic medication is

- Labetalol (Normodyne)

Commonly prescribed norepinephrine depletion sympatholytic medications are

- Guanadrel (Hylorel)
- Guanethidine (Ismelin)

### Vasodilator Medication

**Vasodilator medication** is used to decrease systolic and diastolic BP. There are two classifications of vasodilator medications. These are calcium channel blockers and direct vasodilators. Calcium channel blockers decrease calcium flow into cells resulting in decreased contraction of smooth muscles around the arterioles. Direct vasodilators increase the diameter of blood vessels resulting in decreased peripheral resistance and decreased BP. Vasodilators are used to treat moderate and severe HTN.

Commonly prescribed vasodilator medications are

- Hydralazine (Apresoline)
- Minoxidil (Rogaine)
- Nitroprusside (Nitropress)

## Angiotensin-Converting Enzyme Inhibitor Medication

**ACE inhibitor medication** prevents conversion of angiotensin I to angiotensin II. Angiotensin II is a vasoconstrictor that leads to excretion of aldosterone that retains water and sodium resulting in increased blood volume. By interrupting conversion of angiotensin I to angiotensin II, BP decreases. ACE inhibitors are used to treat HTN and heart failure.

Commonly prescribed ACE inhibitors are

- Benazepril (Lotensin)
- Captopril (Capoten)
- Enalapril (Vasotec)
- Fosinopril (Monopril)
- Lisinopril (Zestril)
- Quinapril (Accupril)
- Ramipril (Altace)

## Medication to Strengthen Cardiac Contractions

Two medications are used to increase cardiac contractions and treat heart failure. These are cardiac glycoside medications and phosphodiesterase (PED) inhibitor medication.

### Cardiac Glycoside

**Cardiac glycoside** medication strengthens cardiac contractions by decreasing the electrical impulse between the SA and AV node, resulting in decreased cardiac rate. Cardiac glycoside medications are used for heart failure and supraventricular arrhythmia.

The commonly prescribed cardiac glycoside medication is

- Digoxin (Lanoxin)

### Phosphodiesterase inhibitor

**PDE inhibitor** medication strengthens cardiac contractions by increasing the movement of calcium into the cardiac cells and increasing the storage of calcium. In addition, PED inhibitor medication causes smooth muscles of the peripheral blood vessels to relax resulting in decreased resistance to cardiac output.

Commonly prescribed PED inhibitor medications are

- Inamrinone (Inocor)
- Milrinone (Primacor)

## Diuretic Medication

**Diuretic medication** causes water and electrolytes to be excreted by the kidneys resulting in decreased BP. There are three classifications of diuretics. These are thiazide diuretics, loop diuretics, and potassium-sparing diuretics.

### Thiazide Diuretic Medication

**Thiazide diuretic medication** prevents the reabsorption of sodium by the kidneys resulting in excretion of sodium. As sodium is excreted, water is also excreted, decreasing the volume of plasma and leading to an initial decrease in cardiac output. Cardiac output returns to normal when treatment stabilizes with thiazide diuretic medication. Thiazide diuretic medication also causes excretion of potassium chloride and bicarbonate leading to an electrolyte imbalance. Thiazide diuretic medication is used to treat edema and HTN.

Commonly prescribed thiazide diuretic medications are

- Hydroflumethiazide
- Bendroflumethiazide (Naturetin)
- Chlorthalidone (Hygroton)
- Hydrochlorothiazide (HydroDIURIL)
- Indapamide (Lozol)

### Loop Diuretic Medication

**Loop diuretic medication** increases the secretion of water, sodium, and chloride in the ascending loop of Henle where urine is concentrated in the kidney. Loop diuretic medication produces the most urine of the diuretic medications and therefore can cause an electrolyte imbalance. Loop diuretic medications are used to treat heart failure, edema, and HTN.

Commonly prescribed loop diuretic medications are

- Bumetanide (Bumex)
- Ethacrynate sodium (Edecrin sodium)
- Furosemide (Lasix)
- Ethacrynic acid (Edecrin)

### Potassium-Sparing Diuretic Medication

**Potassium-sparing diuretic medication** increases the secretion of water, chloride, calcium, and sodium but not potassium.

Commonly prescribed potassium-sparing diuretic medications are:

- Amiloride (Midamor)
- Spironolactone (Aldactone)
- Triamterene (Dyrenium)

## Aortic Aneurysm

An aneurysm (see Chapter 8) is a balloon-like bulge in the aorta caused by weakening in the wall of the aorta. The blood flow within the bulging area becomes turbulent and over time can cause the area to increase in size, creating an aneurysm. The aneurysm can rupture causing a disruption in blood flow to every organ below the affected area, and may even result in death. Severe hypotension and syncope (fainting caused by insufficient blood supply to the brain) may indicate rupture.

An aneurysm may be displayed on a routine diagnostic test, such as chest X-ray (CXR), abdominal ultrasound, computed tomography (CT) scan, or magnetic resonance imaging (MRI). Surgery is likely to resect the aortic aneurysm by removing the section containing the aneurysm and replacing it with a graft.

The ED staff must be alert for the following signs:

- Asymptomatic.
- Abdominal pain.
- Back pain that may radiate to posterior legs.
- Abdominal pulsation.
- Diminished femoral pulses.
- Anxiety.
- Restlessness.
- Decreased pulse pressure.
- Increased thready pulse.
- Swishing sound over the abdominal aorta or iliac or femoral arteries because the natural flow of blood is disturbed (bruit).

ED treatment is

- Administer antihypertensives, reducing the force of the pressure within the aorta to decrease the likelihood of rupture.
- Administer analgesics to treat patients who may be having pain from pressure on nearby structures (nerves, etc.) or tearing of the vessel.
- Administer oxycodone or morphine sulfate as needed to decrease oxygen demand.
- Monitor vital signs by looking for changes in BP or elevated pulse and respiratory rates. During aortic dissection, the BP may initially increase due to severity of pain. It may then become difficult to impossible to obtain both the BP and pulse in one or both arms because of blood flow disruption to the arm(s). The patient may go into shock quickly if the aneurysm ruptures.
- Monitor cardiovascular system by checking heart sounds, peripheral pulses (upper and lower extremities), and for abdominal bruits (swishing sounds heard over the blood vessel when flow is disturbed).
- Measure intake and output.
- Hypovolemia is suspected if there is a low urine output and high specific gravity of urine.

- Palpate abdomen for distention or pulsatile mass.
- Abdominal distention, an enlarged abdomen, may signify imminent rupture of the aneurysm.
- BP decreases as less blood circulates. Pulse rate increases as the heart tries to pump the blood faster to meet the oxygen demands of the body. Respiratory rate increases to meet oxygen needs while peripheral pulse sites are harder to find as BP lowers. The farther the pulse is from the heart, the more difficult it will be to find; it will be harder to locate the dorsalis pedis and posterior tibialis pulses earlier than the radial pulses.
- Increased thready pulse.
- Limit patient's activity.

# Angina Pectoris

Angina (see Chapter 8) is chest pain caused by narrowing of blood vessels to the coronary artery leading to an inadequate blood flow to the heart muscle. An episode of angina is typically precipitated by physical activity, excitement, or emotional stress. There are three categories of angina. Angina is caused by arteriosclerosis. Atherosclerotic heart disease occurs when there is a buildup of plaque within the coronary arteries. Angina is often the first symptom that heart disease exists. When the demand for oxygen by the heart muscle exceeds the available supply, chest pain occurs. The patient who presents in the ED with angina is commonly experiencing unstable angina. Unstable angina is when pain occurs at rest; is of new onset; is of increasing intensity, force, or duration; isn't relieved by rest; and is slow to subside in response to nitroglycerin.

The practitioner will likely order the following tests:

- ECG during episode.
  - T wave inverted with initial ischemia, which is reduced blood flow due to an obstructed vessel, usually first sign.
  - ST segment changes occur with injury to the myocardium (heart muscle).
  - Abnormal Q waves due to infarction of myocardium.
- Laboratory tests: Troponins, creatine kinase-MB (CK-MB), which is an enzyme released by damaged cardiac tissue 2 to 6 hours following an infarction, electrolytes.
- CXR to determine signs of heart failure.

- Coronary angiography to determine plaque buildup in coronary arteries.
- Cardiac positron emission tomography (PET) to determine plaque buildup in coronary arteries.
- Echocardiogram or stress echo to determine any abnormality of wall motion due to ischemia.

The ED staff must be alert for the following signs:

- Chest pain lasting 3 to 5 minutes—not all patients get substernal pain; it may be described as pressure, heaviness, squeezing, or tightness. Use the patient's words.
- Can occur at rest or after exertion, excitement, or exposure to cold—due to increased oxygen demands or vasospasm.
- Usually relieved by rest—a chance to reestablish oxygen needs.
- Pain may radiate to other parts of the body such as the jaw or back; angina pain is not always felt in the chest. Ask if the patient has had similar pain in the past.
- Sweating (diaphoresis)—increased work of body to meet basic physiologic needs; anxiety.
- Tachycardia—heart pumping faster trying to meet oxygen needs as anxiety increases.
- Difficulty breathing, shortness of breath (dyspnea)—increased heart rate increases respiratory rate and increases oxygenation.
- Anxiety—not getting enough oxygen to heart muscle, the patient becomes nervous.

ED treatment is

- 2 to 4 L of oxygen. The goal of treatment is to deliver sufficient oxygen to the heart muscle to meet its need. When suspecting chest pain, always give oxygen as the first line of defense.
- Administer beta-adrenergic blocking agents—this class has a cardioprotective effect, decreasing cardiac workload and likelihood of arrhythmia.
  - Propranolol (Inderal), nadolol (Corgard), atenolol (Tenormin), metoprolol (Lopressor)
- Administer nitrates—aids in getting oxygenated blood to heart muscle.
  - Nitroglycerin—sublingual tablets or spray; timed-release tablets.
  - Topical nitroglycerin—paste or timed-release patch.
- Aspirin for antiplatelet effect.

- Analgesic—typically morphine intravenously during acute pain. The medicine is very fast-acting when given this way and will decrease myocardial oxygen demand as well as decrease pain.

- Monitor vital signs—look for change in BP, pulse (P), respiration (R); irregular pulse; pulse deficit; when a discrepancy is found between an atrial rate and a radial rate, when measured simultaneously; pulse oximetry.

- Notify physician if systolic blood pressure (SBP) is below 90 mm Hg.

- **Nitrates** dilate arteries to the heart and increase blood flow. You may have an order to hold nitrates if SBP is below 90 mm Hg to reduce risk of patient passing out from lack of blood flow to brain.

- Notify physician if heart rate is less than 60 beats/min. Beta-adrenergic blocking agents slow conduction through the AV node and reduce the heart rate and contractility. You may have an order to hold beta-blockers if heart rate goes below 60; you should continuously monitor the patient's pulse rate.

- Monitor cardiac status using a 12-lead ECG while the patient is experiencing an angina attack. Each time the patient has pain, a new 12-lead ECG is done to assess for changes, even if one was already done that day.

- Record fluid intake and output. Assess for renal function.

- Place patient in a semi-Fowler's position (semisitting with knees flexed).

## Myocardial Infarction

MI (see Chapter 8) is disruption of blood supply to the myocardium for a prolonged time due to the blockage of coronary arteries, resulting in insufficient oxygen reaching cardiac muscle and leading to cardiac muscle necrosis. The infarction is often caused by a buildup of plaque over time (atherosclerosis). It may also be caused by a clot that develops in association with the atherosclerosis within the vessel. Patients are typically (not always) symptomatic, but some patients will not be aware of the event; they will have what is called a *silent MI*. Treatment is focused on reversing and preventing further damage to the myocardium.

The practitioner will likely order the following tests:

- ECG
  - T-wave inversion—sign of ischemia.
  - ST segment elevated or depressed—sign of injury.
  - Significant Q waves—sign of infarction.

- Decreased pulse pressure because of diminished cardiac output.
- Increased WBC due to inflammatory response to injury.
- Blood chemistry.
  - Elevated CK-MB—usually done serially, the numbers will rise along a predetermined curve to signify myocardial damage and resolution.
  - Elevated troponin I and troponin T proteins elevated within an hour of myocardial damage.
- Less than 25 mL/h of urine output due to lack of renal blood flow.

The ED staff must be alert for the following signs:

- Chest pain that is unrelieved by rest or nitroglycerin, unlike angina.
- Pain that radiates to arms, jaw, back, and/or neck.
- Shortness of breath, especially in the elderly or women.
- Nausea or vomiting possible.
- May be asymptomatic, known as a silent MI, which is more common in diabetic patients.
- Heart rate more than 100 (tachycardia) because of sympathetic stimulation, pain, or low cardiac output.
- Variable BP.
- Anxiety.
- Restlessness.
- Feeling of impending doom.
- Pale, cool, clammy skin; sweating (diaphoresis).
- Sudden death due to arrhythmia usually occurs within first hour.

ED treatment is

- Administer oxygen, aspirin.
- Administer antiarrhythmic because arrhythmias are common, as are conduction disturbances.
  - Amiodarone
  - Lidocaine
  - Procainamide (Pronestyl)
- Electrical cardioversion for unstable VT. In cardioversion, an initial shock is administered to the heart to reestablish sinus rhythm.
- Administer antihypertensive to keep BP low.
  - Hydralazine (Apresoline)

- Percutaneous revascularization.
- Administer thrombolytic therapy within 3 to 12 hours of onset because it can reestablish blood flow in an occluded artery, reduce mortality, and halt the size of the infarction.
  - Alteplase (Activase)
  - Streptokinase (Streptase)
  - Anistreplase (Eminase)
  - Reteplase (Reteplase)
- Heparin following thrombolytic therapy.
- Administer calcium channel blockers because they appear to prevent reinfarction and ischemia but only in non-Q-wave infarctions.
  - Verapamil (Calan)
  - Diltiazem (Cardizem)
- Administer beta-adrenergic blocking agents because they reduce the duration of ischemic pain and the incidence of VF; decreases mortality.
  - Propranolol (Inderal)
  - Nadolol (Corgard)
  - Metoprolol (Lopressor)
- Administer analgesics to relieve pain, reduce pulmonary congestion, and decrease myocardial oxygen consumption.
  - Morphine
- Administer nitrates to reduce ischemic pain by dilation of blood vessels; helps to lower BP.
  - Nitroglycerin

# Cardiac Tamponade

Cardiac tamponade (see Chapter 9) occurs when a large amount of liquid accumulates in the sac around the heart (pericardium), resulting in pressure on the heart that reduces the filling of ventricles with blood. As a result, there is low volume of blood pumped with each contraction and decreased stroke volume and cardiac output. Pressure within the pericardium may be due to fluid, pus, or blood. Cardiac tamponade is a medical emergency requiring immediate intervention, such as drainage of the fluids. Stabilization occurs quickly once the fluid is removed and pressure is alleviated. If fluid recurs, surgery may be necessary.

The practitioner will likely order the following tests:

- Echocardiogram: Ultrasound imaging of the heart to assess the heart's position, structure, and motion. Ventricles and atria are compressed. Fluid found within pericardial sac.
- Cardiac catheterization.
- CXR shows an enlarged heart if large effusion present.
- ECG used to rule out other cardiac problems.

The ED staff must be alert for the following signs

- Neck vein distention—accumulation of fluid within the pericardium causes pressure on the heart, which prevents the venous return from the jugular veins. This causes distention, more pronounced on inspiration.
- Restlessness due to decreased oxygen to the brain.
- Muffled (dull) heart sounds on auscultation because it's harder to hear through fluid.
- Pulsus paradoxus—decrease of 10 mm Hg or more in SBP during inspiration—change in pressure within the chest during inspiration, resulting in decreased ventricular filling, decreased output, fall in SBP.
- Sweating (diaphoresis).
- Difficulty breathing (dyspnea).
- Tachycardia.
- Hypotension.
- Fatigue.

ED treatment is

- Pericardiocentesis—a needle is inserted into the pericardium and fluid is aspirated or drained.
- Administer adrenergic agent—increases heart rate and BP.
- Ensure adequate oxygenation.

# Cardiogenic Shock

Cardiogenic shock (see Chapter 9) occurs when there is decreased blood flow as a result of the heart unable to pump blood. Blood pools in the left ventricle causing a backup of blood into the lungs and resulting in pulmonary edema.

Cardiac contractions increase to compensate for the decreased cardiac output causing an increase in demand for oxygen by the heart. However, the lungs cannot oxygenate sufficient blood due to decreased blood flow, and therefore heart muscles are starved for oxygen. Treatment needs to find a balance between improving cardiac output and reducing oxygen needs and cardiac workload of the myocardium. This balance must be achieved while maintaining perfusion of the heart muscle.

The practitioner will likely order the following tests:

- Chemistry—check electrolytes, kidney function to ascertain kidney perfusion; calcium level is increased or decreased secondary to muscle contractility.
- Echocardiogram—to look for ventricular rupture, pericarditis, or valve dysfunction.
- ECG
  - Enlarged Q wave due to heart failure.
  - Elevation of ST waves is a sign of ischemia.

The ED staff must be alert for the following signs:

- Hypotension, because blood flow decreases below normal.
- Tachycardia, because the heart is trying to pump faster to maintain adequate blood flow to the body, or occasionally bradycardia, where the heart rate is less than 60 beats/min due to myocardial damage.
- Arrhythmias—when the heart muscle does not have enough oxygen, it becomes irritable, making arrhythmias more likely.
- Clammy skin, because oxygenation to tissues is reduced.
- Drop in skin temperature because of reduced circulation as a result of hypotension.
- Urine output less than 30 mL/h (oliguria) because the kidneys are not being perfused.
- Crackles heard in the lungs secondary to pulmonary edema, meaning fluid is building up in lungs.
- Confusion due to poor perfusion.
- Distended jugular veins—sign of fluid overload, inability of heart to manage fluid flowing into heart.
- Narrow pulse pressure.
- Cyanosis of lips, peripheral extremities due to poor perfusion.

Treatment is based on medical support for the heart until the underlying cause can be determined. ED treatment is

- Administer vasodilator—dilates blood vessels (arterial and venous) to decrease the venous return to the heart and reduces the peripheral arterial resistance.
- Administer adrenergic agent—to increase the heart rate and BP.
  - Epinephrine
- Administer inotropes—strengthens the heartbeat, improves contractions, produces peripheral vasoconstriction.
  - Dopamine (Intropin)
  - Dobutamine
  - Inamrinone
  - Milrinone (Primacor)
- Administer vasopressor—decreases blood flow to all organs except the heart and brain.
  - Norepinephrine
- Provide supplemental oxygen—may need to be through intubation.
- Monitor vital signs—look for changes in BP, P, R.
- Monitor heart sounds.
- Test capillary refill.
- Monitor ABG to measure pH, acidosis or alkalosis, bicarbonate level.
- Monitor respiratory status—due to poor perfusion, these patients are in respiratory distress; mechanical ventilation may be needed.
- Place the patient on bed rest.
- Monitor intake and output of fluids—look for adequate renal perfusion. Without sufficient cardiac function, the patient will not have enough blood flow to the kidneys to get adequate filtration.

# Congestive Heart Failure

The heart is unable to pump sufficient blood to maintain adequate circulation, resulting in a backup of blood, and the extra pressure may cause accumulation of fluid into the lungs. In congestive heart failure (CHF) (see Chapter 9), the heart muscle is too weak to adequately push blood forward or the heart isn't able to sufficiently relax and receive enough blood returning back to the heart.

The practitioner will likely order the following tests:

- BNP—elevated levels in CHF; produced when the ventricles are stretched.
- ECG may show signs of ischemia (T-wave inversion), tachycardia, or extra systole (extra beats).
- Complete blood count (CBC) may show anemia—Hgb less than 12 in females, less than 14 in males; hematocrit (HCT); less than three times the Hgb values.
- Chemistry may show renal problems, electrolyte disturbance.
- CXR
  - Pulmonary congestion because of accumulation of fluid in the lungs.
  - Enlarged left ventricle (left ventricular hypertrophy [LVH]) because of the increased stress on the heart to pump blood.
  - Accumulation of fluid in the pleural cavity (pleural effusion).
  - Enlarged heart (cardiomegaly) because of the increased stress on the heart to pump blood.

The ED staff must be alert for the following signs:

- Extra heart sounds
  - $S_3$: Soft sound caused by vibration of the ventricular wall caused by rapid filling. Heard after $S_2$ heart sound. Heard over the apex of the left ventricle, fourth intercostal space along the mid-clavicular line. Best heard when patient lies on left side. Usually indicates heart failure.
  - $S_4$: Vibration of valves and the ventricular walls during the second phase of ventricular filling when the atria contract. Heard before $S_1$, in the same location as $S_3$, usually due to a "stiff heart."
  - **Murmur:** Sounds of turbulence caused by blood flow through the valves. Heard anywhere around the heart.
- Fatigue.
- Syncope.
- Chest pain.
- Basilar rales from fluid overload.
- Exertional dyspnea.

- Fatigue.
- Positive hepatojugular reflux from liver congestion—the distension of the neck veins precipitated by the maneuver of firm pressure over the liver.
- $S_3$ heart sound.
- Cough.
- Orthopnea.
- Discomfort in right upper abdomen due to hepatomegaly.
- Edema.
- Cardiomegaly—enlarged heart.
- Frothy or pink sputum from capillary permeability (late sign).

ED treatment is

- Administer diuretics for symptom control resulting in patient comfort by reducing blood volume.
    - Furosemide (Lasix), bumetanide (Bumex), metolazone (Zaroxolyn), hydrochlorothiazide (HCTZ), spironolactone (Aldactone)—be aware of electrolyte imbalance—these medications may alter the potassium level.
- Administer ACE inhibitors to decrease afterload.
    - Captopril (Capoten), enalapril (Vasotec), lisinopril (Zestril)
- Administer beta-adrenergic blocking agents, which help raise ejection fraction and decrease ventricular size.
- Administer inotrope to strengthen myocardial contractility.
    - Digoxin (Digitalis)
- Administer vasodilator to reduce preload, relieve dyspnea.
    - Nitroprusside (Nitropress), nitroglycerin ointment
- Administer anticoagulants in patients with severe heart failure, as they have a propensity to develop thrombus and emboli; those with concurrent atrial fibrillation will also need anticoagulation.
- Reduce fluids as fluid overload is a causative factor in CHF.
- High Fowler's position to ease breathing and enhance diaphragmatic excursion.
- Supplemental oxygen to meet increased demand of myocardium.
- Monitor vital signs and look for changes.
- Record fluid intake and output.

# Hypertensive Crisis

Hypertensive crisis is an extremely high BP of 180/120 mm Hg or higher that can damage blood vessels, preventing blood to effectively perfuse tissues and organs and leading to tissues necrosis and organ damage. There are two categories of hypertensive crisis

- **Urgent:** BP is extremely high but there are no signs of organ damage.
- **Emergency:** BP is extremely high and there are signs of organ damage.

The practitioner will likely order the following tests:

- Continuous BP monitoring.
- Continuous ECG monitoring.

The ED staff must be alert for the following signs:

- Severe chest pains
- Severe headache
- Confusion
- Blurred vision
- Shortness of breath
- Nausea and vomiting
- Severe anxiety
- Seizures

ED treatment is

- Intravenous BP medication.
    - Sodium nitroprusside (Nitropress), nitroglycerin (Nitro-Bid), hydralazine (Apresoline) (for preeclampsia)
- Treat organ damage.
- Reduce BP slowly over days. Reduce BP no more than 25% of the mean arterial pressure (MAP) within the first 2 hours.
- Pulse oximetry.
- Administer oxygen.
- Monitor fluid output. Normal is 1 mL/kg/h. Critical is <0.5 mL/kg/h.
- Provide quiet, low-lit environment.
- Monitor for thiocyanate toxicity if patient is administered Nitropress.
    - Delirium

- Blurred vision
- Nausea
- Fatigue
- Tinnitus

# Hypovolemic Shock

Hypovolemic shock (see Chapter 8) is the result of rapid fluid loss that leads to inadequate circulation. An insufficient amount of blood is available within the cardiovascular system, depriving tissues and organs of oxygen and nutrients. Hypovolemic shock can be caused by external hemorrhage, fluids moving in the body from vessels into tissue (third spacing), or dehydration.

The practitioner will likely order the following tests:

- BP—low BP.
- Temperature—low body temperature.
- Pulse—rapid, weak, thready pulse.
- CBC.
- Chemistry—creatinine and BUN to assess kidney function.
- Coagulation studies.
- CT scan—identifies suspected area of bleeding.
- Echocardiogram—rule out cardiac disorder.
- Endoscopy—identifies suspected area of bleeding.
- Urinary catheterization—measure urine output.
- Blood type and match.

The ED staff must be alert for the following signs:

- Bleeding from cuts.
- Bleeding from other injuries.
- Internal bleeding, such as in the gastrointestinal (GI) tract.
- Burns.
- Diarrhea.
- Excessive perspiration.
- Vomiting.

- Urine output less than 25 mL/h because less blood is perfusing the kidneys, causing decreased urinary output.
- Heart rate more than 100 (tachycardia), because the heart attempts to compensate for the decreased volume.
- Cold skin, because of peripheral vasoconstriction due to decreased volume.
- Restlessness, agitation; may be seen due to poor perfusion of the brain.
- Confusion.
- Rapid breathing.

ED treatment is

- No fluids by mouth.
- Stabilize the head and neck if spinal injury is suspected.
- Lay the person flat with head down and feet lifted.
- Intravenous using 14-G catheter (16 or 18 G also adequate if 14 cannot be obtained; use largest possible).
- Crystalloid solutions to expand intravascular and extravascular fluid volume.
  - 0.9% normal saline, lactated Ringer solution (contains electrolytes)
- Catecholamines to increase BP.
  - Dopamine, epinephrine, and norepinephrine
- Inotropic agent to increase BP.
  - Dobutamine
- Fresh frozen plasma for clotting.
- 2 to 4 L of 100% oxygen as necessary using nonrebreather face mask.
- Monitor lungs for crackles and dyspnea due to fluid overflow.
- Blood replacement—type-specific or type O negative, which is the universal donor type.
- Monitor BP every 15 minutes.
- Monitor vital signs every 15 minutes.
- Measure urine output each hour with indwelling urinary catheter.
- Increase fluid rate if urine output is less than 30 mL/h. Be alert for signs of fluid overload. These include, but are not limited to, crackles in the lungs and dyspnea.

# Pulmonary Edema

Pulmonary edema (see Chapter 9) occurs when fluid builds up in the lungs due to ineffective pumping of blood by the heart. The left ventricle is overworked and is unable to pump blood received from the lungs. Pressure in the left atrium increases backing up pressure in the veins in the lungs. Fluid is then pushed through the capillary into the alveoli.

The practitioner will likely order the following:

- **Oxygen:** If saturation is less than 90%.
- **CXR:** Alveolar fluid, large heart.
- Echocardiogram to determine ejection fraction percentages in the heart.
- ABGs will show lower levels of oxygen.

The ED staff must be alert for the following signs:

- Difficulty breathing even when sitting upright (because of the fluid in the lungs).
- Rapid breathing: More than 20 breaths/min (tachypnea), because the body is trying to get more oxygen.
- Frothy sputum with a tinge of blood due to capillary permeability.
- Cyanosis.
- Cool, clammy skin because the body is diverting blood flow from the periphery.
- Restlessness and fear due to lack of oxygenation.
- Distended jugular veins due to increased pressure within chest.
- Crackles, wheezing heard in the lungs as the air moves through the fluid.

ED treatment is

- Administer supplemental oxygen, which increases arterial $PO_2$. Mechanical ventilation may be necessary.
- Administer morphine, which lowers left atrial pressure, decreases myocardial oxygen demand, lowers anxiety, and relieves pain.
- Administer diuretics to remove excess fluid.
  - Furosemide (Lasix), bumetanide (Bumex), metolazone (Zaroxolyn)
- Administer cardiac glycosides to increase contractions of the heart.
  - Digoxin (Digitalis)
- Administer cardiac inotropics to strengthen the heart.
  - Dobutamine

- Inamrinone
- Milrinone (Primacor)
- Administer nitrates to decrease BP and left ventricular filling pressures.
  - Isosorbide dinitrate (Isordil)
- Place the patient in full Fowler's position to enhance air exchange and diaphragmatic movement, sitting with legs dangling over side of bed.
- Monitor cardiovascular function for changes in heart sounds, extra sounds, murmurs.
- Monitor respirations for changes in lung sounds, chest expansion.
- Check oxygen saturation (pulse oximetry).
- Record fluid intake and output.
- Record characteristics of sputum.

# Atrial Fibrillation

Atrial fibrillation (see Chapter 4) is when the atria quiver rather than contract, making it nearly impossible for the atria to pump blood into the ventricle. Multiple cells in the atria send uncoordinated electrical impulses up to 600/min, each trying to move through the AV node. Non-SA node electrical impulses bypass the AV node and enter the ventricles resulting in irregular contractions by the ventricles and leading to an irregular, rapid heart rate.

The practitioner will likely order the following test:

- **ECG:** An ECG records the electrical activities of the heart.

The ED staff must be alert for the following signs:

- Shortness of breath
- Dizziness
- Fainting
- Palpitations of the heart
- Chest discomfort
- Feeling tried

ED treatment is

- Antiarrhythmic medication to maintain normal sinus rhythm.
  - Flecainide acetate (Tambocor), propafenone (Rythmol), sotalol (Betapace), dofetilide (Tikosyn), and amiodarone (Cordarone)

- Digitalis glycoside slows the contractions of the ventricles.
  - Digitalis glycoside is digoxin (Lanoxin).
- Beta-blockers slow the contractions of the ventricles.
  - Metoprolol (Toprol, Lopressor)
- Calcium channel blocker slows the contractions of the ventricles too.
  - Verapamil (Calan) and diltiazem (Cardizem)
- Anticoagulant medication reduces the risk that blood clots will form.
  - Heparin, enoxaparin (Lovenox), dalteparin (Fragmin), argatroban, bivalirudin (Angiomax), fondaparinux (Arixtra), lepirudin (Refludan), warfarin (Coumadin), and dabigatran (Pradaxa)
- Electrical cardioversion is a procedure that delivers an electrical shock through electrodes placed on the patient's chest. The shock stops the heart for a fraction of a second. The SA node then automatically starts sending normal impulses throughout the heart. The patient is anesthetized during the procedure.
- Catheter ablation is a procedure where tissues of the heart that cause the extra impulses are destroyed by radiofrequency energy applied to the area by a catheter that the practitioner inserts into a blood vessel. In some cases, the practitioner ablates the AV node to prevent impulses from the atria from reaching the ventricles. The patient then requires a permanent pacemaker to maintain ventricle contractions.
- The Maze procedure is a surgical procedure where a series of incisions are made in both atria to prevent the abnormal impulses.
- Temporarily limit the patient's activities to decrease stress on the heart.
- Monitor for
  - Heart rate.
  - Signs of stroke related to risk for blood clots.

## Atrial Flutter

Atrial flutter (aflutter) (see Chapter 4) occurs when the atria contract too fast to permit each impulse to move through the AV node and into the ventricles. The atria contract twice as fast as the ventricles. You can differentiate between atrial fibrillation and atrial flutter by contraction of the atria. There are no contractions with atrial fibrillation. There are coordinated contractions between both atria.

The practitioner will likely order the following tests:

- ECG
  - **Rate:** There will be more P waves than QRS complexes because there are more atrial contractions or quivers than ventricle contractions.
  - **P pulmonale:** The point of the P wave is >2.5 mm, indicating an enlarged right atrium.
  - **P mitrale:** The P wave is notched, indicating an enlarged left atrium.
  - **Wavy baseline:** The rhythm is irregular indicating atrial fibrillation
  - **Saw tooth:** The saw tooth wave indicates atrial flutter.
  - **Inverted P wave:** The inverted P wave indicates that the ectopic pacemaker is located at the atrioventricular (AV) junction near the AV node.
  - **P wave superimposed on T wave:** The P wave superimposed on the preceding T wave indicates paroxysmal atrial tachycardia, which is a regular fast heartbeat starting in the atria that begins and ends suddenly.

The ED staff must be alert for the following signs:

- Shortness of breath
- Dizziness
- Fainting
- Palpitations of the heart
- Chest discomfort
- Feeling tried

ED treatment is

- Antiarrhythmic medication to maintain normal sinus rhythm.
  - Flecainide acetate (Tambocor), propafenone (Rythmol), sotalol (Betapace), dofetilide (Tikosyn), and amiodarone (Cordarone)
- Digitalis glycoside slows the contractions of the ventricles.
  - Digitalis glycoside is digoxin (Lanoxin).
- Beta-blockers slow the contractions of the ventricles.
  - Metoprolol (Toprol, Lopressor)
- Calcium channel blocker slows the contractions of the ventricles too.
  - Verapamil (Calan) and diltiazem (Cardizem)

- Anticoagulant medication reduces the risk of formation of blood clots.
  - Heparin, enoxaparin (Lovenox), dalteparin (Fragmin), argatroban, bivalirudin (Angiomax), fondaparinux (Arixtra), lepirudin (Refludan), warfarin (Coumadin), and dabigatran (Pradaxa)
- Electrical cardioversion is a procedure that delivers an electrical shock through electrodes placed on the patient's chest. The shock stops the heart for a fraction of a second. The SA node then automatically starts sending normal impulses throughout the heart. The patient is anesthetized during the procedure.
- Catheter ablation is a procedure where tissues of the heart that cause the extra impulses are destroyed by radiofrequency energy applied to the area by a catheter that the practitioner inserts into a blood vessel. In some cases, the practitioner ablates the AV node to prevent impulses from the atria from reaching the ventricles. The patient then requires a permanent pacemaker to maintain ventricle contractions.
- The Maze procedure is a surgical procedure where a series of incisions are made in both atria to prevent the abnormal impulses.
- Temporarily limit the patient's activities to decrease stress on the heart.
- Monitor for
  - Heart rate.
  - Signs of stroke related to risk for blood clots.

## Asystole

Asystole (see Chapter 4) occurs when there isn't any ventricular depolarization, resulting in absent perfusion of the vital organs. The patient is unresponsive, not breathing, with no pulse or BP (Figure 10–1).

The practitioner will likely order the following tests:

- ECG
  - **P wave:** Absent (flat line) but may be present if the patient was in AV block such as Mobitz II or third-degree block.
  - **QRS complex:** None.
  - **PR interval:** Not measurable.

The ED staff must be alert for the following signs:

- No pulse.

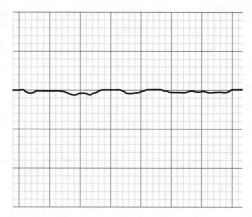

**FIGURE 10–1 ·** Asystole.

- Breathing is stopped (apnea).
- No palpable BP.
- Cyanosis.

ED treatment is

- Begin cardiopulmonary resuscitation (CPR) (see Basic Life Support).
- Begin advanced cardiac life support (see Advanced Cardiac Life Support).

## Ventricular Fibrillation

VF (see Chapter 4) is the quivering of the ventricles and can cause sudden cardiac death. There is no cardiac output and no perfusion of tissues and organs. The patient is pulseless without BP, unresponsive, and death is imminent (Figure 10–2).

The practitioner will likely order the following tests:

- ECG
  - **P wave:** None
  - **QRS complex:** None
  - **PR interval:** Not measurable
  - Wave
    - Fine wave requires antiarrhythmic medication before defibrillation.
    - Coarse wave is likely to respond to defibrillation because it is a new onset.

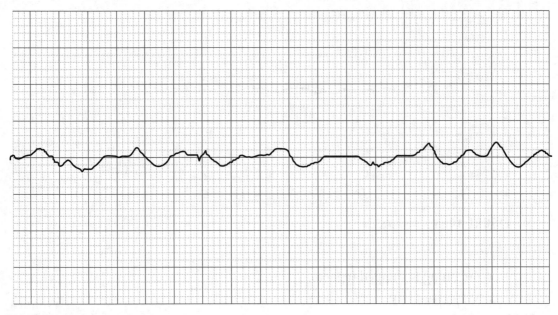

**FIGURE 10−2** · Ventricular fibrillation.

The ED staff must be alert for the following signs:

- No pulse.
- Breathing is stopped (apnea).
- No palpable BP.

ED treatment is

- Begin CPR (see Basic Life Support).
- Begin advanced cardiac life support (see Advanced Cardiac Life Support).

## Ventricular Tachycardia

VT (see Chapter 4) is an impulse rate of 120 beats/min or greater that is generated from one or multiple ectopic sites in the ventricles. Monomorphic VT is from one ectopic site and polymorphic VT is from multiple ectopic sites.

The practitioner will likely order the following tests:

- ECG
  - **P wave:** The P wave is hidden within the QRS complex and might be occasionally seen between QRS complexes.

- **PR interval:** Not measurable.
- **QRS complex:** Wide, distorted, and bizarre.
- **Rhythm:** Regular but can be irregular.
- Torsade de pointes waveform R-on-T phenomenon as a result of hypomagnesemia and prolonged QT intervals.

The ED staff must be alert for the following signs:

- The patient is aware of his/her heartbeat.
- Dizziness.
- Shortness of breath.
- Chest pain (angina).
- Palpitations.
- Weak pulse or no pulse.

ED treatment is

- Begin CPR (see Basic Life Support) if there is no pulse.
- Begin advanced cardiac life support (see Advanced Cardiac Life Support).
- Stable monomorphic VT
  - Administer antiarrhythmic medication such as amiodarone, lidocaine, and procainamide.
  - Cardioversion or defibrillation.
  - Rebalance electrolytes (potassium, magnesium, calcium).
- Unstable monomorphic VT caused by hemodynamic instability
  - Cardioversion or defibrillation
- Polymorphic VT (torsade de pointes) (Figure 10–3)
  - Rebalance electrolytes (potassium, magnesium, calcium).
  - Defibrillation.

# Cardiac Arrest

Cardiac arrest is a condition when cardiac muscles malfunction resulting in ineffective circulation leading to profusion of tissues and organs throughout the body. Cardiac arrest can be the result of many underlying conditions such as MI, overdose of medication, trauma, respiratory arrest, and VF or VT.

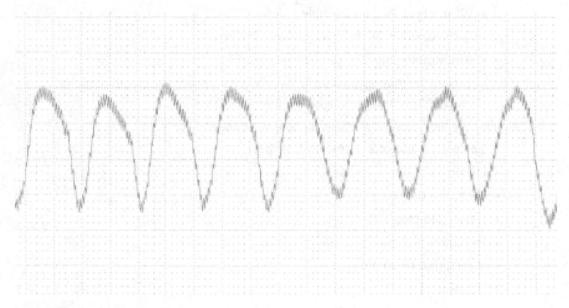

**FIGURE 10-3** · Ventricular tachycardia.

The practitioner will likely order the following tests:

- ECG
  - VF
    - **P wave:** None
    - **QRS complex:** None
    - **PR interval:** Not measurable
    - Wave
      - Fine wave requires antiarrhythmic medication before defibrillation.
      - Coarse wave is likely to respond to defibrillation because it is a new onset.
  - Asystole
    - **P wave:** Absent (flat line) but may be present if the patient was in AV block such as Mobitz II or third-degree block.
    - **QRS complex:** None.
    - **PR interval:** Not measurable.
  - VT
    - **P wave:** The P wave is hidden within the QRS complex and might be occasionally seen between QRS complexes.

- **PR interval:** Not measurable.
- **QRS complex:** Wide, distorted, and bizarre.
- **Rhythm:** Regular but can be irregular.
- Torsade de pointes waveform R-on-T phenomenon as a result hypomagnesemia and prolonged QT intervals.

The ED staff must be alert for the following signs:

- No pulse.
- Breathing is stopped (apnea).
- No palpable BP.

ED treatment is

- Begin CPR (see Basic Life Support) if there is no pulse.
- Begin advanced cardiac life support (see Advanced Cardiac Life Support).
- Treat the underlying causes commonly referred to the *Hs* and *Ts* (Table 10–3).

## Basic Life Support

Basic life support requires the following algorithm (Table 10–4) be performed when presented with a patient who had a sudden loss of consciousness and respirations are absent. This algorithm is provided by the American Heart Association. Consult with the American Heart Association for updates on this algorithm.

Be sure to push hard and fast, at least 100 compressions per minute, allowing full chest recoil. One cycle is 30 compressions to two breaths if there is no advanced airway. There should be five cycles every 2 minutes. Rotate with another person every five cycles.

| TABLE 10–3 Common Causes of Cardiac Arrest | | | | |
|---|---|---|---|---|
| Acidosis | Hypovolemia | Hypoxia | Hypo/ hyperkalemia | Hypoglycemia |
| Hypothermia | Toxins | Cardiac tamponade | Tension pneumothorax | Thrombosis |
| Trauma | | | | |

| TABLE 10–4 Basic Life Support Algorithm |
|---|
| **Step 1** |
| Try arousing the patient by calling him/her by name and rubbing the upper portion of the sternum. |
| **Step 2** |
| Call 911 or send someone to activate the emergency response system and to get an AED. |
| **Step 3** |
| If no response, quickly check for breathing and a pulse. |
| Lightly feel the carotid artery for minimum of 5 s and maximum of 10 s. |
| **Step 4** |
| Bare the patient's chest and position hands for CPR. |
| **Step 5** |
| Deliver first cycle of compression, at least 100 compressions per minute at depth of at least 2 in. Allow complete recoil between compressions. Rotate compressions every 2 min. Limit interruptions to less than 10 s. |
| **Step 6** |
| Open the airway. |
| Tilt the head back if there is no sign of trauma. If there is a sign of trauma, then use a jaw thrust to open the airway. |
| **Step 7** |
| Administer two breaths per 30 compressions. Each breath every 6-8 s. |
| Make sure the chest rises. |
| **Step 8** |
| Attach AED leads to patient and follow AED's voice instructions. Don't stop CPR until the AED's voice tells you to do so. Start CPR immediately after shock is given. |

Abbreviations: AED, automated external defibrillator; CPR, cardiopulmonary resuscitation.

## Advanced Cardiac Life Support

Advanced cardiac life support (ACLS) is used when the patient experiences cardiac arrest and requires external electric stimulation and/or medication to reestablish cardiac function. ACLS is performed by staff that are ACLS certified and who are permitted to perform ACLS within their scope of practice.

Table 10–5 shows the ACLS algorithm used when a patient is in VT or V-Tach. Table 10–6 is the algorithm used when the patient is in VF or V-Fib.

**TABLE 10–5** Advanced Life Support Algorithm for Ventricular Tachycardia

| Ventricular Tachycardia | | |
|---|---|---|
| Pulse | | No pulse |
| Stable (SBP >90) | Unstable (SBP <90) | Defibrillate 200 J |
| Amiodarone drip 150 mg/10 min | Cardioversion 100 J | CPR 2 min |
| Repeat once | Check for pulse | |
| | Cardioversion 200 J | |

Abbreviations: CPR, cardiopulmonary resuscitation; SBP, systolic blood pressure.

**TABLE 10–6** Advanced Life Support Algorithm for Ventricular Fibrillation

| Ventricular Fibrillation |
|---|
| Defibrillate 200 J |
| • Epinephrine 1 mg rapid IV push |
| • CPR 2 min |
| Defibrillate 200 J |
| • Amiodarone 300 mg rapid IV push |
| • CPR 2 min |
| Defibrillate 200 J |
| • Epinephrine 1 mg OR  vasopressin 40 units (vasopressin can be administered once) rapid IV push |
| • CPR 2 min |
| Defibrillate 200 J |
| • Amiodarone 150 mg rapid IV push |
| • CPR 2 min |
| Defibrillate 200 J |
| • Epinephrine 1 mg rapid IV push |
| • CPR 2 min |
| Defibrillate 200 J |
| • Lidocaine 1-1.5 mg/kg rapid IV push |
| • CPR 2 min |
| Defibrillate 200 J |
| • Epinephrine 1 mg rapid IV push |
| • CPR 2 min |

*(Continued)*

| TABLE 10–6   Advanced Life Support Algorithm for Ventricular Fibrillation (Continued) |
|---|
| **Ventricular Fibrillation** |
| Defibrillate 200 J |
| • Lidocaine 0.5-0.75 mg/kg rapid IV push |
| • CPR 2 min |
| Defibrillate 200 J |
| • Epinephrine 1 mg rapid IV push |
| • CPR 2 min |
| Defibrillate 200 J |
| • Lidocaine 0.5-0.75 mg/kg rapid IV push |
| • CPR 2 min |
| Defibrillate 200 J |
| • Epinephrine 1 mg rapid IV push |
| • CPR 2 min |

Abbreviations: CPR, cardiopulmonary resuscitation; IV, intravenous.

Table 10–7 is the algorithm for pulseless electrical activity (PEA) and asystole. PEA is when a patient has cardiac activity but does not have a pulse. These algorithms are provided by the American Heart Association. Consult with the American Heart Association for updates on these algorithms.

| TABLE 10–7   Advanced Life Support Algorithm for Pulseless Electronically Activity and Asystole |
|---|
| **Pulseless Electrical Activity/Asystole** |
| CPR 2 min |
| • Epinephrine 1 mg |
| • Revaluate |
| CPR 2 min |
| • Epinephrine 1 mg OR  vasopressin 40 units (vasopressin can be administered once) rapid IV push |
| • Revaluate |
| CPR 2 min |
| • Epinephrine 1 mg rapid IV push |
| • Revaluate |
| CPR 2 min |
| • Epinephrine 1 mg rapid IV push |

Abbreviations: CPR, cardiopulmonary resuscitation; IV, intravenous.

**TABLE 10–8** Advanced Life Support Algorithm for Bradycardia

| Bradycardia | | |
|---|---|---|
| Stable (SBP >90) | | Unstable (SBP <90) |
| Asymptomatic | Symptomatic | Epinephrine 2-10 µg/min drip OR Dopamine 2-10 µg/kg/min drip OR Atropine 0.5 mg bolus every 3-5 min for a maximum of 3 mg |
| Monitor and transport the patient to the cardiac care unit | Monitor with a 12-lead ECG | Subcutaneous pacing, if medication works |
| | Administer atropine 0.5 mg | |
| | Assess after 3-5 min | |
| | Repeat administration of atropine 0.5 mg every 3-5 min for a maximum of 3 mg | |

Abbreviations: ECG, electrocardiograph; SBP, systolic blood pressure.

# Bradycardia

Bradycardia is a condition when the heart beats slowly, reducing circulation and resulting in deceased oxygenation of tissues and organs. A common underlying cause of bradycardia is a heart block that interrupts the path of the electrical impulse within the heart. The American Heart Association recommends the interventions listed in Table 10–8 when treating bradycardia.

# Fibrinolytic Therapy

Fibrinolytic therapy is used to remove all or a portion of an existing blood clot resulting in normal blood flow 50% of the time using tissue plasminogen activator (tPA), reteplase, tenecteplase, or streptokinase. Table 10–9 lists the

| TABLE 10−9   Fibrinolytic Checklist | | |
|---|---|---|
| **Administer Fibrinolytic Therapy** | **Don't Administer Fibrinolytic Therapy** | |
| Ischemic chest pain | Patient presents more than 12 h after onset of symptoms. | INR >1.7 PT >15 Platelet count >100,000 SBP >185 |
| Persistent ST segment elevation more than 1 mm in two or more contiguous chest or limb leads | Arterial puncture at a noncompressible site within the past 7 d | Warfarin in use by patient |
| Onset of symptoms within 12 h of presentation and positive ECG waves | Active internal bleeding | Patient received heparin within the past 48 h |
| Onset of symptoms within 12 h and positive posterior MI (ST segment depression in early precordial leads) | Witnessed seizure at time of stroke | Acute trauma |
| 18 y or older | Intracranial hemorrhage assessed with noncontrast head CT | Subarachnoid hemorrhage |
| Ischemic stroke with measurable neurologic deficit | History of intracranial hemorrhage | Arteriovenous malformation |
| Less than 3 h last time when patient seemed normal | | |

Abbreviations: CT, computed tomography; ECG, electrocardiograph; INR, international normalized ratio; MI, myocardial infarction; PT, prothrombin time; SBP, systolic blood pressure.

fibrinolytic checklist used to determine if the patient is a candidate for fibrinolytic therapy.

# Acute Stroke

A stroke is referred to as a *cerebrovascular accident* (CVA) that occurs when there is disturbance in blood supply to the brain resulting in a neurological disturbance. The disturbance can be caused by a blockage that leads to an ischemia, a hemorrhage, or from unknown cause. Decreased blood flow can result in tissue damage in the affected area of the brain.

A patient can experience a transient ischemic attack (TIA) commonly called a *mini stroke*. A TIA is a brief disturbance of the blood supply. Symptoms resolve once blood supply returns. There is no tissue necrosis (infarction). A patient can also experience a silent stroke where there are no outward symptoms of a stroke. A silent stroke causes lesions on the brain, which are identified using an MRI. An acute stroke occurs when the patient suddenly shows signs of a stroke. It is critical that the patient receives treatment immediately in order to minimize the effect of the stroke and reduce tissue necrosis. There are two prehospital stroke assessments.

The ED staff must be alert for the following signs:

- Weakness in the face, arm, or leg, typically on one side of the body.
- Confusion.
- Difficulty speaking.
- Difficulty understanding.
- Vision problems.
- Dizziness.
- Coordination problems.
- Severe headache from unknown cause.

Assess the patient using the Cincinnati Pre-Hospital Stroke Scale (CPSS) (Table 10–10) and the Los Angeles Pre-Hospital Stroke Scale (LAPSS) (Table 10–11).

ED treatment is to follow the algorithm (Table 10–12) recommended by the American Heart Association to treat an acute stroke.

| TABLE 10–10 Cincinnati Pre-Hospital Stroke Scale | | |
|---|---|---|
| **Three Signs Indicate an Acute Stroke** | | |
| Sign | Test | Positive Result |
| Facial droop | Patient shows teeth | One side of the patient's face doesn't move as well as other side of the face. |
| Arm drift | Extend both arms palms up for 10 s | One arm moves down. |
| Abnormal speech | The patient says, "you can't teach old dog new tricks." | The patient is unable to speak or words are slurred. |

**TABLE 10–11** Los Angeles Pre-Hospital Stroke Scale

| All Signs Present Indicate an Acute Stroke | |
|---|---|
| Category | Sign |
| Age | >45 y of age |
| History | No history of epilepsy or seizures. |
| Duration | Symptoms started within the past 24 h. |
| Ambulatory | Patient is not bedridden or in wheelchair. |
| Blood glucose | Between 60 and 400. |
| Face | Droop. |
| Grip | Weak or no grip. |
| Arms | Drift down. |

**TABLE 10–12** Stroke Algorithm

| Start | | |
|---|---|---|
| • Make sure airway, breathing, and circulation are patent. <br> • Assess vital signs. <br> • Administer oxygen. <br> • Open IV access. <br> • Gather blood samples. <br> • Assess blood glucose levels. <br> • Review patient's history. <br> • Determine when symptoms first presented. <br> • Administer an ECG. | | |
| Perform CT scan of the brain | | |
| No hemorrhage | | Hemorrhage |
| Assess if patient is a candidate for fibrinolytic therapy (see Fibrinolytic Therapy) | | • Consult neurologist/neurosurgeon |
| Yes | No | |
| • Administer tPA or appropriate fibrinolytic <br> • Do not administer anticoagulants or antiplatelet treatment for 24 h | • Administer low-dose aspirin <br> • Transfer to stroke unit for follow-up care | |

# Acute Coronary Syndrome

An acute coronary syndrome is reported by the patient as chest discomfort described as uncomfortable pressure that may have extended to the jaw, neck, between the shoulder blades, shoulders, and arms. The patient may experience shortness of breath, nausea, sweating, and light-headedness that may result in fainting. The acute coronary syndrome may or may not result in chest pain. Based on these signs and symptoms, the American Heart Association recommends treatment using the following algorithm (Table 10–13).

| TABLE 10–13   Responses to symptoms of stroke |
| --- |
| Start |
| • Monitor airway, breathing, and circulation. |
| • Monitor vital signs. |
| • Administer oxygen 4 L/min to maintain oxygen saturation level >90%. |
| • If the patient shows no evidence of recent GI bleed, then |
|   • If the patient does not have nausea, vomiting, or peptic ulcer, then administer aspirin 160-325 mg orally and ask the patient to chew the aspirin tablet to increase absorption time. |
|   • If the patient has nausea, vomiting, or peptic ulcer, then administer aspirin 160-325 mg rectally. |
| • If the patient is not hypotensive, bradycardic, or tachycardic and has not taken Viagra or Levitra within the past 24 h or Cialis within 48 h, and if the patient is hemodynamically stable, then administer nitroglycerin sublingually three doses each 3 min apart. |
| • If the patient is unresponsive to nitroglycerin, then administer morphine to reduce the left ventricular preload and cardiac oxygen requirements. |
| • Administer a 12-lead ECG. |
| • Open IV access. |
| • Administer IV fluids if patient is hypotensive. |
| • Perform fibrinolytic checklist (see Fibrinolytic Therapy). |
| • Draw blood sample for cardiac marker levels, electrolytes, and coagulation studies. |
| • Administer a chest X-ray within 30 min of the patient's arrival. |
| Review ECG |
| STEMI<br>or<br>LBBB |

*(Continued)*

**TABLE 10–13** Responses to symptoms of stroke (Continued)

### Administer

- Beta-adrenergic receptor blockers
- Plavix
- Heparin
- If more than 12 h from onset, then admit patient to the cardiac care unit.
- If 12 h or less from onset, then
  - Fibrinolytic therapy (within 30 min)
  - PCI to restore blood to the heart (within 90 min)
  - ACE inhibitors/ARB (within 24 h)
  - HMG CoA reductase inhibitor

### UA/NSTEMI

### Administer

- Nitroglycerin.
- Beta-adrenergic receptor blockers.
- Glycoprotein IIb/IIIa inhibitor.
- Plavix.
- Admit patient to the cardiac care unit.

### Normal ST or T waves

- If troponin is positive, then administer
  - Nitroglycerin
  - Beta-adrenergic receptor blockers
  - Glycoprotein IIb/IIIa inhibitor
  - Plavix
- If troponin is negative, then
  - If symptoms of ischemia or infarction persist, then
    - Continue ECG monitoring.
    - Admit patient to the cardiac care unit.
  - If no symptoms of ischemia or infarction, then discharge patient with appropriate follow-up care.

Abbreviations: ACE, angiotensin-converting enzyme; ARB, angiotensin receptor blocker; ECG, electrocardiograph; GI, gastrointestinal; LBBB, left bundle branch block; PCI, percutaneous coronary intervention; STEMI, ST elevation myocardial infarction; UA/NSTEMI, unstable angina non-ST elevation myocardial infarction.

# Cardiac Contusion

A cardiac contusion is a blunt trauma injury to the chest that results in bruising of the myocardium, typically the right ventricle.

The practitioner will likely order the following tests:

- **Echocardiograph:** To assess ejection fraction and ventricular viability.
- **Cardiac enzyme level:** To assess CK-MB levels and injury to cardiac muscle.
- **Cardiac troponin I levels:** To assess injury to cardiac muscle.
- **ECG:** To assess cardiac rhythm.

The ED staff must be alert for the following signs:

- **Precordial chest pain:** Due to bruising
- **Bruising around the sternum:** Due to blunt trauma
- **Shortness of breath:** Due to cardiac irritability
- **Cardiac arrhythmias:** Due to cardiac irritability
- **Bradycardia:** Due to cardiac irritability
- **Tachycardia:** Due to cardiac irritability
- **Murmurs:** Due to cardiac irritability
- **Hemodynamic Instability:** Due to cardiac irritability

ED treatment is

- IV fluids to provide hemodynamic stability (systolic BP above 90 mm Hg).
- Digoxin for signs of cardiac failure.
- Lidocaine for ventricular arrhythmias.
- Inotropic medication to increase cardiac output.
- Oxygen.
- Assess vital signs each hour until patient is stable looking for decreased peripheral tissue perfusion.
- Assess respiration looking for signs of congestion.
- Assess urine output (1 mL/kg/h).
- Raise head of bed 30°.

## CASE STUDY

### CASE 1

A 66-year-old man is taken by ambulance to the ED and is bradycardic with a SBP of 94. You realize that the patient is in crisis. Using ACLS, answer the following questions with your best response.

QUESTION 1. What is your next decision?
ANSWER: Determine if the patient is asymptomatic or has symptoms.

QUESTION 2. What would you do if the patient becomes unresponsive?
ANSWER: Monitor the patient with a 12-lead ECG, call for the code team, and prepare to administer atropine 0.5 mg rapid IV push.

QUESTION 3. The patient's SBP is now 85. What would you do?
ANSWER: The patient has become unstable. Prepare to administer epinephrine 2 to 10 µg/min drip or dopamine 2 to 10 µg/kg/min drip or atropine 0.5 mg rapid IV push depending on what the practitioner orders.

QUESTION 4. The patient becomes responsive. SBP returns to 94. The patient asks what happened. What do you do next?
ANSWER: Monitor the patient and transport the patient to the cardiac care unit.

## FINAL CHECKUP

1. **A 32-year-old man presents in the ED in respiratory distress. A staff member says, "Start CPR." What is your best response?**

   A. Start CPR.
   B. Ask the patient to lay flat on a hard surface.
   C. Begin rescue breathing.
   D. Bring the crash cart.

2. **A 53-year-old woman is brought in by ambulance to the ED following an episode of dehydration and fever. Her husband asks, "Will the practitioner fix what is wrong with her?" What is your best response?**

   A. The practitioner will do her best.
   B. The practitioner will stabilize her and then discharge her to the next appropriate level of care.
   C. The practitioner will treat her and then ask that she visits her primary practitioner tomorrow.
   D. She must be admitted to the hospital.

3. **A 48-year-old woman reported chest pains. The practitioner ordered a cardiac marker test. The patient asks you to describe why the test was ordered. Which is your best response?**

   A. Cardiac marker tests determine if cardiac muscle enzymes appear in your blood.

   B. Cardiac marker tests determine if cardiac muscle enzymes appear in your heart.

   C. Cardiac marker tests determine if cardiac muscle enzymes appear in your muscles.

   D. Cardiac marker tests determine if cardiac muscle enzymes appear anywhere in your body.

4. **An 80-year-old woman arrived in the ED with very high BP. The practitioner ordered the renin assay test. The patient asks why the test was ordered. What is your best response?**

   A. The kidneys cause secretion of the renin enzyme when BP is low. The renin enzyme constricts blood vessels and results in increased BP. The practitioner is determining if renin enzyme level is the cause of your high BP.

   B. The kidneys cause secretion of the renin enzyme when BP is high. The renin enzyme constricts blood vessels and results in decreased BP. The practitioner is determining if renin enzyme level is the cause of your high BP.

   C. The liver causes secretion of the renin enzyme when BP is low. The renin enzyme constricts blood vessels and results in increased BP. The practitioner is determining if renin enzyme level is the cause of your high BP.

   D. The kidneys cause secretion of the aldosterone enzyme when BP is low. The renin enzyme constricts blood vessels and results in increased BP. The practitioner is determining if renin enzyme level is the cause of your high BP.

5. **A 45-year-old patient was told that he has atrial fibrillation and the practitioner wants to perform a cardioversion. He asks you to explain this procedure. What is your best response?**

   A. Cardioversion is a nonsurgical procedure that uses a low energy level shock that is administered and is synchronized with the patient's heart cycle, causing interruption of the reentry circuit and enabling control to resume by the AV node.

   B. Cardioversion is a surgical procedure that uses a low energy level shock that is administered and is synchronized with the patient's heart cycle, causing interruption of the reentry circuit and enabling control to resume by the SA node.

   C. Cardioversion is a nonsurgical procedure that uses a low energy level shock that is administered and is synchronized with the patient's heart cycle, causing interruption of the reentry circuit and enabling control to resume by the SA node.

   D. Cardioversion is a nonsurgical procedure that uses a low energy level shock to let your heart restore a normal heart rhythm. You'll be asleep during this procedure.

6. **A 42-year-old man was diagnosed with angina. He asks you why the practitioner ordered him to take nitroglycerin. What is your best response?**

   A. Nitroglycerin tightens smooth muscle around coronary arteries, increasing the flow of oxygenated blood to the heart and decreasing chest pain.

   B. Nitroglycerin relaxes smooth muscle around coronary arteries, increasing the flow of oxygenated blood to the heart and decreasing chest pain.

   C. Nitroglycerin relaxes smooth muscle around coronary arteries, decreasing the flow of oxygenated blood to the heart and decreasing chest pain.

   D. Nitroglycerin relaxes smooth muscle around coronary arteries, increasing the flow of deoxygenated blood to the heart and decreasing chest pain.

7. **A 54-year-old man is concerned that the practitioner ordered lidocaine for his irregular heartbeat. He said he received lidocaine as an anesthetic when he received stitches years ago. What is your best response?**

   A. Tell the patient that you will double-check the order with the practitioner.

   B. Tell him that he received Xylocaine for the stitches.

   C. Tell him that lidocaine also decreases the time between contractions of the heart and may restore a normal heart rhythm.

   D. Tell him that lidocaine also increases the time between contractions of the heart and may restore a normal heart rhythm.

8. **A 54-year-old woman, who is a nurse, was brought to the ED with chest pains. A 12-lead ECG is used to monitor her. She asks you if the ST segment is elevated. Why is she asking this question?**

   A. Elevated ST segment indicates severe damage to the heart.

   B. Elevated ST segment indicates mild damage to the heart.

   C. Elevated ST segment indicates minor damage to the heart.

   D. Elevated ST segment indicates no damage to the heart.

9. **A 55-year-old man was brought into the ED with hypotension, difficulty breathing, muffled heart sounds, and sweating. The practitioner tells you to prepare for a pericardiocentesis. What is the patient's likely diagnosis?**

   A. Chronic angina

   B. Acute angina

   C. Congestive heart failure

   D. Cardiac tamponade

10. **A 41-year-old man came to the ED in hypertensive crisis. What is your immediate objective?**

    A. Complete the registration process quickly.

    B. Call the rapid response team.

    C. Get the crash cart and prepare for a cardiac arrest.

    D. Lower the patient's BP.

# CORRECT ANSWERS AND RATIONALES

1. C. Begin rescue breathing.
2. B. The practitioner will stabilize her and then discharge her to the next appropriate level of care.
3. A. Cardiac marker tests determine if cardiac muscle enzymes appear in your blood.
4. A. The kidneys cause secretion of the renin enzyme when BP is low. The renin enzyme constricts blood vessels and results in increased BP. The practitioner is determining if renin enzyme level is the cause of your high BP.
5. D. Cardioversion is a nonsurgical procedure that uses a low energy level shock to let your heart restore a normal heart rhythm. You'll be asleep during this procedure.
6. B. Nitroglycerin relaxes smooth muscle around coronary arteries, increasing the flow of oxygenated blood to the heart and decreasing chest pain.
7. C. Tell him that lidocaine also decreases the time between contractions of the heart and may restore a normal heart rhythm.
8. A. Elevated ST segment indicates severe damage to the heart.
9. D. Cardiac tamponade.
10. D. Lower the patient's BP.

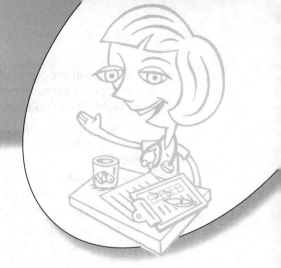

# *Final Exam*

1. **A 59-year-old woman was admitted to the unit for symptoms of lethargy, confusion, weakness, and swelling. The practitioner suspects an electrolyte imbalance but orders a renal panel. Why would a renal panel be ordered?**

   A.  These tests are to determine how well the patient urinates.

   B.  The practitioner must know if kidneys are functioning before ordering medication to treat the patient's condition.

   C.  The levels of electrolytes are maintained by the kidneys.

   D.  The practitioners want to know if the patient has an electrolyte imbalance.

2. **You notice Osler's nodes when assessing a new patient. Should you be concerned?**

   A.  Yes. A stroke or heart attack is imminent.

   B.  Yes. The patient requires a workup for endocarditis.

   C.  Yes. The patient requires a workup for myocarditis.

   D.  Yes. The patient requires a workup for pericarditis.

3. **A 48-year-old man diagnosed with multiple myeloma researched on the Internet that multiple myeloma doesn't affect white blood cells (WBCs). He questions why he was told that his immune system is weakened. What is your best response?**

   A. Multiple myeloma is a malignancy of WBCs. WBCs create antibodies that fight invading microorganisms such as bacteria. There are decreased antibodies in your blood.

   B. Multiple myeloma is a malignancy of plasma cells. Plasma cells create antibodies that fight invading microorganisms such as bacteria. There are decreased antibodies in your blood.

   C. Multiple myeloma is a malignancy of red blood cells (RBCs). RBCs create antibodies that fight invading microorganisms such as bacteria. There are decreased antibodies in your blood.

   D. Plasma makes antibodies.

4. **A 38-year-old woman has neck vein distention, is restless and sweating, has and difficulty breathing during your assessment in the emergency department. Her systolic pressure dropped greater than 10 mm Hg during inspiration. What do you suspect is happening?**

   A. Cardiac tamponade

   B. Pulsus paradoxus

   C. Acute myocardial infarction

   D. Acute heart failure

5. **Which of the follow is the more serious conduction of a premature heartbeat according to the Lown Grading System?**

   A. Grade 5

   B. Grade 4

   C. Grade 7

   D. Grade 6

6. **A patient diagnosed with myocarditis experiences arrhythmia. Why does this occur?**

   A. Angiotensin-converting enzyme (ACE) inhibitors prescribed to treat myocarditis may cause arrhythmia.

   B. Rubbing of layers of the myocardium causes extra impulses that contract the heart.

   C. Rubbing of layers of the myocardium causes extra irritation that contracts the heart.

   D. Inflammation disrupts the conduction paths in the heart.

7. **A 34-year-old man who travels by air many hours every week reports swelling of the lower right leg. The right leg is warm to the touch. What is your best response?**

   A. Lay down and bend your left foot toward your face.

   B. Call 911.

C. Lay down and bend your right foot toward your face.

D. Tell him not to move and call 911.

8. **A 62-year-old woman is to undergo emergency coronary artery bypass grafting (CABG) and asks you to explain the procedure. What is your best response?**

A. This is a nonsurgical procedure in which a long tube with a small balloon is passed through blood vessels into the narrowed artery. The balloon is inflated, causing the artery to expand.

B. This is a small, stainless steel mesh tube that is placed within the coronary artery to keep it open.

C. This is a nonsurgical procedure in which a vein from a leg or an artery from an arm or the chest is removed and grafted to coronary arteries, bypassing the blockage and restoring free flow of blood to heart muscles.

D. This is a surgical procedure in which a vein from a leg or an artery from an arm or the chest is removed and grafted to coronary arteries, bypassing the blockage and restoring free flow of blood to heart muscles.

9. **A 32-year-old man who was diagnosed with deep vein thrombosis (DVT) following a round the world flight, which he takes frequently, asks why he developed a DVT. What is your best response?**

A. The clot occurred because you played football in college and were repeatedly tackled.

B. You smoked two packs of cigarettes a day for the past year.

C. It was likely caused by your immobility during your very long flight.

D. You should start taking shorter flights.

10. **A 22-year-old woman presents in respiratory distress. What is your best response?**

A. Begin rescue breathing.

B. Start cardiopulmonary resuscitation (CPR).

C. Ask the patient to lay flat on a hard surface.

D. Bring the crash cart.

11. **A 45-year-old woman diagnosed with mitral valve stenosis understands that if symptoms do not improve she will undergo a commissurotomy. What is a commissurotomy?**

A. Commissurotomy is an open-heart surgery during which the mitral valve is cleared of scar tissue or calcium deposits, increasing blood flow through the mitral valve.

B. Commissurotomy is a nonsurgical procedure during which the mitral valve is cleared of scar tissue, increasing blood flow through the mitral valve.

C. Commissurotomy is a nonsurgical procedure during which the mitral valve is cleared of calcium deposits, increasing blood flow through the mitral valve.

D. Commissurotomy is an open-heart surgery during which the ring around the mitral valve is replaced.

12. **What is measured by the PR interval?**

    A. The time the electrical impulse takes to travel to the atria after ventricular repolarization.
    B. The time the electrical impulse takes to travel from the left atrium to the right atrium.
    C. The time the electrical impulse takes to travel to the ventricles after atrial repolarization.
    D. The time the electrical impulse takes to travel from the right atrium to the left atrium.

13. **A 4-year-old girl is seen with her legs drawn up near her chest and she sobs constantly and is not speaking. Which is your best assessment of the patient?**

    A. The patient is experiencing a pain rating of 2 on the FLACC Pain Scale.
    B. The patient is looking for attention.
    C. The patient is experiencing discomfort associated with a gastrointestinal (GI) disorder.
    D. The patient is experiencing a pain rating of 2 on the Wong-Baker Pain Scale.

14. **Is the absence of a U wave significant?**

    A. Artifact
    B. No
    C. Loose electrode lead
    D. Fast heart rate

15. **What causes constriction in constrictive pericarditis?**

    A. Coronary blood vessels narrow because of plaque.
    B. Tissues in the pericardium can become damaged from chronic pericarditis, resulting in scar tissues replacing tissues in the pericardium.
    C. Coronary blood vessels narrow because of a clot.
    D. The pericardium loses lubrication.

16. **A 56-year-old man presents with very high blood pressure (BP). A renin assay test is ordered and the patient asks why the test was ordered. What is your best response?**

    A. The kidneys cause secretion of the renin enzyme when BP is high. The renin enzyme constricts blood vessels and results in decreased BP. The practitioner is determining if renin enzyme level is the cause of your high BP.
    B. The liver causes secretion of the renin enzyme when BP is low. The renin enzyme constricts blood vessels and results in increased BP. The practitioner is determining if renin enzyme level is the cause of your high BP.
    C. The kidneys cause secretion of the aldosterone enzyme when BP is low. The renin enzyme constricts blood vessels and results in increased BP. The practitioner is determining if renin enzyme level is the cause of your high BP.

D. The kidneys cause secretion of the renin enzyme when BP is low. The renin enzyme constricts blood vessels and results in increased BP. The practitioner is determining if renin enzyme level is the cause of your high BP.

17. **A 73-year-old man recently diagnosed with leukemia asks you what is happening with him. What is the best response?**

    A. Abnormal and immature WBCs enter the circulatory system and do not function properly, increasing the risk to other disorders.

    B. There is an unregulated proliferation of immature RBCs that do not function properly.

    C. Leukemia is a form of cancer.

    D. This is a blood condition that makes you susceptible to infection.

18. **Why is Lopressor prescribed for a patient diagnosed with myocarditis?**

    A. Lopressor is an ACE inhibitor that prevents blood vessels from narrowing.

    B. Lopressor reduces fluid retention.

    C. Lopressor is a beta-blocker that slows the contractions of the ventricles.

    D. Lopressor increases BP.

19. **What is the rationale for palpating the dorsalis pedis?**

    A. The dorsalis pedis is located at the upper thigh and is the farthest peripheral artery from the heart. You are assured that the patient's legs are receiving sufficient arterial blood flow if the dorsalis pedis can be palpated.

    B. The dorsalis pedis is located at the back of the knee and is the farthest peripheral artery from the heart. You are assured that the patient's legs are receiving sufficient arterial blood flow if the dorsalis pedis can be palpated.

    C. The dorsalis pedis is located at the top of the foot and is the farthest peripheral artery from the heart. You are assured that the patient's legs are receiving sufficient arterial blood flow if the dorsalis pedis can be palpated.

    D. The dorsalis pedis is located at the top of the foot and is the farthest peripheral artery from the heart.

20. **A 44-year-old man is being treated for ventricular fibrillation. As his primary nurse, the patient tells you that his primary practitioner told him to take himself to the hospital any time he had symptoms. What is the best response?**

    A. Ask the patient if he was prescribed warfarin and the last time he had a prothrombin time/international normalized ratio (PT/INR) performed.

    B. Immediately place the patient on a heart monitor and begin intravenous (IV) administration of lidocaine.

    C. Prepare to give amiodarone 300 mg intravenously.

    D. Rush the patient into the emergency department (ED) and get the crash cart.

21. **A 46-year-old woman diagnosed with an aneurysm says that she feels fine and questiones the diagnosis. What is your best response?**

    A. It is best to speak with the practitioner about your concerns.
    B. You are lucky they caught it in time because you can die from an aneurysm.
    C. Aneurysms are common. You shouldn't be concerned unless you experience symptoms.
    D. Some patients have aneurysms for months before a diagnosis is made because they don't have any symptoms.

22. **A 76-year-old woman must undergo an embolectomy and asks you to explain this procedure. What is your best response?**

    A. Embolectomy is the surgical removal of a blood clot from the affected artery.
    B. A catheter containing a grinding tool is inserted into the affected artery and is used to grind plaque from the artery wall.
    C. A metal mesh tube is inserted into the affected artery to keep the artery open.
    D. A vessel from another part of the body is removed and grafted to the affected artery, permitting blood to bypass the blockage.

23. **A 36-year-old man who is having chest pains is ordered a cardiac marker test and asks you to describe the test. Which is your best response?**

    A. Cardiac marker tests determine if cardiac muscle enzymes appear in your heart.
    B. Cardiac marker tests determine if cardiac muscle enzymes appear in your muscles.
    C. Cardiac marker tests determine if cardiac muscle enzymes appear in your blood.
    D. Cardiac marker tests determine if cardiac muscle enzymes appear anywhere in your body.

24. **A 42-year-old man tells you that his B-type natriuretic peptide (BNP) was elevated. He asks whether he should be concerned. What is your best response?**

    A. BNP is secreted by ventricles of your heart when the ventricles are excessively stretched. Elevated BNP may indicate heart failure with symptoms indicating a condition other than heart failure.
    B. It is best to ask your practitioner that question.
    C. BNP is an electrolyte found inside cells. Elevation of BNP may indicate increased cell necrosis.
    D. BNP is secreted by ventricles of your heart when the ventricles are excessively stretched. Elevated BNP may indicate heart failure.

25. **A 41-year-old man was brought to the ED bleeding from an open wound on his arm. The front of his clothes is covered in blood; vital signs are stable. What infusion will the practitioner order next?**

    A. No fluid replacement. Treat the wound and monitor the patient. The patient has a class I hemorrhage.
    B. Normal saline IV because the patient has a class III hemorrhage.

C. Blood transfusion because the patient has a class II hemorrhage.

D. Blood transfusion and lactated Ringer solution because the patient has a class III hemorrhage.

26. **Is paroxysmal atrial tachycardia life-threatening for some patients diagnosed with Wolff-Parkinson-White syndrome?**

A. Yes. The heart rate decreases to critical levels.

B. Yes. The pacemaker wanders around the atria.

C. Yes. The pacemaker wanders around the ventricles.

D. Yes. Wolff-Parkinson-White syndrome is a heart disorder where there is an abnormal extra electrical pathway in the heart.

27. **A patient diagnosed with pericarditis reports sharp, cutting pain over the chest. What causes the pain?**

A. The pain is due to layers of the pericardium rubbing against each other.

B. The patient is experiencing a heart attack.

C. This is a side effect of the medication prescribed to treat pericarditis.

D. The pain is due to layers of the pericardium rubbing against the heart.

28. **A 53-year-old man diagnosed with mitral valve regurgitation (MVR) is always fatigued. He asks why this is happening. What is your best response?**

A. MVR disrupts normal blood flow, resulting in decreased circulation of oxygenated blood, which can make you feel tired.

B. MVR disrupts normal blood flow, resulting in increasing circulation of oxygenated blood, which can make you feel tired.

C. MVR disrupts normal blood flow, resulting in decreased circulation of carbon dioxide in the blood, which can make you feel tired.

D. Your fatigue is a side effect of warfarin, which is prescribed for MVR.

29. **A 23-year-old man was taken to the ED with multiple internal injuries following a motor vehicle accident. Which of the following conditions needs to be ruled out?**

A. Hypovolemic shock

B. Raynaud disease

C. Coronary artery disease

D. Atherosclerosis

30. **A 49-year-old man has atrial fibrillation and needs to undergo cardioversion. He asks you to explain this procedure. What is your best response?**

A. Cardioversion is a nonsurgical procedure that uses a low energy level shock that is administered and synchronized with the patient's heart cycle, causing interruption of the reentry circuit and enabling control to resume by the atrioventricular (AV) node.

B. Cardioversion is a nonsurgical procedure that uses a low energy level shock to let your heart restore a normal heart rhythm. You'll be asleep during this procedure.

C. Cardioversion is a surgical procedure that uses a low energy level shock that is administered and synchronized with the patient's heart cycle, causing interruption of the reentry circuit and enabling control to resume by the sino-atrial (SA) node.

D. Cardioversion is a nonsurgical procedure that uses a low energy level shock that is administered and synchronized with the patient's heart cycle, causing interruption of the reentry circuit and enabling control to resume by the SA node.

31. **A 46-year-old woman who is diagnosed with leukemia tells you that she has too many RBCs. What is your best response?**

A. You have a mix of abnormal RBCs, immature RBCs, and mature RBCs (good RBCs). However, there are more abnormal and immature RBCs than there are normal RBCs.

B. A bone marrow transplant will fix this problem.

C. You have a mix of abnormal WBCs, immature WBCs, and mature WBCs (good WBCs). However, there are more abnormal and immature WBCs than there are normal WBCs.

D. Let's focus on finding a bone marrow match for you.

32. **What is measured by the ST segment?**

A. Isoelectric line artifact

B. The time between the end of ventricular depolarization and ventricular repolarization

C. Atrial repolarization

D. The time between the end of ventricular repolarization and ventricular depolarization

33. **A 36-year-old woman reported being tired recently and unable to get up from bed. She tells you that her practitioner said her RBC count is low. The patient asks you what is happening to her. What is your best response?**

A. You have anemia. There aren't sufficient RBCs to carry oxygen throughout your body.

B. You need to eat more green leafy food.

C. You must take an iron supplement so your body can create more RBCs.

D. You need a $B_{12}$ injection.

34. **A 46-year-old man tells you he has a strange heartbeat. His practitioner told him he has sick sinus syndrome. What is sick sinus syndrome?**

A. Sick sinus syndrome is the decrease in the heart rate due to increased pressure in the sinus cavity.

B. Sick sinus syndrome is a condition that prevents the patient from performing the Valsalva maneuver.

C. Sick sinus syndrome is a malfunction of the AV node.

D. Sick sinus syndrome is a malfunction of the SA node.

35. **A patient diagnosed with disseminated intravascular coagulation (DIC) asks what is happening to her body. What is your best response?**

    A. Proteins involved in blood clotting become overactive resulting in excessive blood coagulation and leading to the depletion of platelets.

    B. You are at risk for microthrombi.

    C. This is not a serious condition. Your body is missing an element that you can obtain from the pharmacy.

    D. There is a depletion of platelets preventing your body from coagulating blood, leading to hemorrhaging.

36. **A 52-year-old man diagnosed with pulmonary edema asks you to describe this condition. What is your best response?**

    A. Fluid builds up in the legs due to ineffective pumping of blood by the heart.

    B. Fluid builds up around the heart due to ineffective pumping of blood by the heart.

    C. Fluid builds up in the lungs due to ineffective pumping of blood by the heart.

    D. Fluid builds up in the lungs due to effective pumping of blood by the heart.

37. **A 47-year-old man is in hypertensive crisis. What is your immediate objective?**

    A. Complete the registration process quickly.

    B. Lower the patient's BP.

    C. Call the rapid response team.

    D. Get the crash cart and prepare for a cardiac arrest.

38. **A 28-year-old man created a 12-day log of his BP. All were within normal range. During his routine physical, his BP is high in both arms using both the automatic and manual BP machines. He asks what is happening. What is your best response?**

    A. You might have "white coat syndrome." Your BP increases

    B. BP taken at home is a better measurement than if taken in the practitioner's office.

    C. The practitioner may ask to you come to the office once a week to monitor your BP.

    D. Three BP readings taken in the office are necessary to determine a diagnosis of hypertension (HTN).

39. **If more than one cardiac rhythm appears on the same strip, what would you do?**

    A. Repeat the electrocardiogram (ECG).

    B. Reposition all leads.

    C. Analyze the first cardiac rhythm.

    D. Analyze each cardiac rhythm.

40. A 46-year-old man diagnosed with tricuspid valve stenosis asks you why he is prescribed treatment but no treatment was given to his friend who has the same diagnosis. What is your best response?

    A. Your friend probably was diagnosed with mitral valve stenosis.

    B. You friend likely had a different diagnosis.

    C. Some practitioners prefer to monitor the patient regularly without prescribing treatment.

    D. Some patients diagnosed with tricuspid valve stenosis don't have any symptoms, and therefore, the practitioner monitors the patient regularly without prescribing treatment.

41. A 60-year-old woman is considering percutaneous transluminal coronary angioplasty and asks you to describe that procedure. What is the best response?

    A. This is a nonsurgical procedure that uses X-rays to expand narrowed arteries.

    B. This is a nonsurgical procedure in which a long tube is passed through the urethra into the narrowed artery. The balloon is inflated, causing the artery to expand.

    C. This is a nonsurgical procedure in which a long tube with a small balloon is passed through blood vessels into the narrowed artery. The balloon is inflated, causing the artery to expand.

    D. This is a surgical procedure in which a long tube with a small balloon is passed through blood vessels into the narrowed artery. The balloon is inflated, causing the artery to expand.

42. A 48-year-old woman diagnosed with angina asks you why she must take nitroglycerin. What is your best response?

    A. Nitroglycerin tightens smooth muscle around coronary arteries, increasing the flow of oxygenated blood to the heart and decreasing chest pain.

    B. Nitroglycerin relaxes smooth muscle around coronary arteries, decreasing the flow of oxygenated blood to the heart and decreasing chest pain.

    C. Nitroglycerin relaxes smooth muscle around coronary arteries, increasing the flow of deoxygenated blood to the heart and decreasing chest pain.

    D. Nitroglycerin relaxes smooth muscle around coronary arteries, increasing the flow of oxygenated blood to the heart and decreasing chest pain.

43. A 43-year-old woman reports chest pains at night when resting and asks you what might be going on. What is your best response?

    A. You might have vasospastic angina.

    B. Speak with your practitioner.

    C. I'm not permitted to answer your question.

    D. You might have vasospastic angina. Let's speak with your practitioner.

44. **An 11-year-old boy has an episode of sickle cell anemia and asks why you are administering morphine. What is your best response?**

    A. Morphine will ease the pain experienced in severe episodes of sickle cell anemia.

    B. Morphine will prevent the cells from becoming stiff and sticky.

    C. Morphine prevents cells from clumping together.

    D. Morphine dilates smaller vessels allowing cells to pass easily.

45. **The practitioner tells a 56-year-old man that he should be monitored by a Swan Ganz catheter. He asks you about the procedure. Which is your best response?**

    A. Swan Ganz catheter is a catheter placed into the lungs to check for pressures in the heart, vessels, and lungs.

    B. Swan Ganz catheter is a catheter placed into the lungs to check for pressures in the lungs.

    C. Swan Ganz catheter is a catheter placed into the heart to check for pressures in the heart.

    D. Swan Ganz catheter is a catheter placed into the pulmonary artery to check for pressures in the heart, vessels, and lungs.

46. **A 59-year-old man asks why lidocaine is given for his irregular heartbeat since lidocaine is a local anesthetic. What is your best response?**

    A. Tell him that lidocaine also decreases the time between contractions of the heart and may restore a normal heart rhythm.

    B. Tell the patient that you will double-check the order with the practitioner.

    C. Tell him that he received Xylocaine for the stitches.

    D. Tell him that lidocaine also increases the time between contractions of the heart and may restore a normal heart rhythm.

47. **A 42-year-old female patient tells you that her good cholesterol is high and her bad cholesterol is low. What is mistaken about the patient's statement?**

    A. There is no such thing as high or low cholesterol.

    B. Low-density lipoprotein (LDL) is commonly referred to as *good cholesterol* and high-density lipoprotein (HDL) as *bad cholesterol*.

    C. The patient is on statin therapy, which alters the real state of her cholesterol levels.

    D. HDL is commonly referred to as *good cholesterol* and LDL as *bad cholesterol*. These are not cholesterols. HDL and LDL are proteins that carry cholesterol to and from organs and tissues.

48. **What is the first step before administering an ECG?**

    A. Zeroing the ECG.

    B. Measuring the height of the isoelectric line with either calipers or index card.

    C. Zeroing the ECG to the normal wave form.

    D. Measuring the wave tracing using the ECG graph.

49. **A 60-year-old man with an irregular heartbeat is told that he should undergo catheter ablation. He asks about this procedure. What is the best response?**

    A. Catheter ablation is a procedure where tissues of the heart that cause the extra impulses are destroyed by radiofrequency energy applied to the area by a catheter that the practitioner inserts into a blood vessel. In some cases, the practitioner ablates the AV node to prevent impulses from the atria from reaching the ventricles. The patient then requires a permanent pacemaker to maintain ventricle contractions.

    B. Catheter ablation is a procedure that delivers an electrical shock through electrodes placed on the patient's chest. The shock stops the heart for a fraction of a second. The SA node then automatically starts sending normal impulses throughout the heart. The patient is anesthetized during the procedure.

    C. Catheter ablation is a procedure that creates an ectopic pacemaker.

    D. Catheter ablation is an open-heart surgery during which part of the heart is removed and replaced with an internal pacemaker.

50. **Is a patient diagnosed with myocarditis at risk for heart failure?**

    A. Yes. Inflammation of the outer layer of the heart reduces the ability of the heart to contract, preventing the heart from efficiently pumping blood.

    B. Yes. Inflammation causes layers of the myocardium to rub together, decreasing the pumping action of the heart.

    C. Yes. Heart failure is a possible side effect of beta-blockers but has a lower probability of occurrence.

    D. Yes. Myocarditis can weaken the heart, preventing the heart from efficiently pumping blood throughout the body.

51. **A 48-year-old man has an episode of dehydration and fever. His wife tells you, "to fix what is wrong with him so they can continue to the party." What is your best response?**

    A. The practitioner will do her best.

    B. The practitioner will treat him and then ask that he visits his primary practitioner tomorrow.

    C. The practitioner will stabilize him and then discharge him to the next appropriate level of care.

    D. He must be admitted to the hospital.

52. **A 48-year-old woman must undergo laser angioplasty and doesn't understand the procedure. What is your best response?**

    A. A laser-tipped catheter is used to correct your eyesight so you no longer require corrective glasses.

    B. A laser-tipped catheter is inserted into the affected artery to remove the blockage.

C. A laser-tipped catheter is inserted into the affected artery and a balloon is inflated to remove the blockage.

D. A laser-tipped catheter is inserted into the affected artery to install a stent.

53. **A 45-year-old patient was admitted to your unit with 103°F temperature. The practitioner ordered a complete blood count (CBC) test. She calls you asking for the WBC count. You report 15,000 WBC. She then asks you about the number of bands. What is the rationale for asking that question?**

A. Increased band formation indicates a viral infection.

B. Bands are immature lymphocytes and are present when there is a bacterial or viral infection.

C. Bands are immature neutrophils that increase when there is a bacterial infection.

D. The practitioner needs to identify the proper medication to prescribe.

54. **A 45-year-old male nurse with chest pains was placed on a 12-lead ECG and asks you if the ST segment is elevated. Why is he asking this question?**

A. Elevated ST segment indicates mild damage to the heart.

B. Elevated ST segment indicates minor damage to the heart.

C. Elevated ST segment indicates severe damage to the heart.

D. Elevated ST segment indicates no damage to the heart.

55. **A 47-year-old man diagnosed with CHF asks you if he is going to die. What is your best response?**

A. Long-term prognosis can be variable, depending on the severity of the disease and associated conditions.

B. Early treatment usually produces good results.

C. Early treatment usually produces good results. Long-term prognosis can be variable, depending on the severity of the disease and associated conditions. Your practitioner is the best person to speak about your prognosis.

D. Early treatment usually produces good results. Long-term prognosis can be variable, depending on the severity of the disease and associated conditions.

56. **A 43-year-old man diagnosed with thrombophlebitis asks how serious this condition is. What is the best response?**

A. You must avoid all movement until thrombophlebitis is resolved.

B. Prognosis is usually good unless embolization or moving of the clot occurs. It may move to the lung or brain, which can be life-threatening.

C. Prognosis is usually poor because a clot will move to the lung or brain, which can be life-threatening.

D. This is not serious as long as you take your medication.

57. **A patient diagnosed with polycythemia vera asks you about the importance of compliance with treatment. What is your best response?**

    A. You should always follow treatment prescribed by a practitioner.

    B. Following the prescribed treatment will eliminate your blurry vision and ringing in your ears.

    C. Your enlarged spleen will return to normal if you follow the treatment prescribed by the practitioner.

    D. If you follow the treatment prescribed by the practitioner, the average survival time is between 10 and 15 years. Without treatment, survival is less than 2 years.

58. **A 45-year-old man presents with hypotension, difficulty breathing, muffled heart sounds, and sweating. He is to undergo pericardiocentesis. What is the patient's likely diagnosis?**

    A. Chronic angina

    B. Acute angina

    C. Cardiac tamponade

    D. CHF

59. **A 48-year-old man has a suspected blockage in an artery and asks you how the practitioner will confirm that the blockage exists. What is your best response?**

    A. The practitioner will use the ankle-brachial index to confirm the blockage.

    B. The practitioner will perform exploratory surgery under a local anesthetic.

    C. The practitioner may use a Doppler ultrasonography to examine the affected area. If this test indicates there might be a blockage, the practitioner will likely order an arteriography where dye is injected into your arteries and an X-ray of your artery is taken.

    D. The practitioner will perform exploratory surgery under a general anesthetic.

60. **A 63-year-old woman diagnosed with mitral valve prolapse (MVP) asks why she should take antibiotics before every dental procedure. What is your best response?**

    A. Antibiotics lower the risk of a blood clot during the procedure.

    B. MVP puts the patient at risk for infective endocarditis. A dental procedure exposes the patient to bacteria and the antibiotics reduce the risk of infection, building the therapeutic level of antibiotics in the blood before the procedure.

    C. MVP puts the patient at risk for infective endocarditis.

    D. MVP puts the patient at risk for infective endocarditis, and the antibiotics reduce the risk by killing bacteria before the procedure.

61. **A 63-year-old man is diagnosed with premature atrial contraction (PAC). Why does the practitioner tell the patient to press his nostrils together and exhale through his nose?**

    A. This is the Valsalva maneuver used as a nonmedication treatment of PAC.

    B. This is the dive reflex used as a nonmedication treatment of PAC.

    C. This is the carotid sinus massage used as a nonmedication treatment of PAC.

    D. This treatment increases blood flow to the heart.

62. **A 54-year-old man who has smoked two packs of cigarettes per day for 20 years reports mild chest discomfort and is short of breath at times during the day. His practitioner ordered a chest X-ray to rule out a potential heart condition. The patient asks how a chest X-ray could determine the condition of his heart. What is your best response?**

    A. A chest X-ray is used to rule out lung disease.

    B. You should ask your practitioner to answer this question.

    C. A chest X-ray is used to detect the size of the heart.

    D. A chest X-ray shows contractions of your heart.

63. **A 56-year-old woman who has been abusing alcohol for 40 years has a low albumin level. She says, "So what else is new?" Should she be concerned?**

    A. Yes. Albumin controls hydrostatic pressure in blood vessels, which keeps blood from leaking out of blood vessels. A low level can lead to ascites.

    B. Yes. Albumin controls oncotic pressure in blood vessels, which keeps blood from leaking out of blood vessels. A low level can lead to atherosclerosis.

    C. No. A low level can lead to poor distribution of hormones and medications.

    D. Yes. A low level can lead to ascites. Albumin controls oncotic pressure in blood vessels, which keeps blood from leaking out of blood vessels.

64. **A 42-year-old woman tells you that she sleeps with four pillows at night and without a blanket during colder months. What is your best response?**

    A. Do you have difficulty breathing?

    B. Do you get cold when sleeping?

    C. Have you tried sleeping with three pillows?

    D. Are your legs swollen?

65. **A patient with a history of endocarditis asks why he is prescribed antibiotics before receiving dental treatment. What is the best rationale?**

    A. The patient may still have the bacteria that cause endocarditis, and the bacteria may be transmitted to the dentist.

    B. The bacteria are dormant and the procedure may reactivate the bacteria.

    C. The patient does not need to take antibiotics before receiving dental treatment.

    D. Bacteria in the mouth and gums could enter the bloodstream and infect the patient's heart.

66. After several episodes of bleeding, a 48-year-old patient diagnosed with idiopathic thrombocytopenic purpura (ITP) asks if he is dying. What is your best response?

    A. ITP is an autoimmune disorder in which antibodies to the patient's own platelets are developed.

    B. Medication can control the majority of cases of ITP. Remission is common.

    C. ITP is a chronic condition in adults and children, which develops after a viral infection.

    D. Avoid situations where injury might occur.

67. A 47-year-old woman asks why she shouldn't strain during a bowel movement. What is your best response?

    A. Straining during a bowel movement means that you are constipated.

    B. Straining during a bowel movement means that you are constipated. You should take a stool softener daily.

    C. Straining during a bowel movement increases pressure in the chest and slows return of blood to the heart.

    D. Straining during a bowel movement means that you are constipated. You shouldn't take a stool softener daily.

68. A 41-year-old patient diagnosed with primary HTN disorder asks you what caused his HTN. What is your best response?

    A. Primary HTN develops gradually over years without an identifiable cause.

    B. Diabetes.

    C. Kidney disease.

    D. Too much salt.

69. A 48-year-old woman diagnosed with DVT tells you she was told that she needs injections in the stomach daily. She asks why. What is your best response?

    A. You are injecting low-molecular-weight heparin, which will reduce formation of new blood clots.

    B. You are injecting low-molecular-weight heparin, which will dissolve the blood clot.

    C. The injections are subcutaneous injections. You should rotate the injection site with each injection.

    D. You are injecting low-molecular-weight heparin, which will prevent formation of new blood clots.

70. A 56-year-old diagnosed with pulmonary valve regurgitation reports periods of rapid breathing. The patient asks why this happens. What is your best response?

    A. There is a buildup of carbon dioxide in your blood because disruption in blood flow prevents the lung from oxygenating the blood. Your body compensates by breathing rapidly to quickly remove the excess carbon dioxide.

    B. You are experiencing respiratory acidosis.

C. There is a buildup of oxygen in your blood because disruption in blood flow prevents the lung from oxygenating the blood. Your body compensates by breathing rapidly to quickly remove the excess carbon dioxide.

D. There is a buildup of carbon dioxide in your blood because disruption in blood flow prevents the lung from oxygenating the blood. As a result, your body compensates by breathing rapidly to quickly remove the excess oxygen.

71. **Can endocarditis lead to a stroke?**

A. Yes. A patient diagnosed with endocarditis is not at risk for a stroke.

B. Yes. The use of IV street drugs can cause a stroke in a patient diagnosed with endocarditis.

C. Yes. The stroke is caused by constrictive endocarditis.

D. Yes. The microorganisms that clump together at a site in the heart can break loose and float in the bloodstream, possibly blocking a blood vessel and leading to tissue necrosis in the brain.

72. **What is the likely cause of a wandering isoelectric line on the ECG tracing?**

A. Respiration

B. First-degree heart block

C. Dried gel on the electrode

D. Second-degree heart block

73. **What is measured by the P wave?**

A. Atrial repolarization

B. Ventricle depolarization

C. Ventricle repolarization

D. Atrial depolarization

74. **A 37-year-old male patient reports pain in a small area of his chest. Vital signs are within normal range. What is your best response?**

A. Ask the patient what he was doing in the past 24 hours.

B. Ask the patient if he has a history of cardiovascular disease.

C. Ask the patient if he feels tightness around his chest.

D. Ask the practitioner if he/she wants to order stat ECG markers and place the patient on 100% oxygen immediately.

75. A 45-year-old man diagnosed with thrombocytopenia tells you that he is relieved because he thought he had too low of a platelet level and was at risk for bleeding. Should the patient feel relieved?

    A. No because thrombocytopenia is the medical term for low platelet level.
    B. Yes because having a low platelet count places the patient at risk for bruising and bleeding.
    C. No because the patient is at risk for blood clots.
    D. Yes because the practitioner has placed the patient on medication therapy for thrombocytopenia.

76. A 24-year-old man reports "a funny feeling in his chest occasionally"; however, his ECG is within normal range. Why did the practitioner order that the patient wear an event monitor?

    A. An event monitor is a wearable device that records your heart activity for up to 48 hours.
    B. An event monitor is a wearable device that records data only when a cardiac event occurs and will record your heart activity the next time you have a "funny feeling" in your chest.
    C. An event monitor is a wearable device that records data only when a cardiac event occurs and you can wear the event monitor for up to a month.
    D. An event monitor is a wearable device that records your heart activity.

77. Can digoxin toxicity cause accelerated junctional rhythm?

    A. Yes. Digoxin toxicity increases conduction through the AV node, resulting in the AV node assuming the role of the pacemaker
    B. Yes. Digoxin toxicity interferes with operations of the internal pacemaker.
    C. Yes. Digoxin toxicity slows conduction through the AV node, resulting in the AV node assuming the role of the pacemaker
    D. Yes. Digoxin toxicity stimulates the SA node.

78. Would a patient diagnosed with pericarditis experience swelling of the legs?

    A. Yes. Swelling is a sign that fluid is backed up in the lungs.
    B. Yes. Swelling is commonly seen in the legs and abdomen caused by pooling of blood due to decreased ability of the heart to pump blood.
    C. Yes. Fluid retained by the abdomen prevents the heart from contracting normally, resulting in decreased cardiac output.
    D. Yes. Swelling is due to fluid retention caused by Lasix, prescribed to increase cardiac output.

79. **A 53-year-old man diagnosed with mitral stenosis is concerned that after taking Lasix he will urinate. Why is he prescribed Lasix and why does he urinate?**

    A. Mitral stenosis disrupts blood flow to the right ventricle causing a buildup of fluid that leads to swelling. Lasix is a diuretic that causes the kidney to increase production of urine to reduce excess fluid, decreasing swelling.

    B. Mitral stenosis disrupts blood flow to the left ventricle causing a buildup of fluid that leads to swelling. Lasix is a beta-blocker that causes the kidney to increase production of urine to reduce excess fluid, decreasing swelling.

    C. Mitral stenosis disrupts blood flow to the left ventricle causing a buildup of fluid that leads to swelling. Lasix is a diuretic that causes the bladder to increase creation of urine to reduce excess fluid, decreasing swelling.

    D. Mitral stenosis disrupts blood flow to the left ventricle causing a buildup of fluid that leads to swelling. Lasix is a diuretic that causes the kidney to increase production of urine to reduce excess fluid, decreasing swelling.

80. **A 31-year-old woman diagnosed with pulmonary valve stenosis asks you how she caught the disease. What is the best response?**

    A. You likely caught pulmonary valve stenosis by not going to the practitioner the last time you had a throat infection.

    B. You can only catch pulmonary valve stenosis from rheumatic fever.

    C. The cause of pulmonary valve stenosis is unknown.

    D. The most common cause of pulmonary valve stenosis is congenital abnormal development of the pulmonary valve.

81. **A 59-year-old woman must weigh herself daily and call the practitioner immediately if there is a weight gain of 3 lb. She asks you why. What is your best response?**

    A. Weight gain is an early sign that you are retaining fluid.

    B. Weight gain may indicate that you are not adhering to your new diet.

    C. Weight gain may indicate that your new diet needs to be changed.

    D. Weight gain is an early sign that you are retaining fluid. Retaining fluid may indicate a problem with your heart that needs to be addressed immediately.

82. **A 23-year-old man arrives in the ED following a motor vehicle accident. BP is 70/50 with a pulse of 110 beats/min. What do you expect is happening?**

    A. Cardiac tamponade

    B. Pulmonary edema

    C. CHF

    D. Cardiogenic shock

83. **A 56-year-old man is diagnosed with tricuspid valve stenosis. He is told that he should undergo a valvuloplasty. He questions the procedure. What is your best response?**

    A. Valvuloplasty is a surgical procedure during which a balloon-tipped catheter is inserted into a blood vessel and then moved into the tricuspid valve where the balloon is inflated, opening the tricuspid valve.

    B. Valvuloplasty is a surgical procedure during which a balloon-tipped catheter is inserted into a blood vessel in your arm or groin and then moved into the tricuspid valve where the balloon is inflated, opening the tricuspid valve.

    C. Valvuloplasty is a nonsurgical procedure.

    D. Valvuloplasty is a surgical procedure during which a balloon-tipped catheter is inserted into a blood vessel in your arm or groin and then moved into the tricuspid valve where the catheter scrapes excess tissue around the tricuspid valve.

84. **A 76-year-old man diagnosed with hypertrophic cardiomyopathy (HCM) asks you to explain the disorder. What is your best response?**

    A. HCM occurs when the heart muscle becomes stiff and restricts blood from filling ventricles.

    B. HCM occurs when the heart muscle thins and enlarges.

    C. HCM occurs when the ventricular heart muscle thickens, resulting in outflow obstruction or restriction. There is some blood flow present.

    D. HCM occurs when the heart muscle thins and narrows.

85. **A 52-year-old man recently diagnosed with tricuspid valve regurgitation questions why you asked if he had an untreated throat infection. What is your best response?**

    A. An untreated bacterial throat infection can lead to complications for a patient who is diagnosed with tricuspid valve regurgitation.

    B. An untreated bacterial throat infection is always the cause of tricuspid valve regurgitation.

    C. An untreated bacterial throat infection can lead to infective endocarditis, which is an underlying cause of tricuspid valve regurgitation.

    D. The practitioner might have noticed signs of a throat infection during your physical assessment.

86. **Why is an intra-aortic balloon pump implanted in a patient diagnosed with myocarditis?**

    A. The balloon is inflated to block return blood flow.

    B. The balloon filters clots from the blood to prevent a stroke.

    C. A balloon is inserted into the aorta and is then inflated and deflated to increase blood flow throughout the body.

    D. A balloon is inserted into the aorta and is then inflated and deflated to decrease blood flow throughout the body.

87. **On an ECG, what is the difference between unifocal and multifocal premature ventricular contractions (PVCs)?**
    A. Each unifocal PVC looks the different. Each multifocal PVC looks the same.
    B. Each unifocal PVC has a different P wave. Each multifocal PVC has multiple P waves.
    C. There is no noticeable difference on the ECG.
    D. Each unifocal PVC looks the same. Each multifocal PVC looks different.

88. **A 58-year-old woman was brought to the ED complaining of lower jaw pain. Why would the practitioner order a myoglobin test?**
    A. Troponin elevates in blood after muscle injury, including a heart attack, sooner than myoglobin levels.
    B. Myoglobin returns to normal levels 24 hours after the muscle injury.
    C. Myoglobin elevates in blood after muscle injury, sooner than troponin level. This includes a heart attack.
    D. Troponin levels can remain elevated for up to 2 weeks following a heart attack.

89. **A 35-year-old man experienced severe bleeding. Why would the practitioner order an infusion of fresh frozen plasma?**
    A. Fresh frozen plasma causes vasoconstriction that narrows blood vessels, resulting in decreased bleeding.
    B. Plasma contains clotting factors.
    C. Fresh frozen plasma is composed mostly of clotting factors that will stop bleeding.
    D. The practitioner is replacing all the blood that the patient has lost.

90. **If after a short period of monitoring the ECG wave you notice a strangely abnormal cardiac waveform, what should you do first?**
    A. Call the practitioner.
    B. Call the rapid response team.
    C. Ask the patient to sip water.
    D. Assess the electrode connections to the patient.

91. **A 42-year-old man is concerned that he has rheumatic heard disease (RHD). What should you do?**
    A. Ask the patient if he ever had strep throat.
    B. Ask the patient if he ever had strep throat as a child.
    C. Ask the patient if he ever had rheumatic fever or scarlet fever as a child.
    D. Ask the patient if he has had strep throat recently.

92. **A 55-year-old woman diagnosed with mitral valve regurgitation is prescribed warfarin. She is concerned because she has no history of blood clots. What is your best response?**

    A. You should ask the practitioner. I'm not permitted to answer your question.

    B. Mitral valve regurgitation places you at risk for atrial fibrillation, which is an irregular contraction of the atria. As a result, there is a chance that blood might pool leading to blood clots.

    C. Mitral valve regurgitation places you at risk for atrial fibrillation, which is an irregular contraction of the ventricles. As a result, there is a chance that blood might pool leading to blood clots. Warfarin reduces the formation of blood clots.

    D. Mitral valve regurgitation places you at risk for atrial fibrillation, which is an irregular contraction of the atria. As a result, there is a chance that blood might pool leading to blood clots. Warfarin reduces the formation of blood clots.

93. **What does a notched QRS complex indicate?**

    A. First-degree heart block

    B. Bundle branch conduction

    C. Bundle branch block

    D. Atrial repolarization

94. **What is the rationale for comparing right and left peripheral arteries?**

    A. Corresponding peripheral arteries should have relatively the same contour and amplitude when palpated.

    B. You are able to detect any fistula.

    C. Comparing left and right corresponding peripheral arteries is an efficient way of assessing peripheral arteries.

    D. You are able to detect a shunt.

95. **Why is metoprolol prescribed for a patient diagnosed with paroxysmal junctional tachycardia?**

    A. Metoprolol is a beta-blocker that increases contraction of the ventricles.

    B. Metoprolol is a beta-blocker that slows the contractions of the ventricles.

    C. Metoprolol is a calcium channel blocker that slows contraction of the ventricles.

    D. Metoprolol is a calcium channel blocker that increases contraction of the ventricles.

96. **A 79-year-old man diagnosed with aplastic anemia asks you if this was acquired from drinking from plastic cups. What is your best response?**

    A. Drinking from plastic cups does not cause aplastic anemia.

    B. Aplastic means that a part of the body is failing to develop. Aplastic anemia occurs when bone marrow stops producing a sufficient amount of new RBCs.

    C. You can continue to use plastic cups. Plastic cups have no effect on your condition.

D. Aplastic means that a part of the body is failing to develop. Aplastic anemia occurs when bone marrow stops producing a sufficient amount of new WBCs.

97. **What cardiac monitor is used to monitor the heart over a short time period?**

    A. A 12-lead ECG
    B. Cardiac telemetry
    C. A 3-lead cardiac monitor
    D. An 8-lead cardiac monitor

98. **A 52-year-old patient with positive hepatojugular reflux asks you to explain this condition. What is your best response?**

    A. Positive hepatojugular reflux is distension of the neck veins precipitated by the maneuver of firm pressure over the liver by the practitioner.
    B. Positive hepatojugular reflux is distension of the gallbladder precipitated by the maneuver of firm pressure over the liver by the practitioner.
    C. Positive hepatojugular reflux is distension of the hepatic veins precipitated by the maneuver of firm pressure over the liver by the practitioner.
    D. Positive hepatojugular reflux is distension of the liver precipitated by the maneuver of firm pressure over the liver by the practitioner.

99. **A 51-year-old man presents to the ED with swelling in both legs. What question should you ask the patient?**

    A. Are you experiencing shortness of breath?
    B. Do you have dependent rubor?
    C. Do you abuse alcohol?
    D. Do you spend hours on your feet at work?

100. **What is the treatment for grade 1 PVC?**

    A. 24-hour monitoring in the cardiac care unit.
    B. Treat the underlying causes of the PVC.
    C. Administer lidocaine and amiodarone.
    D. No treatment.

## ANSWERS

1. C. The levels of electrolytes are maintained by the kidneys.
2. B. Yes. The patient requires a workup for endocarditis.
3. B. Multiple myeloma is a malignancy of plasma cells. Plasma cells create antibodies that fight invading microorganisms such as bacteria. There are decreased antibodies in your blood.
4. A. Cardiac tamponade.

5. A. Grade 5.

6. D. Inflammation disrupts the conduction paths in the heart.

7. C. Lay down and bend your right foot toward your face.

8. D. This is a surgical procedure in which a vein from a leg or an artery from an arm or the chest is removed and grafted to coronary arteries, bypassing the blockage and restoring free flow of blood to heart muscles.

9. C. It was likely caused by your immobility during your very long flight.

10. A. Begin rescue breathing.

11. A. Commissurotomy is an open-heart surgery during which the mitral valve is cleared of scar tissue or calcium deposits, increasing blood flow through the mitral valve.

12. C. The time the electrical impulse takes to travel to the ventricles after atrial repolarization.

13. A. The patient is experiencing a pain rating of 2 on the FLACC Pain Scale.

14. B. No.

15. B. Tissues in the pericardium can become damaged from chronic pericarditis, resulting in scar tissue replacing tissue in the pericardium.

16. D. The kidneys cause secretion of the renin enzyme when BP is low. The renin enzyme constricts blood vessels, resulting in increased blood pressure. The practitioner is determining if renin enzyme level is the cause of your high BP.

17. A. Abnormal and immature WBCs enter the circulatory system and do not function properly, increasing the risk of other disorders.

18. C. Lopressor is a beta-blocker that slows the contractions of the ventricles.

19. C. The dorsalis pedis is located at the top of the foot and is the farthest peripheral artery from the heart. You are assured that the patient's legs are receiving sufficient arterial blood flow if the dorsalis pedis can be palpated.

20. A. Ask the patient if he was prescribed warfarin and the last time he had a PT/INR performed.

21. D. Some patients have aneurysms for months before a diagnosis is made because they don't have any symptoms.

22. A. Embolectomy is the surgical removal of a blood clot from the affected artery.

23. C. Cardiac marker tests determine if cardiac muscle enzymes appear in your blood.

24. D. BNP is secreted by ventricles of your heart when the ventricles are excessively stretched. Elevated BNP may indicate heart failure.

25. A. No fluid replacement. Treat the wound and monitor the patient. The patient has a class I hemorrhage.

26. D. Yes. Wolff-Parkinson-White syndrome is a heart disorder where there is an abnormal extra electrical pathway in the heart.

27. A. The pain is due to layers of the pericardium rubbing against each other.

28. A. MVR disrupts normal blood flow, resulting in decreased circulation of oxygenated blood, which can make you feel tried.

29. A. Hypovolemic shock.

30. B. Cardioversion is a nonsurgical procedure that uses a low energy level shock to let your heart restore a normal heart rhythm. You'll be asleep during this procedure.

31. C. You have a mix of abnormal WBCs, immature WBCs, and mature WBCs (good WBCs). However, there are more abnormal and immature WBCs than there are normal WBCs.

32. B. The time between the end of ventricular depolarization and ventricular repolarization.

33. A. You have anemia. There aren't sufficient RBCs to carry oxygen throughout your body.

34. D. Sick sinus syndrome is a malfunction of the SA node.

35. D. There is a depletion of platelets preventing your body from coagulating blood, leading to hemorrhaging.

36. C. Fluid builds up in the lungs due to ineffective pumping of blood by the heart.

37. B. Lower the patient's BP.

38. A. You might have "white coat syndrome." Your BP increases

39. D. Analyze each cardiac rhythm.

40. D. Some patients diagnosed with tricuspid valve stenosis don't have any symptoms, and therefore, the practitioner monitors the patient regularly without prescribing treatment.

41. C. This is a nonsurgical procedure in which a long tube with a small balloon is passed through blood vessels into the narrowed artery. The balloon is inflated, causing the artery to expand.

42. D. Nitroglycerin relaxes smooth muscles around coronary arteries, increasing the flow of oxygenated blood to the heart and decreasing chest pain.

43. D. You might have vasospastic angina. Let's speak with your practitioner.

44. A. Morphine will ease the pain experienced in severe episodes of sickle cell anemia.

45. D. Swan Ganz catheter is a catheter placed into the pulmonary artery to check for pressures in the heart, vessels, and lungs.

46. A. Tell him that lidocaine also decreases the time between contractions of the heart and may restore a normal heart rhythm.

47. D. HDL is commonly referred to as *good cholesterol* and LDL as *bad cholesterol*. These are not cholesterols. HDL and LDL are proteins that carry cholesterol to and from organs and tissues.

48. A. Zeroing the ECG.

49. A. Catheter ablation is a procedure where tissues of the heart that cause the extra impulses are destroyed by radiofrequency energy applied to the area by a catheter that the practitioner inserts into a blood vessel. In some cases, the practitioner ablates the AV node to prevent impulses from the atria from reaching the ventricles. The patient then requires a permanent pacemaker to maintain ventricle contractions.

50. D. Yes. Myocarditis can weaken the heart, preventing the heart from efficiently pumping blood throughout the body.

51. C. The practitioner will stabilize him and then then discharge him to the next appropriate level of care.
52. B. A laser-tipped catheter is inserted into the affected artery to remove the blockage.
53. C. Bands are immature neutrophils that increase when there is a bacterial infection.
54. C. Elevated ST segment indicates severe damage to the heart.
55. C. Early treatment usually produces good results. Long-term prognosis can be variable, depending on the severity of the disease and associated conditions. Your practitioner is the best person to speak about your prognosis.
56. B. Prognosis is usually good unless embolization or moving of the clot occurs. It may move to the lung or brain, which can be life-threatening.
57. D. If you follow the treatment prescribed by the practitioner, the average survival time is between 10 and 15 years. Without treatment, survival is less than 2 years.
58. C. Cardiac tamponade.
59. C. The practitioner may use a Doppler ultrasonography to examine the affected area. If this test indicates there might be a blockage, the practitioner will likely order an arteriography where dye is injected in your arteries and an X-ray of your artery is taken.
60. B. MVP puts the patient at risk for infective endocarditis. A dental procedure exposes the patient to bacteria and the antibiotics reduce the risk of infection, building the therapeutic level of antibiotics in the blood before the procedure.
61. A. This is the Valsalva maneuver used as a nonmedication treatment of PAC.
62. C. A chest X-ray is used to detect the size of the heart.
63. D. Yes. A low level can lead to ascites. Albumin controls oncotic pressure in blood vessels, which keeps blood from leaking out of blood vessels.
64. A. Do you have difficulty breathing?
65. D. Bacteria in the mouth and gums could enter the bloodstream and infect the patient's heart.
66. B. Medication can control the majority of cases of ITP. Remission is common.
67. C. Straining during a bowel movement increases pressure in the chest and slows return of blood to the heart.
68. A. Primary HTN develops gradually over years without an identifiable cause.
69. A. You are injecting low-molecular-weight heparin, which will reduce formation of new blood clots.
70. A. There is a buildup of carbon dioxide in your blood because disruption in blood flow prevents the lung from oxygenating the blood. Your body compensates by breathing rapidly to quickly remove the excess carbon dioxide.
71. D. Yes. The microorganisms that clump together at a site in the heart can break loose and float in the bloodstream, possibly blocking a blood vessel and leading to tissue necrosis in the brain.
72. A. Respiration.
73. D. Atrial depolarization.
74. A. Ask the patient what he was doing in the past 24 hours.

75. C. No because the patient is at risk for blood clots.
76. B. An event monitor is a wearable device that records data only when a cardiac event occurs and will record your heart activity the next time you have a "funny feeling" in your chest.
77. C. Yes. Digoxin toxicity slows conduction through the AV node, resulting in the AV node assuming the role of the pacemaker.
78. B. Yes. Swelling is commonly seen in the legs and abdomen caused by pooling of blood due to decreased ability of the heart to pump blood.
79. D. Mitral stenosis disrupts blood flow to the left ventricle causing a buildup of fluid that leads to swelling. Lasix is a diuretic that causes the kidney to increase production of urine to reduce excess fluid, decreasing swelling.
80. D. The most common cause of pulmonary valve stenosis is congenital abnormal development of the pulmonary valve.
81. D. Weight gain is an early sign that you are retaining fluid. Retaining fluid may indicate a problem with your heart that needs to be addressed immediately.
82. D. Cardiogenic shock.
83. C. Valvuloplasty is a nonsurgical procedure.
84. C. HCM occurs when the ventricular heart muscle thickens, resulting in outflow obstruction or restriction. There is some blood flow present.
85. C. An untreated bacterial throat infection can lead to infective endocarditis, which is an underlying cause of tricuspid valve regurgitation.
86. C. A balloon is inserted into the aorta and is then inflated and deflated to increase blood flow throughout the body.
87. D. Each unifocal PVC looks the same. Each multifocal PVC looks different.
88. C. Myoglobin elevates in blood after muscle injury, including a heart attack, sooner than troponin levels.
89. B. Plasma contains clotting factors.
90. D. Assess the electrode connections to the patient.
91. C. Ask the patient if he ever had rheumatic fever or scarlet fever as a child.
92. D. MITRAL VALVE REGURGITATION places you at risk for atrial fibrillation, which is an irregular contraction of the atria. As a result, there is a chance that blood might pool, leading to blood clots. Warfarin reduces the formation of blood clots.
93. C. Bundle branch block.
94. A. Corresponding peripheral arteries should have relatively the same contour and amplitude when palpated.
95. B. Metoprolol is a beta-blocker that slows the contractions of the ventricles.
96. B. Aplastic means that a part of the body is failing to develop. Aplastic anemia occurs when bone marrow stops producing a sufficient amount of new RBCs.
97. C. A 3-lead cardiac monitor.
98. A. Positive hepatojugular reflux is distension of the neck veins precipitated by the maneuver of firm pressure over the liver by the practitioner.
99. C. Do you abuse alcohol?
100. D. No treatment.

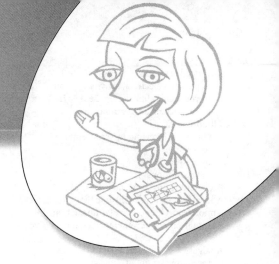

# Index

## A